Treatment and Prognosis in
OBSTETRICS AND
GYNECOLOGY

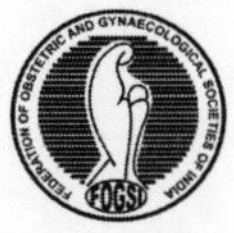

Federation of Obstetric and Gynaecological Societies of India

Treatment and Prognosis in
OBSTETRICS AND GYNECOLOGY

Editors

Manju Gita Mishra
DGO MS FICS FICOG FIAMS FICMCH

Chief Consultant
MGM Hospital and Research Center
Ex-Professor
Department of Obstetrics and Gynecology
Patna Medical College
Patna, Bihar, India
Ex-Chairperson
CME Committee, FOGSI 2007–2009

Hemali Heidi Sinha
MBBS DGO MS (Obs & Gyne) FICMCH

Professor and Head
Department of Obstetrics and Gynecology
All India Institute of Medical Sciences
Patna, Bihar, India

Foreword

Suchitra N Pandit

—— A FOGSI Publication ——

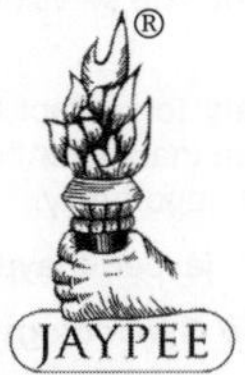

JAYPEE BROTHERS MEDICAL PUBLISHERS (P) LTD
New Delhi • London • Philadelphia • Panama

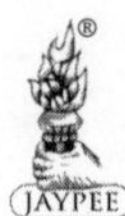 **Jaypee Brothers Medical Publishers (P) Ltd**

Headquarters

Jaypee Brothers Medical Publishers (P) Ltd
4838/24, Ansari Road, Daryaganj
New Delhi 110 002, India
Phone: +91-11-43574357
Fax: +91-11-43574314
Email: jaypee@jaypeebrothers.com

Overseas Offices

J.P. Medical Ltd
83 Victoria Street, London
SW1H 0HW (UK)
Phone: +44-2031708910
Fax: +02-03-0086180
Email: info@jpmedpub.com

Jaypee Medical Inc
The Bourse
111 South Independence Mall East
Suite 835, Philadelphia, PA 19106, USA
Phone: +1 267-519-9789
Email: jpmed.us@gmail.com

Jaypee Brothers Medical Publishers (P) Ltd
Bhotahity, Kathmandu, Nepal
Phone: +977-9741283608
Email: kathmandu@jaypeebrothers.com

Jaypee-Highlights Medical Publishers Inc
City of Knowledge, Bld. 237, Clayton
Panama City, Panama
Phone: +1 507-301-0496
Fax: +1 507-301-0499
Email: cservice@jphmedical.com

Jaypee Brothers Medical Publishers (P) Ltd
17/1-B Babar Road, Block-B, Shaymali
Mohammadpur, Dhaka-1207
Bangladesh
Mobile: +08801912003485
Email: jaypeedhaka@gmail.com

Website: www.jaypeebrothers.com
Website: www.jaypeedigital.com

© 2014, Jaypee Brothers Medical Publishers

The views and opinions expressed in this book are solely those of the original contributor(s)/author(s) and do not necessarily represent those of editor(s) of the book.

All rights reserved. No part of this publication may be reproduced, stored or transmitted in any form or by any means, electronic, mechanical, photocopying, recording or otherwise, without the prior permission in writing of the publishers.

All brand names and product names used in this book are trade names, service marks, trademarks or registered trademarks of their respective owners. The publisher is not associated with any product or vendor mentioned in this book.

Medical knowledge and practice change constantly. This book is designed to provide accurate, authoritative information about the subject matter in question. However, readers are advised to check the most current information available on procedures included and check information from the manufacturer of each product to be administered, to verify the recommended dose, formula, method and duration of administration, adverse effects and contraindications. It is the responsibility of the practitioner to take all appropriate safety precautions. Neither the publisher nor the author(s)/editor(s) assume any liability for any injury and/or damage to persons or property arising from or related to use of material in this book.

This book is sold on the understanding that the publisher is not engaged in providing professional medical services. If such advice or services are required, the services of a competent medical professional should be sought.

Every effort has been made where necessary to contact holders of copyright to obtain permission to reproduce copyright material. If any have been inadvertently overlooked, the publisher will be pleased to make the necessary arrangements at the first opportunity.

Inquiries for bulk sales may be solicited at: jaypee@jaypeebrothers.com

Treatment and Prognosis in Obstetrics and Gynecology

First Edition: **2014**

ISBN 978-93-5152-162-4

Printed at Rajkamal Electric Press, Plot No. 2, Phase-IV, Kundli, Haryana.

Dedicated to

*Our patients in all humility
who have been and will remain to be our greatest teachers*

Contributors

Abha Rani Sinha
Associate Professor
Department of Obstetrics and Gynecology
Patna Medical College
Patna, Bihar, India
Secretary
Bihar Obstetrics and Gynecological Society

Alka Kriplani
Professor and Head
Department of Obstetrics and Gynecology
Director-in-Charge
WHO-HRCC and Family Planning
All India Institute of Medical Sciences
New Delhi, India
President
Gynecological Endocrine Society of India
(2011–continuing)
President
Association of Obstetricians and
Gynecologists of Delhi (2013–2014)
Member
Governing Council ICOG
(2008–continuing)
Editor
Asian Journal of Obstetrics and
Gynecological Practice (1999–continuing)

Alokananda Ray
Department of Obstetrics and Gynecology
Tata Main Hospital
Jamshedpur, Jharkhand, India

Alokendu Chatterjee
Formerly, Head
Department of Obstetrics and Gynecology
NRS Medical College
Kolkata, West Bengal, India

Amrita Sharan
Associate Professor
Department of Obstetrics and Gynecology
Patna Medical College
Patna, Bihar, India

Anita Verma
Senior Medical Officer
Department of Obstetrics and Gynecology
Patna Medical College
Patna, Bihar, India

Archana Jha
Department of Obstetrics and Gynecology
Jawahar Lal Nehru Medical College
Bhagalpur, Bihar, India

Archana Kumari
Assistant Professor
Department of Obstetrics and Gynecology
Rajendra Institute of Medical Sciences
Ranchi, Jharkhand, India

Charu Modi
Consultant Obstetrician and Gynecologist
Modi Nursing Home
Patna, Bihar, India

Deependra Kumar Rai
Assistant Professor
Department of Pulmonary Medicine
All India Institute of Medical Sciences
Patna, Bihar, India

Dipika Deka
Professor and Unit Head
Chief, Fetal Medicine Division
Department of Obstetrics and Gynecology
All India Institute of Medical Sciences
New Delhi, India
Past Chairperson
Genetics and Fetal Medicine
Committee, FOGSI

DN Sharma
Additional Professor
Department of Radiation Oncology
BRA Institute Rotary Center Hospital
All India Institute of Medical Sciences
New Delhi, India

Esa Bose
Ex-Registrar
Department of Obstetrics and Gynecology
Kurji Holy Family Hospital
Patna, Bihar, India

Garima Kacchawa
Assistant Professor
Department of Obstetrics and
Gynecology
All India Institute of Medical Sciences
New Delhi, India

Hemali Heidi Sinha
Professor and Head
Department of Obstetrics and
Gynecology
All India Institute of Medical Sciences
Patna, Bihar, India

Hiralal Konar
Professor
Department of Obstetrics and Gynecology
Calcutta National Medical College
Kolkata, West Bengal, India
Chairman
Indian College of Obstetrics and
Gynecology (ICOG)

Jagdishwari Mishra
Ex-Professor and Head
Department of Obstetrics and Gynecology
Patna Medical College
Chief Consultant
JM Maternity and Child Welfare Clinic and
Research Center
Patna, Bihar, India

JB Sharma
Additional Professor
Department of Obstetrics and Gynecology
All India Institute of Medical Sciences
New Delhi, India

K Aparna Sharma
Assistant Professor
Department of Obstetrics and Gynecology
All India Institute of Medical Sciences
New Delhi, India

Kumari Mamta
Consultant Obstetrician and Gynecologist
Mahavir Vaatsalya Aspataal
Patna, Bihar, India

Kusum Gopal Kapoor
Consultant Obstetrician and Gynecologist
Ex-Professor and Head
Department of Obstetrics and Gynecology
Nalanda Medical College
Patna, Bihar, India
Ex-Chairperson
Rural Obstetric Committee, FOGSI

Mamta Singh
Consultant Obstetrician and Gynecologist
Patna, Bihar, India

Manila Jain
Department of Obstetrics and Gynecology
MGM Medical College
Indore, Madhya Pradesh, India

Manju Gita Mishra
Ex-Professor
Department of Obstetrics and Gynecology
Patna Medical College
Chief Consultant
MGM Hospital and Research Center
Patna, Bihar, India
Ex-Chairperson
CME Committee, FOGSI 2007–2009

Manisha Yadav
Senior Resident
Department of Obstetrics and Gynecology
All India Institute of Medical Sciences
New Delhi, India

Meena Samant
Senior Consultant and Head
Department of Obstetrics and Gynecology
Kurji Holy Family Hospital
Patna, Bihar, India

Monica Chouhan
Department of Obstetrics and Gynecology
NSCB Medical College
Jabalpur, Madhya Pradesh, India

N Palaniappan
Associate Professor
Department of Obstetrics and Gynecology
Ramachandra Medical College
Porur, Chennai, Tamil Nadu, India

Navneet Magon
Head
Department of Obstetrics and Gynecology
Air Force Hospital
Jorhat, Assam, India

Neelam
Consultant
'SANTATI' Fertility Clinic and ART Center
Arvind Hospital
Patna, Bihar, India

Nisha Singh
Professor
Department of Obstetrics and Gynecology
King George Medical University
Lucknow, Uttar Pradesh, India

Pankaj Desai
Ex-Associate Professor and Unit Chief
Department of Obstetrics and Gynecology
Medical College
Baroda, Gujarat, India

Pankaj Hans
Assistant Professor
Department of Medicine
Patna Medical College
Patna, Bihar, India

Partha Mukherjee
Professor
Department of Obstetrics and Gynecology
Medical College
Kolkata, West Bengal, India

Picklu Chaudhuri
Associate Professor
Department of Obstetrics and Gynecology
Nilratan Sircar Medical College and
Hospital
Kolkata, West Bengal, India

Prachi Renjhen
Senior Consultant
Obstetrics and Gynecology
Alchemist Hospital
Gurgaon, Haryana, India

Pragya Mishra Choudhary
Consultant Obstetrician, Gynecologist and
Infertility Specialist
Nu Life Test Tube Baby Center
MGM Hospital and Research Center
Patna, Bihar, India

Pramila Modi
Senior Consultant Obstetrician and
Gynecologist
Modi Nursing Home
Honorary Consultant Obstetrician and
Gynecologist
Arogya Mandir Hospital
Patna, Bihar, India

Purvi Patel
Associate Professor
Department of Obstetrics and Gynecology
Medical College
Baroda, Gujarat, India

Rakhee R Sahu
Consultant Obstetrician and Gynecologist
Dr HL Hiranandani Hospital
Ex-Associate Professor
Nowrosjee Wadia Maternity Hospital
Mumbai, Maharashtra, India
MOGS Youth Council Member 2013

Reeti Mehra
Department of Obstetrics and
Gynecology
Government Medical College and
Hospital
Chandigarh, India

Rita Kumari Jha
Assistant Professor
Department of Obstetrics and Gynecology
Patna Medical College
Patna, Bihar, India

Rita Sinha
Associate Professor
Department of Obstetrics and Gynecology
Nalanda Medical College
Patna, Bihar, India

Roza Olyai
Consultant
Department of Obstetrics and Gynecology
Olyai Hospital
Gwalior, Madhya Pradesh, India
National Vice-President Elect, FOGSI 2014
Fellow and Member
Governing Council, ICOG 2012–2015
Who Consultant
Expert Panel Adolescent Reproductive
Sexual Health, Geneva 2010

SN Tripathy
Ex-Professor and Head
Department of Obstetrics and Gynecology
SCB Medical College
Cuttack, Odisha, India

Sandeep Mathur
Additional Professor
Department of Pathology
All India Institute of Medical Sciences
New Delhi, India

Sebanti Goswami
Associate Professor
Department of Obstetrics and Gynecology
Medical College
Kolkata, West Bengal, India

Seema Pandey Choudhary
Consultant Obstetrician and Gynecologist
Bengaluru, Karnataka, India

Shanti HK Singh
Ex-Associate Professor
Department of Obstetrics and Gynecology
Patna Medical College
Patna, Bihar
Consultant Obstetrician and Gynecologist
Sundari Devi Hospital
Patna, Bihar, India

Shobha Chakravorty
Ex-Professor
Department of Obstetrics and Gynecology
Rajendra Medical College
Consultant Obstetrician and Gynecologist
Ranchi, Jharkhand, India

Sindhu Nandini Tripathy
Ex-Professor and Head
SCB Medical College
Cuttack, Odisha, India

Smita Kumari
Consultant Obstetrician and Gynecologist
Patna, Bihar, India

Smriti Modi
DNB Trainee (F Medicine)
Apollo Gleneagles Hospitals
Kolkata, West Bengal, India

Suchitra N Pandit
Specialist
Department of Obstetrics and Gynecology
Kokilaben Dhirubhai Ambani Hospital and
Research Center
Mumbai, Maharashtra, India
President Elect, FOGSI 2014
President, MOGS 2013
Vice-Chairman, ICOG 2012–2013
Fellow of Executive Council West Zone
RCOG
Vice-President, FOGSI 2008–2009

Sujata Misra
Associate Professor
Department of Obstetrics and Gynecology
SCB Medical College
Cuttack, Odisha, India
Ex-Chairperson
Medical Disorders in Pregnancy
Committee, FOGSI
Vice-President Elect, FOGSI 2015

Suneeta Singh
Department of Obstetrics and Gynecology
Military Hospital
Mhow, Madhya Pradesh, India

Sunesh Kumar
Professor
Department of Obstetrics and Gynecology
All India Institute of Medical Sciences
New Delhi, India

Sushma Pandey
Professor and Head
Department of Obstetrics and Gynecology
Patna Medical College
Patna, Bihar, India

Sushma Singh
Department of Obstetrics and Gynecology
Patna Medical College
Patna, Bihar, India

Tripti Sinha
Specialist Obstetrician and Gynecologist
Bihar State Health Services
Patna, Bihar, India

Usha Didwania
Consultant Obstetrician and Gynecologist
Patna, Bihar, India

Vinita Sahay
Senior Resident
Department of Obstetrics and Gynecology
Patna Medical College
Patna, Bihar, India

Foreword

This book *Treatment and Prognosis in Obstetrics and Gynecology* represents a contemporary resource on obstetrics and gynecology to all individuals in training as well as already established obstetricians.

Patient safety is paramount in the field of operative obstetrics and gynecology, and it is hoped that this book will provide both practical and timely information to reduce the risk.

The editors have attempted to gather experts from their fields and present an integrated management approach with topics ranging from the initial clinical diagnosis, management, new treatment options, and scientific rational for the various approaches.

I hope this text will serve as a clinically useful reference guide for periodic review to all.

I would like to acknowledge all the authors and the publishers whose efforts and work helped lay the foundation for this text.

I am grateful for the opportunity to write this Foreword.

Suchitra N Pandit
Specialist in High-risk Pregnancy Adolescent and Menopausal Problems
Nondescent Vaginal Hysterectomy and Pelvic Floor Surgery
Kokilaben Dhirubhai Ambani Hospital and Research Center
Mumbai, Maharashtra, India
President, MOGS 2013
President, FOGSI Elect 2014
Vice-Chairman, ICOG (2012–2013)
Organizing Secretary, AICOG 2013, Mumbai
West Zone Coordinator, ISOPARB (2009–2011)
Fellow of Executive Council West Zone RCOG
Vice-President, FOGSI (2008–2009)
Chairperson-Young Talent Promotion Committee, FOGSI (2003–2008)
Joint Secretary-President, FOGSI (2001–2002)

Preface

Obstetrics and gynecology is an ever-changing dynamic discipline. It is challenging for the busy practitioners to keep abreast of all the new developments. Management of medical problems has seen a sea change over the years.

Each one of us has faced situations where we feel we have failed to deliver the desired result. Though we have a myriad of information available to us through computer programs and the Internet, it is the books we go back to, for learning new lessons and relearning old ones.

This book has been written to help clinicians, postgraduate students and teachers to turn to for easy reference. The topics that have been covered are those conditions commonly seen in a busy clinic.

We acknowledge the contribution of each author and would like to thank each one of them, for their meticulous contribution.

We also take this opportunity to thank Shri Jitendar P Vij (Group Chairman), Mr Ankit Vij (Managing Director) and Mr Tarun Duneja (Director-Publishing) of M/s Jaypee Brothers Medical Publishers (P) Ltd, New Delhi, India, especially Ms Samina Khan and Mr Sabyasachi Hazra and their team, for sparing no effort in bringing this book together in such a short time and for bearing with us.

It was a pleasure editing the text, as well as a great learning experience.

Manju Gita Mishra
Hemali Heidi Sinha

Contents

PART II – GYNECOLOGY

SECTION 1: PEDIATRIC AND ADOLESCENT GYNECOLOGICAL PROBLEMS

SECTION 2: MENSTRUAL PROBLEMS

SECTION 3: REPRODUCTIVE ENDOCRINOLOGY

PLATE 1

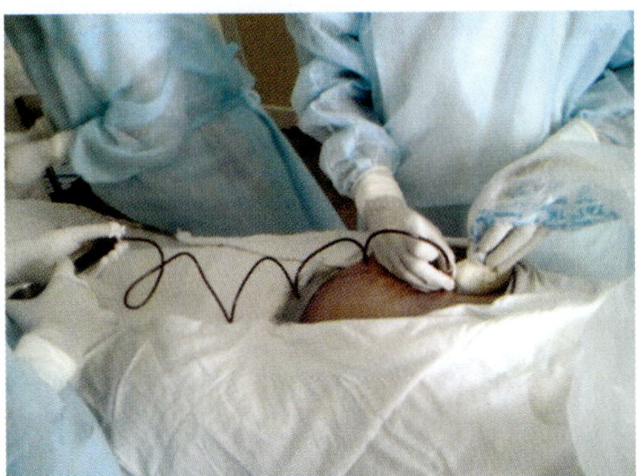

Fig. 3: Packed cells being transfused through needle *(Chapter 18)*

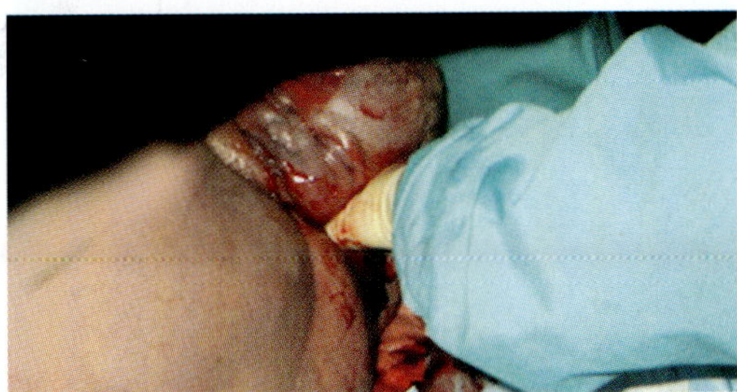

Fig. 1: Turtle sign *(Chapter 23)*

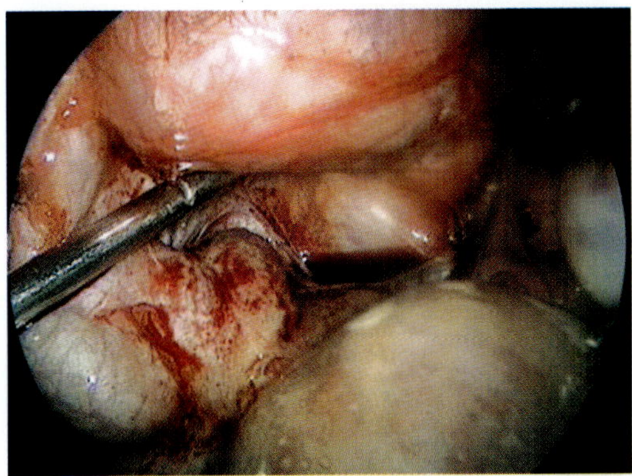

Fig. 1: Laparoscopic view showing hematometra, hematosalpinx
and endometriosis *(Chapter 27)*
Courtesy: Dr Alka Kriplani

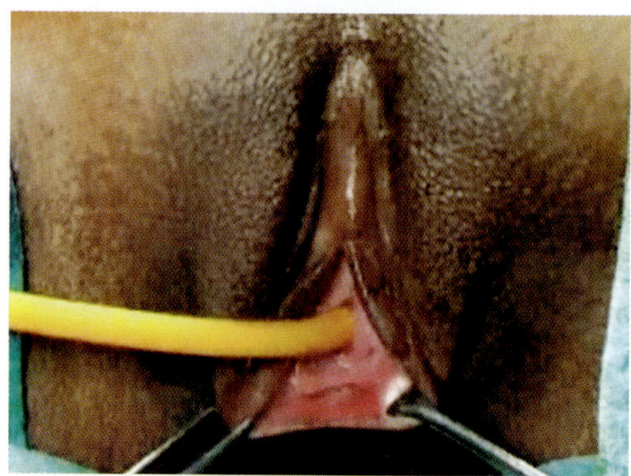

Fig. 2: Vaginal agenesis (Mayer Rokitansky Kustner Hauser syndrome) *(Chapter 27)*

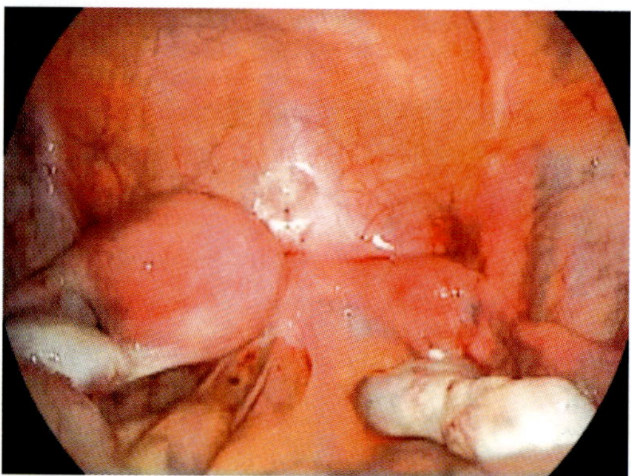

Fig. 4: Laparoscopic view showing unicornuate uterus (left horn) with rudimentary horn (right horn) *(Chapter 27)*
Courtesy: Dr Alka Kriplani

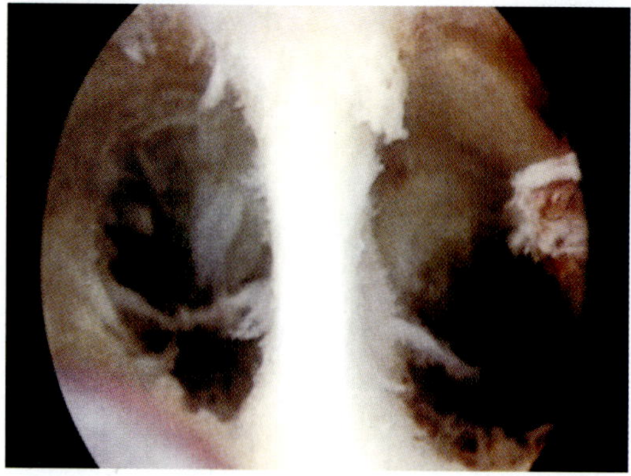

Fig. 5: Hysteroscopic view of a complete uterine septum *(Chapter 27)*
Courtesy: Dr Alka Kriplani

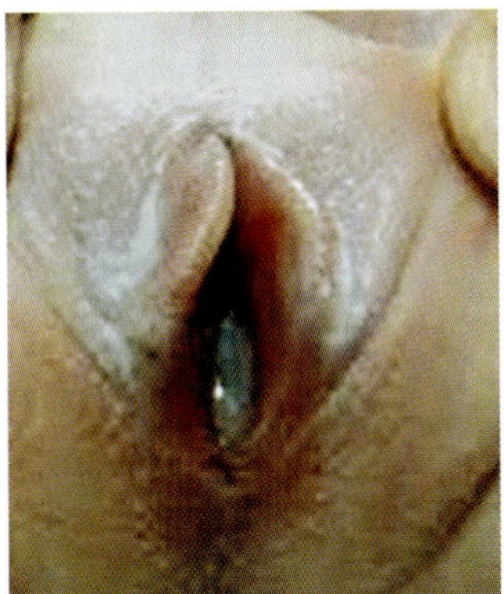

Fig. 2: Imperforate hymen with typical bluish discoloration behind the hymen suggestive of collected blood *(Chapter 29)*

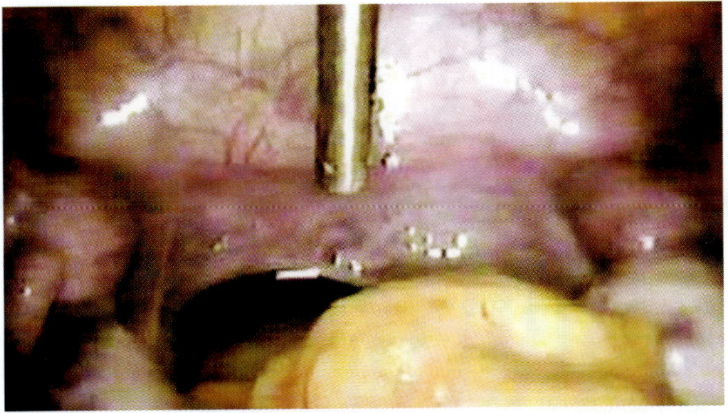

Fig. 3: Absent uterus in a subject with primary amenorrhea at laparoscopy *(Chapter 29)*

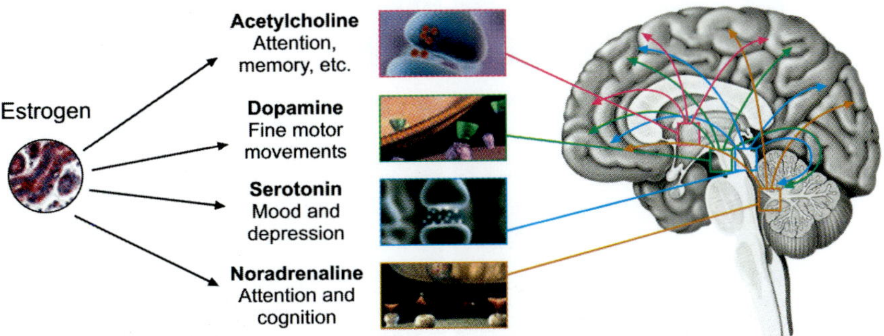

Fig. 2: Mental symptoms in postmenopausal women *(Chapter 35)*
(Source: http://www.34-menopause-symptoms.com/difficulty-concentrating-causes.htm)

PLATE 4

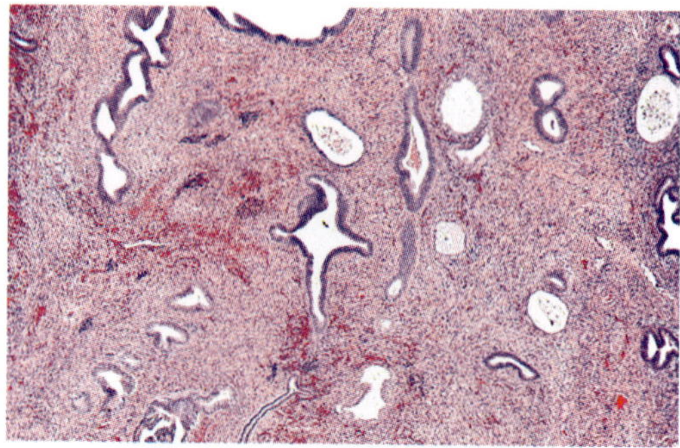

Fig. 1: Histological section of endometrial polyp *(Chapter 37)*

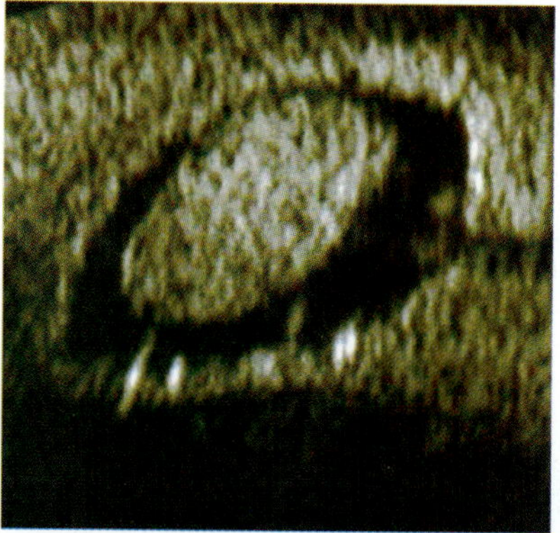

Fig. 2: Endometrial polyp on saline infusion sonography *(Chapter 37)*

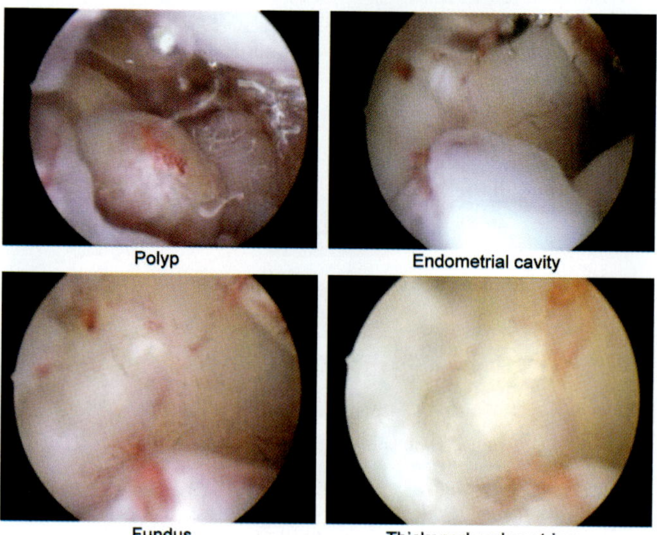

Fig. 3: Endometrial polyp on hysteroscopy *(Chapter 37)*

PLATE 5

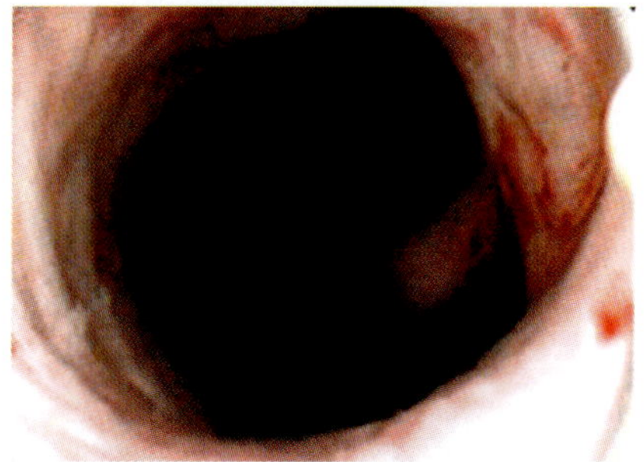

Fig. 4: Multiple polyps on hysteroscopy *(Chapter 37)*

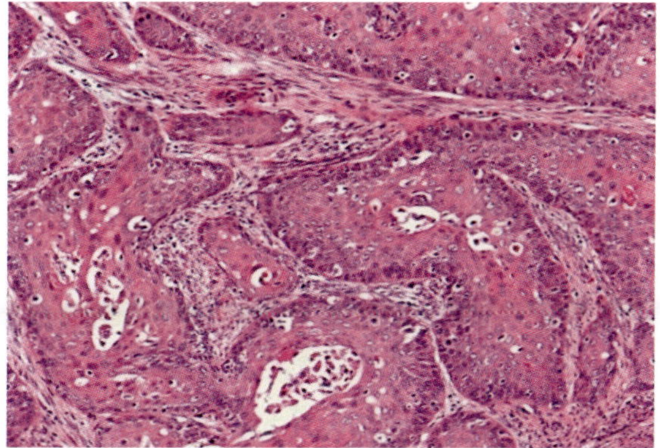

Fig. 1: Keratinizing squamous cell carcinoma *(Chapter 48)*

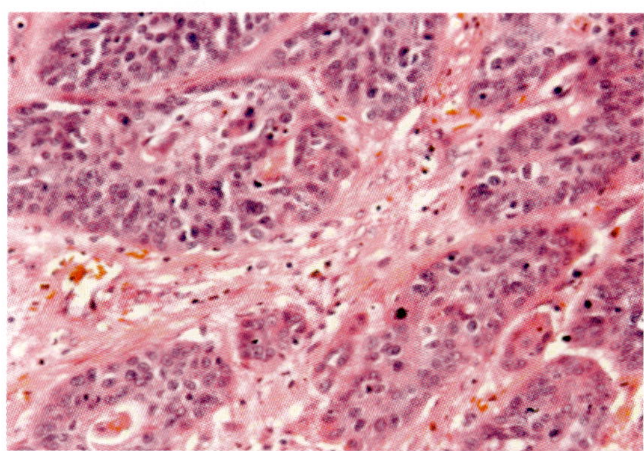

Fig. 2: Basaloid squamous cell carcinoma composed of islands of
smaller basaloid cells *(Chapter 48)*

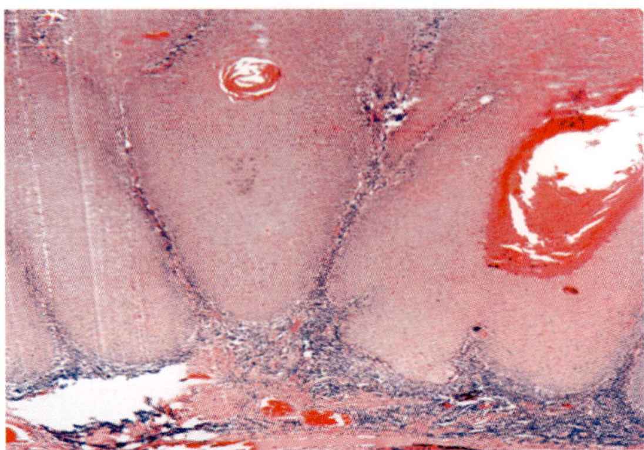

Fig. 3: Verrucous carcinoma displaying broad based rete ridges *(Chapter 48)*

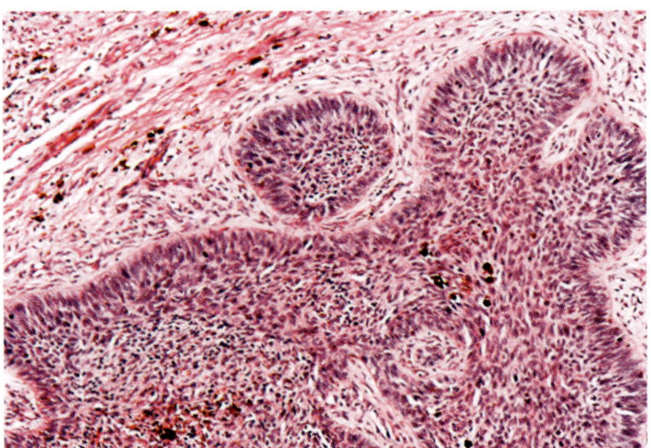

Fig. 4: Basal cell carcinoma composed of islands of basaloid cells with peripheral palisading of nuclei and scant pigment *(Chapter 48)*

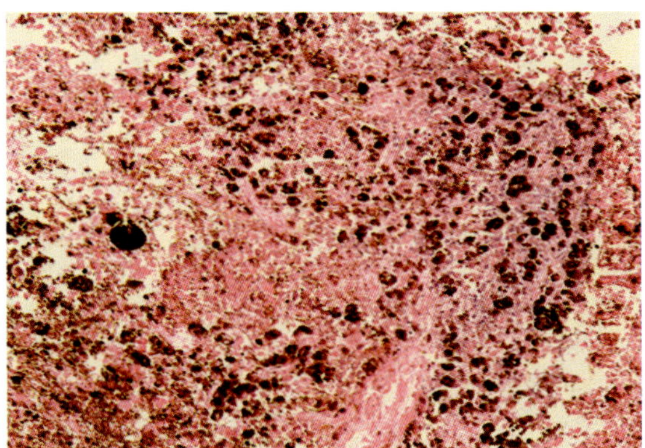

Fig. 5: Malignant melanoma composed of islands of densely pigmented tumor cells *(Chapter 48)*

PLATE 7

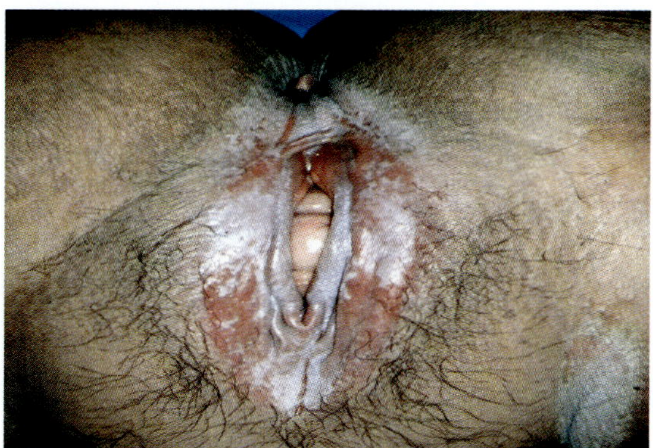

Fig. 6: Vulval intraepithelial neoplasia *(Chapter 48)*

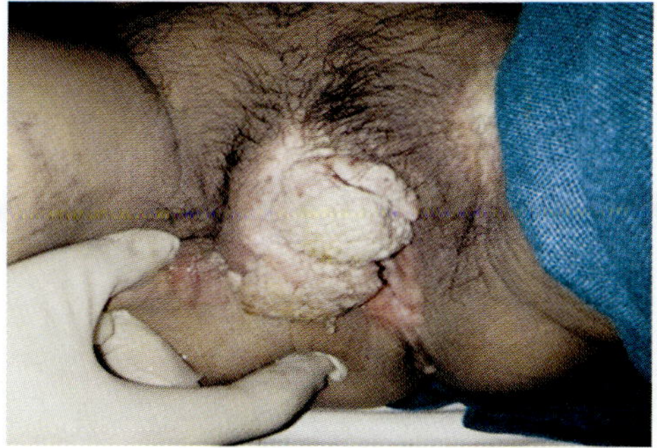

Fig. 7: Carcinoma vulva *(Chapter 48)*

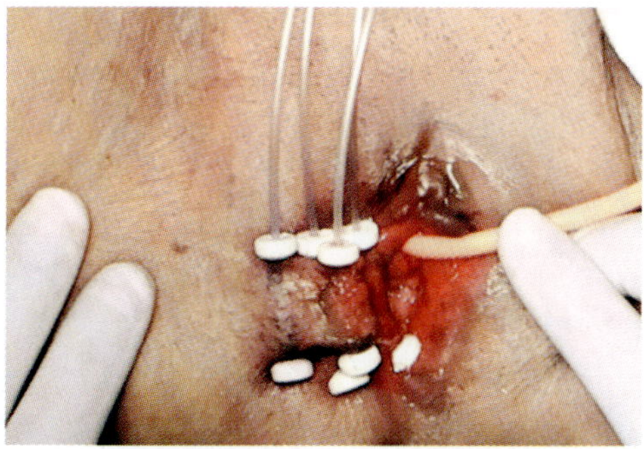

Fig. 11: Clinical image showing the brachytherapy implant for vulvar carcinoma *(Chapter 48)*

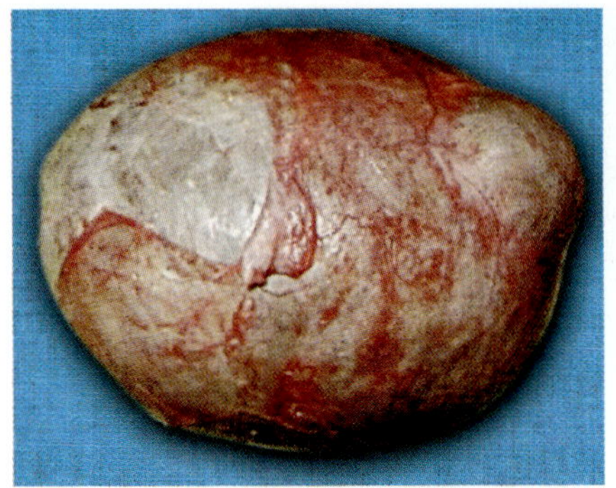

Fig. 1: Benign serous cystadenoma *(Chapter 50)*

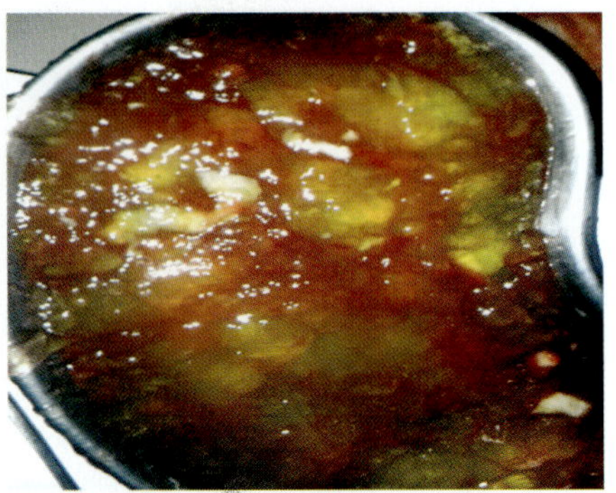

Fig. 2: Mucin from a benign mucinous cystadenoma *(Chapter 50)*

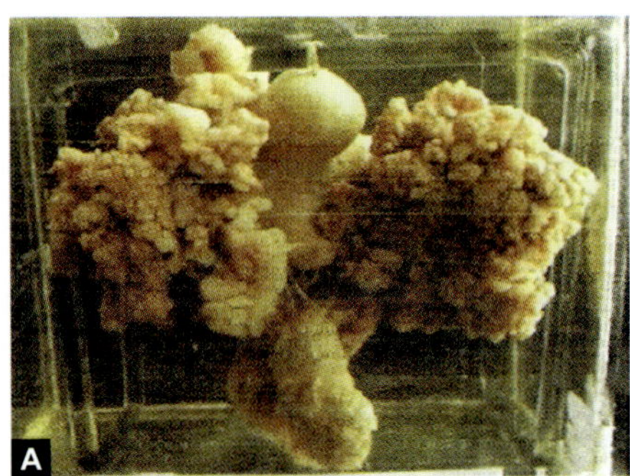

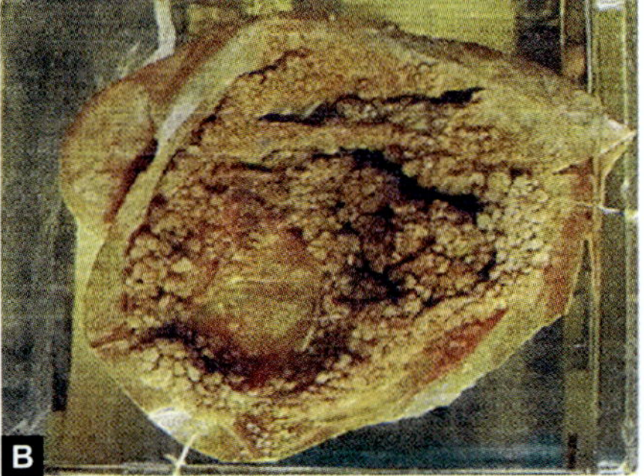

Figs 1A and B: (A) Specimen of uterus and ovaries covered with papillary excrescences. (B) Papillary projections within the cyst on cut section *(Chapter 51)*

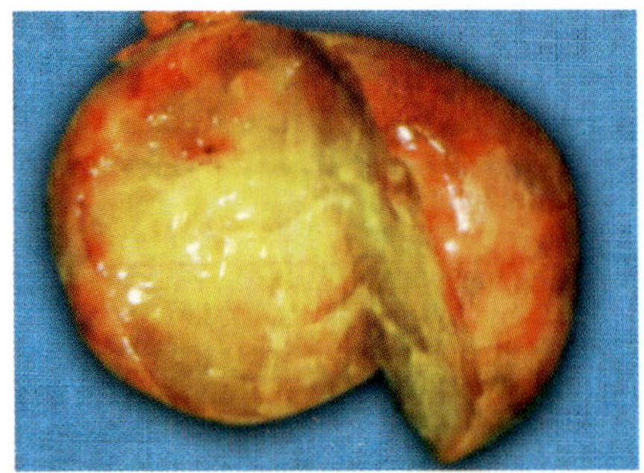

Fig. 2: Dysgerminoma *(Chapter 51)*

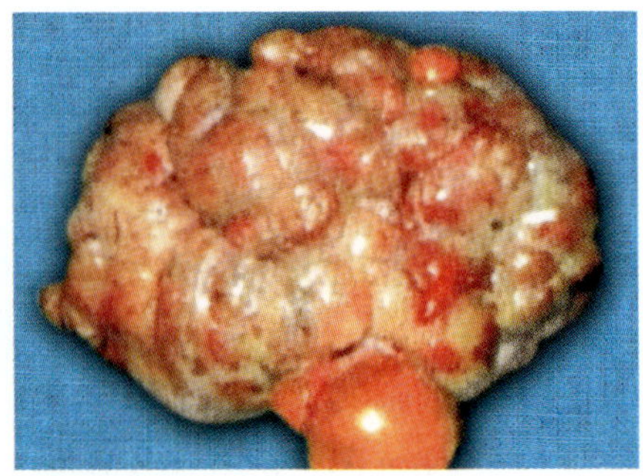

Fig. 3: Immature Teratoma *(Chapter 51)*

PART-I

OBSTETRICS

Chapter
1
Hyperemesis Gravidarum

Hemali Heidi Sinha

INTRODUCTION

Nausea and vomiting are very common symptoms in pregnancy, affecting about 70–85% pregnant women. The usual onset is around the 4th to 7th week of pregnancy, with a peak between 8th and 12th week. Most cases resolve by 20th week of gestation, persistence beyond which may point toward a medical condition.

Hyperemesis gravidarum is a severe form of nausea and vomiting which affects between 0.3 and 2.0% of all pregnancies. Pernicious vomiting may affect homeostasis, electrolyte imbalance, and kidney function and may have adverse fetal consequences.

Uncontrolled vomiting requiring hospitalization, severe dehydration, associated with ketonuria and weight loss of more than 5% body weight is a common clinical feature. Most of these patients also suffer from hyponatremia and hypokalemia. Ptyalism is also a typical symptom.

PATHOGENESIS

The exact pathogenesis of hyperemesis gravidarum remains unknown, though a number of hypotheses have been postulated. Many studies have suggested hormonal changes in pregnancy as a cause. Molar pregnancy and trisomy gestation are associated with elevated human chorionic gonadotrophin (hCG) levels. However, hCG levels do not correlate well with the severity of hyperemesis. hCG has thyrotropic action and hyperemesis gravidarum is more common in pregnancies with high hCG levels exhibiting transient self-limiting hyperthyroidism. Antithyroid drugs are not required.

Chronic *Helicobacter pylori* infection may play a role in hyperemesis. However, seropositivity does not correlate with gastrointestinal symptoms. *H. pylori* infection has been found in cases of persistent vomiting. Some researchers also postulate that psychological factors might be responsible. Olfactory sensitivity may play a role in the pathogenesis of hyperemesis. Women with vomiting in pregnancy also commonly have a positive family history of hyperemesis.

COMPLICATIONS

Maternal Complications

Persistent severe vomiting can lead to dehydration, electrolyte imbalance and ketosis. More serious conditions include esophageal tear or rupture, pneumothorax and peripheral neuropathy due to vitamin B_6 and B_{12} deficiency. Wernicke's encephalopathy has been associated with treatment of hyperemesis gravidarum with intravenous dextrose replacement without thiamine supplement. Central pontine myelinolysis associated with Wernicke's encephalopathy has been reported.

Fetal Complications

Uncontrolled hyperemesis gravidarum is associated with fetal growth retardation and fetal death. Infants maybe born prematurely or be small for gestational age. Hyperemesis has a detrimental effect on the weight of newborns. In a study by Veenendaal et al, it was found that women with hyperemesis gaining less than 7 kg weight during pregnancy when compared with women who gained 7 kg or more, the risk of small gestational age infants increased odd ratio (OR) I.5; 95% confidence interval (CI) 1.0–2.2.

Also, babies of women with less than 7 kg weight gain had an increased risk of having babies with a 5 minute APGAR score of less than 7 (OR 5.0, 95% CI 2.6–9.6) compared with babies from a control group.

Hyperemesis by itself is not a risk factor for adverse outcome, but these outcomes are the consequences of low weight gain associated with hyperemesis. With minimal weight gain, adverse outcomes for the newborn are invariably noted. If a mother does have significant weight loss during pregnancy, it creates further complications. In retrospective analysis, patients who had more than 5% weight loss and were malnourished, experienced adverse pregnancy outcomes. These were low birth weight, antepartum hemorrhage, preterm delivery and an association with fetal anomalies. Congenital malformations associated include undescended testicles, hip dysplasia and Down's syndrome. Vomiting is not teratogenic, but untreated electrolyte disturbances, malnutrition and maternal weight loss maybe harmful. There is restriction of activities, and decreased quality of life.

CLINICAL EVALUATION

History

Hyperemesis occurs commonly in primigravida. When this condition is seen in multipara, it may have occurred in previous pregnancies. There is no associated fever, chills, rigor, headache and visual disturbance in hyperemesis gravidarum.

In the presence of these symptoms, other acute medical or surgical conditions should be excluded.

Physical Examination

A thorough general examination including hydration status, pulse and blood pressure should be performed. A patient with dry lips and tongue, decreased skin turgor and reduced urine output, suggesting dehydration should be admitted for resuscitation and observation. The thyroid should be examined to look for goiter and to elicit signs of thyrotoxicosis. The abdomen should be palpated for uterine size. If the uterus is larger than the period of gestation, and fetal parts are not palpable, molar pregnancy should be ruled out. The pregnancy is best confirmed by ultrasonography. Other conditions that require exclusion are acute pyelonephritis, and acute surgical conditions like renal colic and acute appendicitis.

Investigations

The most important immediate investigation is serum electrolyte estimation, because hypokalemia and hyponatremia are common complications in severe hyperemesis gravidarum. These may lead to metabolic alkalosis. Blood should also be tested for urea levels. Urine should be tested for specific gravity and ketone bodies on a daily basis, till specific gravity returns to normal and ketone bodies are negative for at least two days. Daily weight measurement and intake—output records should be maintained.

Other routine investigations for pregnancy if not done earlier should be completed. These include hemoglobin level estimation, ABO grouping and Rh typing, venereal disease research laboratory (VDRL) testing, HIV serology, Hepatitis B and Hepatitis C serology testing.

When the diagnosis is unclear and symptoms persist for more than three days despite treatment, other investigations are required. These are thyroid function tests, complete liver function tests, serum amylase level estimation, and complete renal function test.

TREATMENT

Nonpharmacologic Management

The management of hyperemesis gravidarum depends on the severity of the patient and should be individualized according to the patient. These range from explanation, emotional support, dietary modification, and antiemetics to more aggressive treatment including hospitalization to correct fluid and electrolyte imbalances. Though there is a range of options from routine changes to medications, alterations in maternal diet and lifestyle can have dramatic effect.

Family members need to be informed that the pregnant mother suffers from hyperemesis gravidarum, and may need to alter her meal times and may require dietary modification, besides tender, love, care and emotional support.

A large number of patients recover with temporary change in environment, and hospitalization for a short period is beneficial. Patients must be encouraged to rest when symptomatic. These mothers should receive appropriate support from family members.

Diet

Modification of the amount and size of meals consumed, may help relieve symptoms. Lesser amounts of food and fluid help to prevent mild cases from getting worse. Meals should contain more carbohydrates than fat. Protein rich diet also relieves symptoms. Drinks should be rich in electrolytes. Citrus drinks are better tolerated than plain water and may be used for rinsing the mouth.

Lifestyle

Stress should be avoided and periods of rest increased. Supportive counseling and crisis intervention may be necessary.

Acupressure

Some studies have shown that acupressure causes significant reduction in nausea and vomiting. Pressure is applied on a point situated three fingerbreadths above the wrist on the volar surface.

Ginger

Root of ginger—*Zingiber officinale*—has been used for treatment of nausea and vomiting and is considered as an effective antiemetic. In one study, ginger powder in the dose of 1 g per day was more effective than a placebo in reducing nausea and vomiting. Effectiveness is dependent on its aroma, carminative and absorbent characteristics. It acts on the gastrointestinal tract, increasing motility.

Its absorbent property decreases stimuli to the chemoreceptor zone in the medulla inhibiting stimuli to the emetic center of the brain stem. Ginger also blocks the gastrointestinal responses and consequently the nausea feedback.

Despite earlier misgivings on its effect on sex steroid differentiation in the fetus, no teratogenic effects have been found.

Pharmacotherapy

In the initial period of severe vomiting, parenteral antiemetics should be administered along with intravenous fluids. The gut requires to be kept empty for the first 24 hours in hyperemesis gravidarum. When vomiting stops and the patient is able to tolerate orally, antiemetics can be prescribed orally.

Intravenous Fluid Therapy

Persistent vomiting with ketonuria and dehydration requires admission to hospital and intravenous fluid therapy to replenish the lost intravenous volume.

Rehydration along with replacement of electrolytes is important in treatment. Normal saline or Ringer's lactate are the mainstay of fluid therapy. If dextrose solution is used, prior administration of thiamine is necessary to prevent Wernicke's encephalopathy. While replacing electrolytes, care must be taken to consider the risks of rapid infusion to prevent central pontine myelinolysis.

Thiamine

The dose for routine supplementation in patients with protracted vomiting is 1.5mg/day. If oral dose is not tolerated, 100 mg of thiamine is diluted in 100 mL normal saline and infused over 30 minutes to one hour weekly.

Antiemetics

Commonly used drugs are not advisable prior to 12–14 weeks to prevent detrimental effect to the fetus.

In the 2004 guidelines on vomiting in pregnancy, the American Congress of Obstetrics and Gynecology, recommended that the first line antiemetic medication be intravenous metoclopramide or promethazine. In a double blind study in 2010, it was found that though the therapeutic effects of both drugs were similar, less drowziness was seen with metoclopramide. The dose of metoclopramide is 10 mg and 25 mg of promethazine every 8 hours for 24 hours.

Combination treatment of droperidol and diphenhydramine significantly shortens hospital stay, as well as fewer readmissions compared to those not receiving droperidol or diphenhydramine as primary therapy. The dose of droperidol is 1.0–2.5 mg depending on the severity of symptoms. This dose is administered over 15 minutes. Continuous infusion is started at 1.0 mg/hour and if symptoms persist, the rate is increased to 1.25 mg/hour. The doses are increased by 0.25 mg every 4 hours. No abnormal fetal or neonatal outcomes are noted; neither is any maternal adverse effect including hypotension seen.

Ondansetron is a selective 5-hydroxytryptamine (5HT3) receptor antagonist and acts on central and peripheral nervous system. It delays gastric emptying and decreases vomiting after the first dose, with subsequent decrease in nausea. Patients are able to tolerate a light diet after two days of therapy.

Steroids

They act by direct effect on the vomiting center of the brain. It has been found that vomiting ceases within three hours of administration of the first dose of IV hydrocortisone. Maintenance doses range from 15–45 mg/day.

Steroids are used only after all other causes of vomiting have been excluded, or vomiting continues for more than four weeks. Steroids are more effective than promethazine. The dose of methylprednisolone is 16 mg thrice a day.

MANAGEMENT DURING SPECIAL CIRCUMSTANCES

Nasogastric Enteral Feeding

With nasogastric enteral feeding, symptoms improve within 24 hours. This treatment has potential complications like pneumothorax, aspiration, infection, and venous thrombosis. It is cheaper than total parenteral nutrition (TPN) and is useful in patients whose nausea and vomiting is associated with consumption of food.

Total Parenteral Nutrition

In severe hyperemesis, there is lack of adequate nutrients. TPN provides utilizable nitrogen, electrolytes, trace elements, water and fat-soluble vitamins. It is a non-protein calorie source, generally glucose or lipid emulsion. This source of calories prevent ketosis, which develops from metabolism of fatty acids and may have adverse effect on the fetus.

Complications of the TPN catheter include pneumothorax, puncture of adjacent blood vessel or air embolism. Use of large amounts of glucose may lead to hyperglycemia, leading to fetal anomalies and the risk of macrosomia.

TPN is discontinued when enteral feeding is tolerated.

CONCLUSION

Hyperemesis gravidarum is a multifactorial neurohormonal disorder of early pregnancy. It can lead to maternal and fetal complications if not treated early and aggressively. Acute medical and surgical conditions presenting with vomiting should be excluded. A complete history, physical examination and investigations help to establish the diagnosis. Pharmacotherapy along with non-pharmacological treatment successfully controls the symptoms.

SUGGESTED READING

1. Loh KY, Sivalingam N. Understanding Hyperemesis Gravidarum. Med J Malaysia. 2005;60(3):394-9.
2. Wegrzynick LJ, Repke JT, Ural SH. Treatment of Hyperemesis Gravidarum. Rev Obstet Gynecol. 2012;5(2):78-84.

Bleeding in Early Pregnancy

Rita Sinha, Hemali Heidi Sinha

DEFINITION

Any vaginal bleeding before 20 weeks of gestation is known as early pregnancy bleeding.

INCIDENCE

Vaginal bleeding occurs in 15–25% of early pregnancies. 50% of women who have vaginal bleeding in early pregnancy have a viable pregnancy.

Bleeding in first trimester is not always a problem, it may be caused by:

- Sexual Intercourse
- An infection
- The fertilized egg implanting in the uterus
- Hormonal changes during pregnancy.

More serious cause of bleeding in early pregnancy is related to pregnancy, and maybe pre-existing or aggravated during pregnancy. These are:

- Abortion
- Cervical lesions
- Ectopic pregnancy
- Vascular erosions
- Hydatidiform mole
- Polyp.

Implantation bleeding: The process of implantation takes place 6–8 days postovulation or fertilization. Vaginal bleeding can occur as a result of the burrowing of the blastocyst into the uterine endometrium (invasion of the decidua basalis by chorion). The resulting bleeding is characterized by spotting or light bleeding for a day or two. This may be bright red in appearance.

In addition to creating anxiety for the women, vaginal bleeding may create a confusing clinical picture. Unusual vaginal bleeding in a woman who is sexually active especially if she is not using contraception, must be considered pregnancy related until proven otherwise.

Although abortions, ectopic pregnancy and Gestational Trophoblastic Disease (GTD) are key differential diagnoses, others should not be overlooked (cervicitis, cervical lesion, polyp, cervical/vaginal trauma, secondary to sexual activity, vaginitis/vaginosis and sexually transmitted infections including pelvic inflammatory disease (PID)).

Uterine fibroids are also associated with vaginal bleeding during pregnancy.

ABORTION

Any fetal loss from conception until the time of fetal viability at 20 weeks of gestation or expulsion of a fetus or embryo weighing 500 g or less which is not capable of independent survival is abortion.

Incidence

15–20% pregnancy.

Classification

- Spontaneous abortion—occurs without medical or mechanical means.
- Induced abortion.

Pathology—necrotic changes occur in the decidual tissues near the placental site which result in hemorrhage into this area.

As bleeding continues, the sac and the placenta become detached from the uterine wall and are expelled by uterine contractions.

Common Causes of Abortion, Trimester-wise

First Trimester

- Genetic factors
- Endocrine disorders
- Immunological disorders
- Infections
- Unexplained.

Second Trimester

- Anatomical abnormalities
- Cervical incompetence
- Mullerian fusion defects
- Uterine synechiae
- Uterine fibroids
- Maternal medical illness
- Unexplained.

Types of Spontaneous Abortion and Clinical Features

- *Threatened abortion*
  - Symptoms and signs of pregnancy coincide with its duration

- Vaginal bleeding maybe slight or mild, bright red in color
- Pain is slight or absent
- On pelvic examination—cervical os is closed.

Prognosis—If the blood loss is less than normal menstrual flow and is not accompanied by the pain of uterine contractions, there is reasonable chance for pregnancy to continue. This occurs in 50% cases while other half will proceed to inevitable or missed abortion.

- *Inevitable abortion*
  - Symptoms and signs of pregnancy coincide with its duration
  - Vaginal bleeding is excessive and may accompanied with clots
  - Abdominal pain is colicky felt in the suprapubic region, radiating to the back
  - Pelvic examination—internal os of the cervix is dilated and products of conception may be felt through it.
- *Incomplete abortion*
  - Retention of a part of the products of conception inside the uterus. The whole or part of the placenta may be retained
  - The patient usually notices the passage of a part of the products of conception
  - Bleeding is continuous
  - Uterus is less than the period of amenorrhea, but still large in size
  - On pelvic examination—cervical os is opened and retained products maybe felt through it.
- *Complete abortion*
  - All products of conception have been expelled from the uterus
  - Bleeding is slight and gradually diminishes
  - The pain ceases
  - Uterus is slightly larger than normal
  - Cervical os is closed.
- *Missed abortion*
  - Retention of dead products of conception for four weeks or more
  - Regression of pregnancy symptoms such as nausea, vomiting and breast symptoms
  - Uterine size does not increase and may even decrease in size
  - The fetal movements are not felt or cease if previously felt
  - A dark brown vaginal discharge may occur (prune juice discharge)
  - Complication—disseminated intravascular coagulation (DIC) may occur if the dead conceptus is retained for more than four weeks.
- *Septic abortion*
  - Any type of abortion which is complicated by infection
  - *E. coli*, bacteroids, anaerobic *Streptococcus*, *Clostridia* and *Staphylococci* are among the common causative organisms.
- *Recurrent abortion:* Three or more successive spontaneous abortion

Ectopic pregnancy: Ectopic means "out of place". Ectopic pregnancy is defined as the implantation of fertilized ovum outside endometrial cavity.

The fertilized ovum settles in the fallopian tubes in more than 95% of ectopic pregnancies. This is the reason that ectopic pregnancies are commonly called tubal pregnancies. Other sites are uterine cornua, undeveloped horn of a bicornuate uterus, cervix, ovum and the abdominal cavity.

Ectopic pregnancy can be difficult to diagnose because symptoms often mirror those of a normal early pregnancy like missed periods, nausea, vomiting, frequent urination or breast tenderness. First warning sign of an ectopic pregnancy is pain or vaginal bleeding.

Hydatidiform mole: Hydatidiform mole is an abnormal conception resulting in hydropic swelling of the chorionic villi and trophoblastic hyperplasia leading to the formation of grape like vesicles. Gestational trophoblastic disease is the term used for the spectrum of diseases resulting from abnormal proliferation of trophoblasts. The diseases are vesicular mole, invasive mole, and choriocarcinoma.

Hydatidiform mole can be divided into two types, on the basis of gross morphology, histopathology and karyotype—complete mole and partial mole.

By the end of third month, women experience vaginal bleeding from spotting to excessive bleeding.

Sometimes, grape like cluster of cells are shed with blood.

Other symptoms are severe nausea and vomiting, high blood pressure. As pregnancy progresses, fetal movements are not perceived and there is no fetal heart beat.

CLINICAL APPROACH TO A PATIENT WITH BLEEDING IN EARLY PREGNANCY

History

- ➲ Vaginal bleeding—slight and bright red, associated with passage of fleshy mass or clots. Discharge may be serosanguinous or dark colored with foul smell and passage of grape like vesicles. This is commonly referred as "White Currant in Red Currant Juice." There is often abdominal pain which is colicky or agonizing
- ➲ Shoulder pain, may be a sign of ruptured ectopic
- ➲ Symptoms of early pregnancy—history of amenorrhea, morning sickness, frequency of micturition, breast discomfort, fatigue, hyperemesis, breathlessness, thyrotoxic features, syncopial attack
- ➲ Careful menstrual history—previous cycles, last menstrual period (LMP)
- ➲ Past history—similar episodes, infertility, details of contraceptive use
- ➲ History of inserting something into the vaginal (suggestive of an illegal abortion).

Examination

- ➲ General look
    - Lies quiet and conscious, perspires and looks blanched
    - Looks more ill than accounted for—Molar pregnancy.

- Vital signs—temperature, pulse, blood pressure and respiratory rate.
- Look for pallor.
- Abdominal examination
  Auscultate for bowel sounds—absent in peritonitis due to septic abortion
  - Assess presence, location and severity of pain, check whether the abdomen is distended
  - Palpate for abdominal rigidity and guarding (peritonitis, ectopic pregnancy)
  - Palpate for rebound tenderness
  - Assess the abdominal mass (molar/ectopic pregnancy).
- Pelvic examination
  - External pelvic and digital vaginal examination
    - Inspection for laceration outside the vagina or over the external genitalia
    - Assessment of the amount of bleeding per vaginam
    - POC lying outside the vaginal orifice.
  - Per speculum examination—look for:
    - Any visible product of contraception (POC) protruding from the cervical os or visible in the vaginal canal
    - Foul swelling vaginal/cervical discharge
    - Cervical laceration (indicative of instrumentation, may be suggestive of illegal abortion)
    - Foreign body in the vagina.
  - Digital vaginal examination:
    - Assess the amount of bleeding
    - Check whether the cervical os is open or closed (to determine the stage of abortion).
  - Bimanual examination—look for:
    - Size of the uterus
    - Any pelvic pain (severity, location and what causes the pain, whether present at rest, increase with touch and pressure, increase on moving the cervix)
    - Any adnexal mass—ectopic pregnancy.

Investigation

- Complete blood count, ABO grouping and Rh typing, thyroid function test, urine pregnancy test, serum beta human chorionic gonadotropin (hCG) level
- Ultrasonography (USG)—transabdominal and transvaginal.

DIAGNOSIS

- Threatened abortion
  - Positive urine pregnancy test
  - On USG (ultrasonography), intrauterine viable fetus
- Incomplete abortion
  - Positive uterine pregnancy test
  - On USG—nonviable fetus, POC in situ

- ⊃ Complete abortion
  - Positive urine pregnancy test
  - On USG—empty uterine cavity
- ⊃ Ectopic pregnancy
  - Positive urine pregnancy test
  - On USG—POC not seen in uterus, some adnexal mass may be seen
- ⊃ Molar pregnancy
  - Positive urine pregnancy test
  - On USG—snow storm appearance.

GENERAL MANAGEMENT OF VAGINAL BLEEDING IN EARLY PREGNANCY

Universal

Monitor the woman's vital signs and general condition. When complications exist, it is important to take steps to continue stabilizing the woman's condition, before giving specific management for abortion. If the condition of the patient suddenly worsens, reassess for shock or other complications, and treat as appropriate.

Oxygen

If the woman is stable and there are no life-threatening complications (she is not in shock and the vital signs are normal), oxygen is not required. If woman is in shock, manage accordingly.

Fluids

If the woman is stable and there are no complications (she is not in shock and the vital signs are normal), IV fluids are NOT required. If woman is in shock, manage accordingly.

Medicines

Oral medicines may be given if the woman is stable and there are no life threatening complications. The IV or IM routes of administration are the only acceptable routes for giving medicines if the woman is in shock. If she is also being treated for a life-threatening condition, follow the treatment guidelines for that condition.

Antibiotics

Antibiotics should preferably be given intravenously. If an evacuation is needed, start antibiotics before carrying out the evacuation. In case of a septic abortion, give the woman an antibiotic cover for at least 48 hours before carrying out uterine evacuation.

Tetanus Toxoid

If there is a possibility that the woman was exposed to tetanus (if the abortion was not performed with sterile instruments and/or if there was any contamination of the instruments or wound with dirt, as may be the case in an unsafe abortion, there is a chance of exposure to tetanus) and her vaccination history is uncertain, give her tetanus toxoid injection (0.5 mg IM) and tetanus antitoxin.

MANAGEMENT OF THREATENED ABORTION

- Rest in bed until one week after bleeding stops
- Women are advised to avoid strenuous exercise, sexual intercourse, as it may disturb pregnancy by the mechanical effects and effects of semen prostaglandins on the uterus
- If bleeding stops, follow up in antenatal clinic. Reassess, if bleeding occurs
- If bleeding persists, assess for fetal viability or ectopic pregnancy. Persistent bleeding particularly in the presence of a uterus larger than expected, may indicate twins or molar pregnancy
- Hormonal treatment and local agents are contraindicated.

MANAGEMENT OF INEVITABLE ABORTION

- Any attempt to maintain pregnancy is useful
- If the pregnancy is less than 12 weeks, plan for evacuation of the contents of the uterus. 400 µg misoprostol should be given and it should be repeated once after 4 hours, if necessary
- Arrange for evacuation as soon as possible
- If the pregnancy is of more than 12 weeks, we should wait for spontaneous expulsion of the POC and then evacuate the uterus to remove any retained POC
- If necessary, uterine contractions should be augmented to expel the POC with oxytocin 20 units in 500 mL of Ringer's lactate at the rate of 40 drops/minute.
- 800 µg misoprostol tablet is administered transvaginally again after four hours. Two tablets can be given if the woman has not aborted till then.

MANAGEMENT OF INCOMPLETE ABORTION

- If the bleeding is light to moderate and the pregnancy is less than 12 weeks, fingers or sponge forceps should be used to remove the POC protruding through the dilated cervix.
- If the bleeding is heavy and the pregnancy is less than 12 weeks, uterus should be evacuated
  - Manual vacuum aspiration is the preferred method of evacuation. Sharp curettage should not be done

- If evacuation is not immediately possible, 400 µg misoprostol should be given orally (it should be repeated once after 4 hours, if necessary).
- If the pregnancy is more than 12 weeks
  - Oxytocin drip should be started, 20 units of oxytocin in 500 mL of Ringer's lactate at the rate of 40 drops/minute until the POC are expelled
  - 200 µg misoprostol can be given vaginally every 4 hours, if necessary until the POC are expelled. More than 800 µg should not be administered.
- After 12 weeks of pregnancy, fetus is usually expelled completely.

MANAGEMENT OF COMPLETE ABORTION

- Evacuation of the uterus is not necessary as all the POC have been expelled
- Observe for heavy bleeding
- Ensure follow-up of woman after treatment.

Follow-up after abortion
- Counsel that spontaneous abortion is common
- Reassure woman that chances for subsequent successful pregnancy are good
- Advise contraception.

MANAGEMENT OF MISSED ABORTION

- We should wait for four weeks for spontaneous expulsion.
- Evacuation of the uterus is indicated in the following conditions:
  - Spontaneous expulsion does not occur within 4 weeks
  - Profuse bleeding
  - Infection or disseminated intravascular coagulation (DIC).
- Management done according to the size of the uterus
  - Uterine size less than 12 weeks—suction evacuation
  - Uterine size more than12 weeks—evacuation be done by:
    - Prostaglandins—intravaginal (PgE2) intravenous, intra- or extra-amniotic (PGF2 alpha)
    - Oxytocin drip
    - Combination of drugs.

MANAGEMENT OF SEPTIC ABORTION

- Blood, cervical swabs and urine are sent for culture and sensitivity. This helps in identifying the infecting organism and appropriate antibiotics may then be administered
- If bleeding is minimal, treat infection with broad-spectrum antibiotics
  - Dilatation and curettage is done.
- If bleeding is severe,
  - POC from the cervix are removed with a sponge holding forceps
  - Intravenous broad spectrum antibiotics should be given
  - When infection is controlled—dilatation and curettage is done.

MANAGEMENT OF HABITUAL ABORTION

- Rest
- Increased intake of vitamin B, vitamin C and vitamin E
- Medical treatment
    - Hypofunction of corpus luteum—progesterone is added
- Surgical treatment
    - Correction of congenital anomalies of uterus: removal of myoma
    - Repair of incompetent cervix—12–20 weeks.

CONCLUSION

Bleeding in early pregnancy is common, affecting about 15% of confirmed pregnancies. The pregnancy may remain viable in spite of bleeding (threatened abortion) or bleeding may be a feature of non viability (missed abortion/blighted ovum). The pregnancy may be partly (inevitable/incomplete abortion) or completely expelled (complete abortion).

Though the term abortion has been used throughout the chapter, the term miscarriage is preferred, to distinguish spontaneous from induced pregnancy losses.

SUGGESTED READING

1. Guidelines: Define a non viable pregnancy. NEJM: 2013;369:1443-51.
2. James DK, Steer PJ, Weiner CP, Gonik B. High-risk Pregnancy: Management Options. Elsevier Inc. 4th Edition, 2011.

Ectopic Pregnancy

Sushma Singh, Shanti HK Singh

DEFINITION

The blastocyst normally implants in the endometrial lining of the uterine cavity. Implantation may occur anywhere outside the normal uterine cavity, the subsequent gestation being called ectopic.

FREQUENCY

Ectopic pregnancy is seen in about 2 percent of all pregnancies in USA, 3–4 percent worldwide incidence. Ruptured ectopic pregnancy accounts for 10–15 percent of all maternal deaths.

The incidence of rupture and case fatality rate declined from 35.5 deaths per 10,000 ectopic pregnancies in 1970 to 3.8 per 10,000 in 1989, after the advent of transvaginal ultrasonography and beta subunit of human chorionic gonadotropin tests.

SITES OF ECTOPIC PREGNANCY

The possible sites can be classified according to frequency:
1. Fallopian tubes   95–98 percent
2. Uterine cornua   2–2.5 percent
3. Ovary, cervix and abdominal cavity   < 1 percent

Lately ectopic pregnancy over the cesarean scar has been reported. Primary abdominal pregnancy is indeed a very rare phenomenon, but secondary abdominal pregnancies have been reported.

RISK FACTORS

1. Pelvic inflammatory diseases (6-fold increased risk)
2. Raised *Chlamydia* antibody titer (2-fold increased risk)
3. Use of IUCDs (3–5% increased risk)
4. Smoking (2–5%) increased risk
5. ART pregnancies (3–5 % increased risk)
6. Tubal surgery (5–8% increased risk), e.g. sterilization and reconstruction

7. Prior ectopic pregnancy (10-fold increased risk)
8. Age risk of ectopic is 3-fold greater in women of 35–44 years as compared to 18–24 years.
9. Endometriosis
10. In utero diethylstilbestrol exposure
11. Overdevelopment of ovum and external migration.

ETIOLOGY

The cause of ectopic pregnancy is tubal damage or altered motility that results in the blastocyst being improperly transported and abnormally implanted. The commonest cause is acute salpingitis in almost 50 percent of cases. In almost 40 percent cases no risk factor is apparent.

Pelvic inflammatory disease: The most common cause is previous salpingitis due to sexually transmitted disease such as gonococcal and chlamydial infection, or salpingitis that follows septic abortion and puerperal sepsis. 40% of women with ectopic pregnancy show evidence of PID.

USE OF IUCDs

IUCDs prevent intrauterine pregnancy; hence, the ratio of ectopic to intrauterine pregnancies is much higher.

Ectopic pregnancy is more likely with progesterone IUCD.

Smoking:

Cigarette smokers, who smoke > 20 cigarettes per day, have a relative risk of 2.5 times compared to the non-smokers.

Nicotine is thought to alter tubal motility, ciliary activity and blastocyst implantation.

ASSISTED REPRODUCTION TECHNIQUES

There is a higher incidence of ectopic pregnancy after in vitro fertilization.

TUBAL SURGERY

Ectopic pregnancy is seen following surgery for blocked tubes and reversal of sterilization and is also higher following cauterization procedures.

PRIOR ECTOPIC PREGNANCY

Women, who have one ectopic pregnancy, are likely to have a 10-fold increased risk of having an ectopic pregnancy again and this risk is due to the fact that PID and salpingitis is a bilateral disease and the risk factor will be the same for the other side even after being ectopic on one side.

PATHOGENESIS OF ECTOPIC IMPLANTATION

The fallopian tube is by far the most common site of ectopic implantation, accounting for more than 98% of all ectopic pregnancies. Overall 70% of ectopic pregnancies are located in the tubal ampulla, 12% in the isthmus, 11% in the fimbria and 2% in the interstitial cornual segment.

Reactions in the Tube

The histopathology of ectopic pregnancy varies with the site of implantation. In approximately half of the ampullary ectopic pregnancies, trophoblastic proliferation occurs entirely within the tubal lumen and the muscularis remains intact.

In the remainder, the trophoblast penetrates the tubal wall and proliferates in the loose connective tissues between the muscularis and the serosa.

In most cases, the characteristic segmental dilation of the tubal ampulla is comprised mostly of coagulated blood rather than trophoblastic tissue.

In contrast, ectopic implantation in the tubal isthmus typically penetrates the tubal wall early probably because the most muscular segment is less distensible. All the ectopic pregnancies are not destined to rupture. In fact, many will resolve without intervention, presumably by spontaneous regression in site or tubal absorption (expulsion via the fimbria).

Reactions of the Uterus

The uterus itself is under the influence of the hormones of the corpus luteum and of the trophoblast. So, it responds by generalized enlargement, increased vascularity, hypertrophy of all tissues and decidual reaction in the endometrium.

A special appearance of the endometrial glands (the Arias Stella reaction) is seen in 10–15 percent of the cases. This is chacterized by mixed patterns of atypical proliferative and secretory activity.

Pregnancy Outcome

Course of ectopic pregnancy is shown in Flow chart 1.

CLINICAL MANIFESTATIONS

Tubal pregnancy present as a chronic or an acute illness, or as acute-on-chronic. The first is much more common but the acute picture is so dramatic that is tends to receive more attention.

SYMPTOMS AND SIGNS

1. Normal symptoms and sign of pregnancy (amenorrhea and uterine softening)

Flow chart 1: Pregnancy outcome—course of ectopic pregnancy

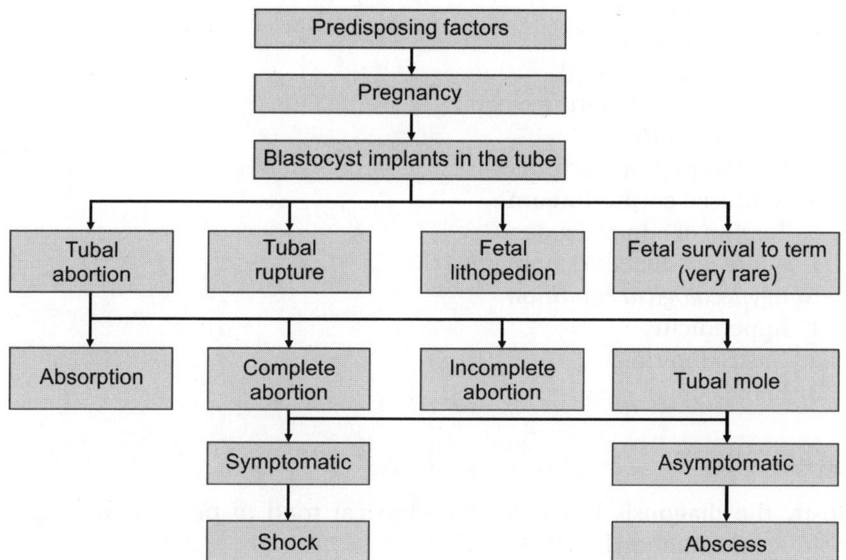

2. Acute abdominal pain (dull, crampy or colicky pain in 95% of women)
3. Evidence of hemodynamic instability (hypotension, collapse, signs and symptoms of shock)
4. Adnexal mass (with or without tenderness) and cervical motion tenderness
5. Abnormal vaginal bleeding (60 to 80% of women)
6. Signs of peritoneal irritation (shoulder-tip pain)
7. Absence of gestational sac on ultrasound with a β–hCG of $\geq$ 2500 mIU/mL.

CLASSICAL TRIAD

A patient with amenorrhea, pain and vaginal bleeding should always be suspected to have an ectopic pregnancy.

DIFFERENTIAL DIAGNOSIS

The picture of ectopic pregnancy is extremely variable and can mimic any intra-abdominal disease. It should be kept in mind here that in ectopic pregnancy, the clinical diagnosis is more on symptoms rather than signs (Negative physical signs should not be allowed to overrule the symptoms).

The following conditions are most likely to be confused with ectopic pregnancy. These may be pelvic disease or nongynecological, nonobstetric disease.

A. *Obstetric disease*
   1. Abortion of an early intrauterine pregnancy
   2. Abortion followed by salpingitis
   3. Early pregnancy C-pelvic tumors

    4. Retroverted gravid uterus
    5. Septic abortion
B. *Gynecological disease*
    1. Degenerated fibroid
    2. Dysfunctional uterine bleeding
    3. Endometriosis
    4. Ovulation (Mittelschmerz)
    5. Ruptured corpus luteum
    6. Torsion of adnexal mass
    7. Acute or subacute salpingitis
C. *Nongynecological condition*
    1. Appendicitis
    2. Gastroenteritis
    3. Renal colic.

DIAGNOSIS

Mostly the diagnosis based on the classical triad of pelvic pain, vaginal spotting and amenorrhea (5–9 weeks).

Other classical symptoms are dizziness, pregnancy symptoms and vaginal passage of clot.

The most common classical finding is pelvic pain with manipulation of the cervix and adnexal mass (cervical excitation pain).

Ruptured ectopic may present as shock (tachycardia with hypotension). Shoulder pain due to diaphragmatic irritation is a late sign of hemoperitoneum.

Tests and Aids to Diagnosis

1. *Urine pregnancy test:* It is positive in about 50 percent of cases. Current serum and urine pregnancy tests that use ELISA for beta hCG are sensitive to the levels of 10 to 20 mIU/mL and are positive in > 99% of ectopic pregnancies (Kaminski and Guss, 2002).
2. *β-hCG levels:* In ectopic pregnancy, the production of β-hCG is less as compared to normal pregnancy. A subnormal rise in Beta hCG in early pregnancy (< 66% in 48 hours) suggests pregnancy is not viable (early pregnancy failure or ectopic pregnancy).
3. *Serum progesterone:* It may be helpful as an adjunct to β-hCG in evaluating ectopic pregnancy. A progesterone level to > 25 ng/mL is associated with an intrauterine pregnancy in 97.5%. Value below 5 ng/mL suggests either an ectopic pregnancy or missed abortion.
4. *Transvaginal ultrasound:* It is a valuable diagnostic tool. The presence of an intrauterine pregnancy generally excludes ectopic pregnancy (Heterotrophic ectopic should be kept in mind).
   A gestational sac is visualized in almost 100% cases at a β-hCG level above the discriminatory zone >2400 mIU/mL (with the use of transabdominal USG, the value of discriminatory zone is 6500 mIU/mL)

The following transvaginal ultrasound findings may be seen in an ectopic pregnancy:

 i. Empty uterus
 ii. Thickened endometrium
 iii. Pseudogestational sac (Nyberg and Associates, 1987, Hilland co-workers, 1990)
 iv. Adnexal ring sign
 v. Complex adnexal mass
 vi. Free fluid in POD.

Color Doppler will classically identify "ring of fire" round the ectopic on the same side as corpus luteum.

The blood flow is low resistant trophoblastic flow pattern.

5. *Laparoscopy:* A laparoscopic confirmation of diagnosis is useful. Today, operative video laparoscopy has revolutionized the surgical management of ectopic and will prevent over 40% laparotomies as well.

Therefore, TVS followed by quantitative β-hCG testing is an optimal and cost-effective strategy for diagnosing ectopic pregnancy.

MANAGEMENT OF ECTOPIC PREGNANCY

Management of the acutely ill women differs from the more common presentation of a woman, who is clinically stable, in which situation there are a number of treatment options available.

Acute Ectopic

Laparotomy is called for as soon as the diagnosis of ruptured ectopic pregnancy is made and resuscitation and operation at the same time can be life-saving.

- Immediate laparotomy and clamping of the bleeding vessel
- When the donated blood is not available, an autotransfusion of blood, ladled from peritoneal cavity and filtered through gauze gives excellent results. But it should be fresh and not old blood
- The opposite tube and ovary should be examined before deciding the surgical treatment of the affected tubes
- Salpingectomy has long been considered the gold standard treatment for ectopic pregnancy.

However, considerable recent emphasis has been placed on the conservation of the fallopian tubes.

The Royal College of Obstetricians and Gynecologists recommends that surgical treatment by laparoscopic salpingectomy is the preferred method of treatment for an ectopic pregnancy when the fallopian tube on the other side is normal.

In the management of an ectopic pregnancy, removal of the fallopian tube (salpingectomy) is considered to be the safest, most clinically effective and most cost effective. Ipsilateral ovary and its vascular supply are preserved.

Oophorectomy is done only if the ovary is pathological or damaged beyond salvage.

Laparoscopic salpingostomy should be considered in the presence of contralateral tubal disease and the desire for future fertility.

Unruptured Tubal Pregnancy

It can be managed by laparotomy and operative laparoscopy. The Royal College of Obstetricians and Gynecologists (May 2004) recommends that management must be tailored medically and occasionally by observation alone, according to the clinical condition and future fertility requirements of the woman.

1. Expectant management
2. Medical management
3. Surgically administered medical management
4. Surgical management
    a. Conservative surgery includes:
        i. Salpingostomy
        ii. Salpingotomy
        iii. Segmental resection and anastomosis
    b. Radical surgery (Salpingectomy).

Expectant Management

Expectant Management is between 47 and 82% effective in managing ectopic pregnancy. A good candidate for expectant management has:
- A β-hCG level less that 1,000 mIU/mL and decreasing
- Tubal pregnancy only
- An ectopic mass < 3.5 cm
- No fetal heartbeat
- Has agreed to comply with the follow-up requirement.

Medical Treatment

Methotrexate, a folic acid antagonist, is a well studied medical therapy.

Methotrexate deactivates dihydrofolate reductase, which reduces tetrahydrofolate levels (a cofactor for deoxyribonucleic acid and ribonucleic acid synthesis), thereby rapidly dividing the trophoblastic cell.

Other therapeutic agents include hyperosmolar glucose, prostaglandins and mifepristone.

Indications:
1. Hemodynamically stable patients.
2. No contraindications to methotrexate.
3. Able to return for follow-up care for several weeks.
4. Nonlaparoscopic diagnosis of ectopic pregnancy.
5. Unruptured adnexal mass <3.5 cm in size on scan.
6. No fetal cardiac activity on scan
7. hCG level does not exceed 3000 IU/L.

Methotrexate Therapy Protocol

Regimen	Surveillance
Single dose Methotrexate, 50 mg/m² IM	Measure β-hCG levels, days 4 and 7: if difference > 15%, repeat Weekly until undetectable ❖ if difference > 15% between day 4 and 7 levels, repeat methotrexate dose ❖ if fetal cardiac activity present on day 7, repeat methotrexate dose ❖ surgical treatment if β-hCG levels are not decreasing or fetal cardiac activity persists after three doses of methotrexate
Double dose Methotrexate 50 mg/m² IM, days 0 and 4	Follow-up as for single dose regimen
Variable dose (up to four doses) Methotrexate, 1 mg/kg IM, days 1, 3, 5 and 7 Leucovorin, 0.1 mg/kg IM, days 2, 4, 6 and 8	Measure β-hCG levels day 1, 3, 5 and 7. Continue alternate-day injections until β-hCG levels decrease ❖ 15% in 48 hours or four doses of methotrexate given. Then, weekly β-hCG until undetectable

Persistent Ectopic

Incomplete removal of trophoblast may result in persistent ectopic pregnancy and can be identified by persistent or rising hCG levels. Usually, β-hCG levels fall quickly and are at about 10% of preoperative values by day 12 (Hajenius and colleagues, 1995).

According to Seifer (1997), factors that increase the risk of persistent ectopic pregnancy includes:
1. Small pregnancies, that is less than 2 cm
2. Early therapy before 42 menstrual days
3. Serum β-hCG levels exceeding 3000 mIU/mL
4. Implantation medial to the salpingostomy site. In the face of persistent or increasing β-hCG, additional surgical or medical therapy is necessary.

Surgically Administered Medical Treatment

Methotrexate, potassium chloride (20%) and RU486 can be administered laparoscopically into the gestational sac or transvaginally under ultrasonic guidance, provided the sac measures <3.5 cm. It is successful in 90% of the cases.

Surgical Management of Unruptured Tubal Pregnancy

A laparoscopic approach to the surgical management of tubal pregnancy, in hemodynamically stable patient, is preferable to an open approach.

In the presence of a healthy contralateral tube, salpingectomy is the preferred method of treatment.

Laparoscopic salpingostomy should be considered as the primary treatment when managing tubal pregnancy in the presence of contralateral tubal disease and the desire for future fertility.

Tubal surgery is considered conservative when there is tubal salvage. Examples include salpingotomy, salpingostomy and fimbrial expression of ectopic pregnancy. Radical surgery is defined by salpingectomy. Conservative surgery may increase the rate of subsequent uterine pregnancy but is associated with higher rates of persistently functioning trophoblast (Bangsgaard and colleagues, 2003).

Laparoscopy has similar tubal patency and future fertility rates as medical treatment. Salpingostomy has an estimate 8 to 9% failure rate, which can be managed with methotrexate.

- In Rh-negative women not sensitized to Rh antigen, anti-D gammaglobulin should be administered soon after operation to prevent isoimmunization.

Cervical Pregnancy

- When the implantation occurs in cervical canal at or below internal os
- Bleeding is profuse and painless (90%)
- Clinical diagnostic criteria:
    a. Soft enlarged cervix equal to or larger than the fundus
    b. Uterine bleeding without cramping pain
    c. Products of conceptions entirely confined within the endocervix
    d. Closed internal os with partially opened external os.

Diagnosis
- TVS, MRI and 3-D sonography.

Management
- Cerclage, curettage and tamponade
- Arterial embolization.

Abdominal Pregnancy

- Two types—primary [rare] and secondary [1:3000 pregnancies]
- Implantation in the peritoneal cavity excluding tubal, ovarian and intraligamentary implantation
- Presenting complaint—abdominal pain, nausea, vomiting and decreasing to absent fetal movement
- Signs—uterine contour not well defined, fetal parts felt easily.

Diagnosis
- Imaging—sonography
- MRI and CT.

Management
The principal surgical objectives include delivery of fetus and careful assessment of placental implantation. Some advocate leaving the placenta

in place as its removal may precipitate torrential hemorrhage. Postoperative methotrexate can be given.

Ovarian Pregnancy

- Rare
- *Spiegelberg criteria*
    a. Tube on the affected side intact.
    b. Gestation sac must be towards the position of the ovary
    c. Gestation sac connected to the uterus by ovarian ligament
    d. Ovarian tissue found on its wall on hist. examination
- Treatment—salpingo-oophorectomy
- Ovarian cystectomy and wedge resection for small lesions.

Heterotopic Pregnancy

Incidence—1:4000 to 1:7000 pregnancies. IVF centers present the incidence of 1–3% of heterotopic pregnancy.

Treatment is preferably laparoscopic minimal invasive surgery allowing uterine pregnancy to grow.

FUTURE FERTILITY AND RISK OF RECURRENCE

Approximately, 30% of women treated for ectopic pregnancy later have difficulty conceiving.

The overall conception rate is approximately 77% regardless of treatment. The rates of recurrent ectopic pregnancy are between 5 and 20%, but the risk increases to 32% in women who have had two consecutive ectopic pregnancies.

SUGGESTED READING

1. Barnhart K, Esposito M, Coutifaris C. An update on the medical treatment of ectopic pregnancy. Obstet Gynecol Clin North Am. 2000;27:653-67, viii.
2. Della-Giustina D, Denny M. Ectopic pregnancy. Emerg Med Clin North Am. 2003;21:565-84.
3. Gracia CR Barn hart CT. Diagnosing ectopic pregnancy, obstet-gynae. 2001;97:464-70.
4. Lewis G, Drife J, editors. Why Mothers Die 1997–1999? The Fifth Report of the Confidential Enquiries into Maternal Deaths in the United Kingdom. London: RCOG Press;2001.
5. Royal College of Obstetricians and Gynaecologists. Searching for evidence. Clinical Governance Advice No. 3. London: RCOG Press;2001.
6. Royal College of Obstetricians and Gynaecologists. The use of munoglobulin for rhesus prophylaxis. Guideline No. 22. London: RCOG Press; 2002.
7. Sowter M, Frappell J. The role of laparoscopy in the management of ectopic pregnancy. Rev Gynaecol Practice 200;2:73-82. Ankum W. Laparoscopy in

the diagnosis of ectopic pregnancy. In: Grudzinskas JG, O'Brien PMS, editors. Problems in Early Pregnancy: Advances in Diagnosis and Treatment. London: RCOG Press.1997;p.154-9.

8. Tay JI, Moore J, Walker JJ. Clinical review: Ectopic pregnancy [published correction appears in BMJ 2000;321:424]. BMJ. 2000;320:916-9.
9. Tenore JL. Ectopic pregnancy. Am Fam Physician. 2000;61:1080-8.
10. Yao M, Tulandi T. Current status of surgical and nonsurgical management of ectopic pregnancy. Fertil Steril. 1997;67:421-33.
11. Ylöstalo P, Cacciatore B, Korhonen J, Kääriäinen M, Mäkelä P, Sjöberg J, et al. Expectant management of ectopic pregnancy. Eur J Obstet Gynecol Reprod Biol. 1993;49:83-4.

Chapter

4

Epilepsy and Pregnancy

Navneet Magon, Alokananda Ray

INTRODUCTION

Epilepsy is one of the most common neurological disorders to complicate pregnancy. About 0.3 to 0.8% of all pregnancies occur in women suffering from active epilepsy.[1-3] The management of epilepsy in the childbearing age is not straightforward and many factors need to be considered during pregnancy, preconception and perinatal period. The confidential enquiry into maternal death has revealed that maternal mortality rates are increased in women with epilepsy (they are approximately ten times more likely to die during pregnancy than the general population). Poor control of seizures, accidents due to epilepsy and/or SUDEP (sudden unexpected death in epilepsy) may account for this.[4] Women with epilepsy are also at an increased risk of having a child with a major congenital malformation (MCM),[5-8] neurodevelopmental delays[9-12] and fetal anticonvulsant syndrome.[13-15] However, majority of women with epilepsy have uneventful pregnancies with delivery of normal healthy babies.

EFFECTS OF PREGNANCY ON EPILEPSY

A study, which included over 300 countries, indicated that majority of women with epilepsy and a good degree of seizure control prior to conception maintained this control throughout pregnancy in 63.6%, while 5.9% experienced improved control and only 17.9% experienced an increase in seizure frequency.[16] By contrast, mothers who experienced more than one seizure per month prior to pregnancy were more likely to deteriorate throughout pregnancy.[17]

New onset epilepsy during pregnancy is not uncommon and can be explained by the fact that few latent conditions have a tendency to present during pregnancy due to hormonal and physiological changes, and epilepsy may, in such cases, be the presenting feature of the underlying disorder. However, this entity needs to be differentiated from eclampsia, which should be considered as the primary cause of first episode seizure during pregnancy, unless proved otherwise.

Reduced seizure control can occur in pregnancy, due to reduced serum antiepileptic drug (AED) levels as a result of nausea and vomiting or poor compliance with medication (related to fears of teratogenicity) in early pregnancy. Pharmacokinetic changes due to pregnancy-specific physiological changes, lack of sleep towards term, or pain and hyperventilation during labor can also predispose to seizures.[17]

Effects of pregnancy on AEDs deserve a special mention. Several physiological changes that occur during pregnancy may affect drug levels, which may have an impact on maternal seizure control. The maternal blood volume increases to the extent of 30–50% due to an increase in both plasma and red cell volume.[17] This results in reduction in serum drug levels due to the increased volume of distribution. Increased cardiac output and glomerular filtration rates increase renal clearance of the drug.[18] Altered hepatic enzymatic activity during pregnancy can also result in increased drug clearance. The fall in albumin concentration in the maternal plasma, decreases protein binding of antiepileptic drugs with an increase in the free drug level. The effect of decreased protein binding, however, is usually outweighed by the effect of increased drug clearance and volume of distribution, and so overall drug levels during pregnancy tend to fall rather than increase.[17]

The increase in drug clearance during pregnancy, is of more clinical relevance with some drugs than others. The older drugs like carbamazepine and sodium valproate, despite falling levels during pregnancy are associated with adequate seizure control throughout pregnancy.[19,20] On the other hand, newer drugs like lamotrigine have increased clearance with significant reduction in serum levels and loss of seizure control. On an average, a twofold increase in the preconceptual daily dosage is required for adequate seizure control (mean daily dose of 572 mg during pregnancy, in comparison to the mean preconceptual daily dose of 286 mg).[21] Several studies have demonstrated that this observed increase in lamotrigine clearance steadily progress throughout gestation, reaching a peak in the third trimester in approximately the 32nd week of gestation.[22,23] Maximal increase in lamotrigine clearance of as much as 300–330% from baseline has been noted in a few studies.[24,25] However, such pronounced increase in clearance has not been demonstrated in those pregnancies in which the mother was concomitantly receiving sodium valproate.[24] This may be due to the inhibitory effect of valproate on lamotrigine glucuronidation, which reduces clearance of lamotrigine by approximately 50%.[26]

Mono therapy with lamotrigine requires dosage increments, on an average in the order of 315%, hence a three-fold prophylactic increase in lamotrigine dose to maintain seizure control has been advocated by some authors during pregnancy.[27] Owing to this, alternative and newer agents such as levetiracetam are increasingly being adviced during pregnancy. However, more research on use of these newer agents as monotherapy for seizure control during pregnancy are required.

EFFECT OF EPILEPSY ON PREGNANCY

Evidence suggests that most pregnancies complicated with epilepsy have uneventful outcome with birth of healthy and normal babies.

It has been postulated that decrease in placental blood flow during seizure activity or in the postictal phase may lead to hypoxia and acidosis in the fetus.[28-31] Fetal heart rate changes during a maternal seizure indicative of fetal hypoxia, including bradycardia and reduced variability, have been reported.[28-30] It is therefore possible, that maternal seizure disorder could lead to adverse pregnancy outcomes, such as intrauterine growth restriction (IUGR) and stillbirth, through recurrent hypoxic insults to the fetus. Several studies have reported an increased risk of adverse pregnancy outcomes in women with seizure disorders such as, IUGR, preeclampsia, eclampsia, preterm labor, antepartum hemorrhage (APH) and increased perinatal mortality; however, this risk was based primarily on birth certificate data and retrospective case-control studies.[1-3] More recent prospective studies on the other hand suggest women with a seizure disorder are not at increased risk of IUGR, stillbirth, preeclampsia, or preterm birth.[32]

There is no evidence that simple partial, complex partial, absence seizures, myoclonic seizures or tonic-clonic seizure adversely affect the pregnancy or the developing fetus in anyway other than through the coincidental effects of trauma. There is some recent evidence, however, linking frequent tonic-clonic seizures during pregnancy with cognitive or behavioral changes in childhood.[33]

There is a growing evidence of the potential teratogenic effects of antiepileptic drugs (AEDs) taken during pregnancy. There have been studies from as early as the 1960s suggesting links between major congenital malformations (MCMs) and the use of AEDs during pregnancy.[34-37] Women of childbearing age are routinely excluded from randomized controlled trials, as studies to examine human teratogenic risks are unethical. There are thus no randomized controlled trials of AEDs in pregnancy. Recently, with the advent of a number of prospective population-based epilepsy and pregnancy registers—it is hoped that more accurate information regarding the relative risks of the AEDs when used in pregnancy shall be available for clinical application and care of pregnant women with epilepsy.[19,38-40]

Sodium valproate appears to carry an elevated risk of MCM and neurodevelopmental delay compared with other AEDs.[19,38-40] According to the UK Epilepsy and Pregnancy Register, mothers taking sodium valproate are at increased risk of having a child with a major malformation (6.2%; 95% Cl: 4.6–8.2%) compared with other drugs used as mono therapy.[38] In September 2003, based on a review of available information and evidence, the committee on the safety of medicines recommended that women of childbearing age should not be started on sodium valproate without specialist neurological consultation.[41] The North American Antiepileptic Drug Pregnancy Registry reported a 10.7% (95% CI: 6.3–16.9%) MCMs with sodium valproate use in pregnancy.[42] In a smaller sample size, the Australian registry also suggested an increased risk in mothers taking sodium valproate and reported a dose-effect relationship, in that doses in excess of 1100 mg/day were associated with an increased rate of malformations.[43] The EUROCAT malformation registry has highlighted an over-representation of neural tube defects, facial clefts, hypospadias, atrial septal defects and some skeletal abnormalities in association with in utero exposure to sodium valproate.[44]

Carbamazepine use in pregnancy has a greater safety profile than valproate at a dosage of less than 1000 mg per day with 3-5% MCMs- most commonly cardiac and neural tube defects.[45]

Pregnancy outcome data for lamotrigine has been reassuring in the recent years. The International Lamotrigine Pregnancy Registry has reported 12 MCMs (2.9%; 95% CI: 1.6–5.1%) in 414 first trimester monotherapy with lamotrigine. The UK Epilepsy and Pregnancy Register has also reported similar results with MCMs in 3.2% (95% CI: 2.1–4.9%) of 647 children.[38] The North American registry demonstrated a low teratogenic risk, but suggested an increased risk of cleft palate among infants exposed in utero to lamotrigine[8] (8.9 per 1000 compared to 0.6 per 1000 in the control, giving a relative risk of approximately 15). This association has, however, not been seen in the other available registries or in a recent analysis by the EUROCAT registry.[46] A population-based cohort study of 8,37,795 from Denmark has suggested that all of the newer generation AEDs are associated with a lesser teratogenic risk similar to the unexposed population.[47] The evidence for low teratogenic risk is strongest for lamotrigine, with some studies confirming encouraging preliminary data on levetiracetam.[48] Topiramate one of the newer AEDs has been shown to be teratogenic in animal studies. Both the UK and the North American registry has cautioned on the use of topiramate in pregnancy with a possible association with cleft lip and palate. In line with these findings US FDA has classified topiramate as category D drug.

In utero exposure to AEDs can be associated with neurodevelopmental delays although the overall incidence and relative risk associated with different agents remain controversial with conflicting reports from various studies. Significant cognitive impairment in 10–30% and behavorial disorders such as inattention and hyperactivity have also been reported in various studies.[9-12] Significant percentage of children exposed to sodium valproate in utero have developmental delays and learning difficulties.[49-51] After adjusting for confounding factors, a study from Liverpool UK identified valproate as a drug carrying potential risks for developmental delay with significant lower verbal IQ and cognitive impairment, compared to no exposure or other monotherapy. It was also the first study to suggest that tonic-clonic seizures during pregnancy may have a similar effect.[33]

For the newer AEDs, there is some emerging literature to support the safety of lamotrigine and levetiracetam with respect to neurodevelopment.[52,53]

Fetal anticonvulsant syndrome is a syndrome of dysmorphic features, combined with one or more of six features including neonatal withdrawal symptoms, major malformation, developmental delay, behavioral problems, learning difficulties and general medical problems. This result from the in utero exposure to AEDs and is more commonly seen in children exposed to sodium valproate than to the other AEDs.[14,15]

Maternal mortality rates in women with epilepsy are higher and they are ten times more likely to die during pregnancy than the general population. Poor seizure control, accidents related to the epilepsy and/or sudden unexplained death in epilepsy (SUDEP) may account for this. The exact cause of SUDEP is not known but could be due to cardiac arrhythmias or respiratory failure due to seizure activity. Patients with a good seizure control are at a lower risk of SUDEP.[54]

MANAGEMENT OF PREGNANCY WITH EPILEPSY

Preconception Care

Preconception counseling plays a very important role in the management of women with epilepsy, in the childbearing age group. This should aim at awareness among women with epilepsy, that the best pregnancy outcome may be secured if it is planned in advance. This will allow the necessary time for any changes or discontinuation of antiepileptic treatment to be carried out or if necessary, for optimal seizure control prior to pregnancy.[55,56] Abrupt cessation of AED therapy should be avoided at all cost because it can precipitate uncontrolled epileptic seizures.[57] For women with epilepsy who have been seizure free for 2 years on medication, withdrawal of drug may be considered. In this group of women successful withdrawal from treatment without relapse may be possible.[58] If the risk of complete drug withdrawal is too high it may still be possible to reduce the dose and drug load or reduce the number of AEDs prescribed.

Antiepileptic drugs are known to be teratogenic and this is largely influenced by the type dose and number of drugs being used to control seizures. Carbamazepine, lamotrigine and levetiracetam have the best safety profile whereas sodium valproate and topiramate are best avoided during pregnancy. Since for all AEDs teratogenicity is dose dependant and more for multidrug regime—the lowest possible dose of monotherapy for seizure control should be advised in women contemplating a pregnancy.

Neural tube defects (NTDs) have been associated with exposure to in utero AEDs particularly sodium valproate and carbamazepine.[44] In the general population supplementation with folic acid has been shown to prevent NTD. In the high risk group for NTD such as history of NTD in previous child or first degree relative with a child having NTD higher doses of folic acid 4 mg daily had a 72% protective effect.[59] Extrapolating these results to the epilepsy population a daily dose of 5 mg of folic acid has been recommended for women planning a pregnancy and on AEDs, especially sodium valproate and carbamazepine, starting prior to pregnancy and continuing till the end of the first trimester.[60]

Some recent studies have, however, failed to demonstrate added protective value from folic acid in this population group.[61] However, as there is no evidence of harm, it is still generally recommended that all women with epilepsy planning pregnancy should receive preconceptual folic acid at a dose of at least 0.4 mg daily. There is little evidence to suggest that higher doses of folic acid offer more protective effect than the usual lower doses, but as this may be of benefit and risks are low, many clinicians continue to use the higher dose routinely in women on AEDs.

Antenatal Care

Pregnancies complicated with epilepsy are viewed as high risk pregnancies and require careful management. Ideally such management is best delivered by a joint obstetric-epilepsy clinic, if however, there is no shared service between these specialties, an obstetrician who specializes in high risk and medically complicated pregnancies should be identified and the women referred early in pregnancy.[60]

Seizure control should be optimized with an aim of complete freedom from seizures during pregnancy, as uncontrolled seizures resulting from sudden withdrawal or non-adherence to AEDs can have untoward effect on both the mother and fetus. The primary goal of treatment is seizure control with monotherapy at the lowest possible dose. Adherence to therapy is of utmost importance and women should be advised to this effect as also to protect themselves from getting tired through not having adequate rest and sleep.

In recent years there has been a trend towards prescribing the newer AEDs like lamotrigine and levetiracetam, as they are less teratogenic than the older AEDs, such as valproate and carbamazepine. However, it is possible that such a practice will increase the difficulty in maintaining seizure control as the plasma levels of the newer agents like lamotrigine significantly decrease with increasing gestation—hence dose adjustments maybe required as the pregnancy progresses.[21,23-25,27]

Folic acid supplementation 5 mg daily is recommended by some authors to be started prior to pregnancy and continued till the end of first trimester. Given the high risk of congenital anomalies in women on AEDs—they should be referred early in pregnancy to a maternal-fetal unit, for antenatal screening with ultrasounds, to rule out structural abnormalities and other relevant blood tests or occasionally amniocentesis if required.

Neonatal coagulopathy and hemorrhagic disease of the new born can occur in babies of women on hepatic enzyme inducing AEDs, such as phenytoin, phenobarbitone, primidone and carbamazepine. This is due to a deficiency of vitamin K dependent clotting factors-II, VII, IX and X. It was previously recommended that 10–20 mg of vitamin K should be given orally to the mother in the last month of pregnancy and the baby should be administered intramuscular vitamin K (1 mg at birth and at 28 days postdelivery).[59] However, more recently the maternal recommendation has been dropped and the current advice is simply to give the neonate, the intramuscular dosage at birth.[55]

Management During Labor

About 1–2 % of women with active epilepsy get a tonic-clonic seizure during labor and another 1–2% within 24 hours of delivery.[61]

AEDs should be continued during labor. A tonic-clonic convulsion during labor can result in severe maternal hypoxia, which can lead to fetal distress. CTG tracings have shown evidence of both fetal bradycardia and loss of variability during maternal seizures. Delivery of women with epilepsy, therefore should be in a high risk obstetric unit geared for maternal and fetal resuscitation.

Most women with epilepsy can have normal vaginal delivery and cesarean section is only for obstetric reasons. Hyperventilation, pain, stress and lack of sleep can all increase the risk of seizure during labor. Epidural anesthesia early in labor, can minimize these risk factors. However, pethidine[63] and tramadol can predispose to convulsions and are best avoided for labor analgesia. An elective cesarean section may be planned if frequent tonic-clonic or prolonged complex partial seizures occur in the last weeks of pregnancy. Intravenous lorazepam can be used for acute treatment for repeated seizures during labor.[60]

Peurperium

At birth vitamin K injection 1 mg intramuscularly is advised to the neonate in order to prevent hemorrhagic disease of the new born.

Breastfeeding should be encouraged in women on AEDs because although all AEDs are excreted in breast milk usually the amount is very small.[55] Some newer agents like lamotrigine, however, are found in higher concentrations than other antiepileptic agents.[27] Immature drug metabolism and decreased serum protein binding in the neonate can result in drug accumulation—the main concern for this is sedation and lack of feeding in the newborn. This was especially true for the older drugs like phenobarbitone or primidone and less likely with the conventional and newer AEDs, which are not generally associated with similar degrees of sedation. Studies have shown no adverse cognitive effects of breastfeeding during AED therapy in children who have previously been exposed to AEDs in utero.[64] Another advantage of breastfeeding is that the babies exposed to the AEDs in utero have a further decreasing exposure through breast milk, which may prove a useful way to wean them off the AED, thereby avoiding the potential for any withdrawal symptoms.

Follow-up with the general practitioner and the obstetrician should take place at 6 weeks postpartum and it is good medical practice to advice one specialist epilepsy consultation at 12 weeks after delivery.[54] This is because the dosage of drugs, which might have been increased during pregnancy due to altered drug pharmacokinetics to achieve effective seizure control might have to be gradually tapered to prevent maternal toxicity.[65] However, there is as yet no firm consensus as to when and how the drug should be tapered, as there may be increased risk of seizures during the weeks following delivery (related to a number of factors such as hormonal change, lack of sleep and emotional stress). Therefore, if there is no evidence of any toxic symptoms from the increased dose (despite the probable rise in serum levels after delivery) and there is a sustained benefit on seizure control then the regime may be left unaltered.

Advice regarding precautions to be taken while caring for the baby should be given to all women, for example, women can be advised to sit in a secure position while breastfeeding so as to reduce the risk of trauma should a seizure occur, also they should be encouraged not to bath the baby in water unless another individual is present.

For women opting for oral contraceptive pills for contraception in the immediate postpartum period, progesterone only pill (POP) can be advised. Women on enzyme inducing AEDs require double the dose of POP. Those who are not breastfeeding can be advised OCPs containing 50 µg of estrogen with a shorter pill free interval of four days instead of seven.[66]

SUMMARY AND KEY POINTS

- Epilepsy is the commonest neurological disorder in pregnancy. About 3 to 7 out of 1,000 pregnancies are complicated with active epilepsy across the globe.
- Reduced seizure control during pregnancy can occur due to various reasons—altered drug pharmacokinetics or physiological changes of pregnancy, poor drug compliance, vomiting, sleep deprivation in later weeks of gestation, or pain and hyperventilation during labor can all predispose to seizures.
- Women with epilepsy are at an increased risk of having a fetus with congenital anomalies (3-9%). Sodium valproate carries the highest risk of anomalies especially when used at a dose of greater than 1000 mg per day.
- The newer AEDs like lamotrigine and levetiracetam are safer options and are associated with a much lower incidence of congenital anomalies in the fetus. However, topiramate is associated with a high incidence of cleft lip and cleft palate and is best avoided in pregnancy.
- All women of childbearing age group on AEDs and planning a pregnancy should be advised 5 mg folic acid preconceptually because of the suggested protective effect of folic acid on congenital birth defects. Whether the higher dose of folic acid is more protective than the normal lower dose of 0.4 mg needs to be assessed in future studies.
- In utero exposure to AEDs can be associated with neurodevelopmental delays, cognitive disorders and low verbal IQ. This is especially true for sodium valproate exposure. Uncontrolled tonic-clonic seizures during pregnancy can also be associated with cognitive disorder in the child.
- Reduced seizure control in pregnancy has been noted to be more common in the newer AEDs like lamotrigine, which makes it necessary

to increase the dose almost two to three fold of the preconception dosage as pregnancy progresses.

○ Neonates of women on enzyme inducing AEDs should receive vitamin K injection—1 mg intramuscularly at birth to prevent hemolytic disease of the newborn.

○ Breastfeeding is not contraindicated in women on AEDs. The newer drugs like lamotrigine and levetiracetam are less sedative than the older agents. Exposure to AEDs through breast milk may protect the baby against with drawl symptoms when already exposed to the drug in utero.

REFERENCES

1. Borthen I, Eide MG, Daltveit AK, Gilhus NE. Obstetric outcome in women with epilepsy: A hospital-based, retrospective study. BJOG. 2011;118:956-65.
2. Richmond JR, Krishnamoorthy P, Anderson E, Benjamin A. Epilepsy and pregnancy: an obstetric perspective. Am J Obstet Gynecol. 2004;190:371-9.
3. World Health Organization. Health topics: epilepsy. Available at: http://www.who.int/topics/epilepsy/en/. Accessed. Aug. 1, 2013. 011;118:956-65.
4. National Clinical Audit of Epilepsy-Related Death. ISBN: 1-84257-84173-177. National Institute of Clinical Excellence. London, UK; 2002.
5. Canger R, Battino D, Canevini MP, et al. Malformations in offspring of women with epilepsy: a prospective study. Epilepsia. 1999;40:1231-6.
6. Canger R, Battino D, Canevini MP, et al. Congenital malformations due to antiepileptic drugs. Epilepsy Res. 1999;33:145-58.
7. Samrén EB, van Duijn CM, Christiaens GC, Hofman A, Lindhout D. Antiepileptic drug regimes and major congenital abnormalities. Ann Neurol. 1999;46:739-46.
8. Holmes L, Wyszynski D, Baldwin E, Habecker E, Glassman L, Smith C. Increased risk for non-syndromic cleft palate among infants exposed to lamotrigine during pregnancy. Clin Mol Teratol. 2006;76:318.
9. Hanson JW, Myrianthopoulos NC, Harvey MA, Smith DW. Risks to the offspring of women treated with hydantoin anticonvulsants, with emphasis on fetal hydantoin syndrome. J Pediatrics. 1976;89:662-8.
10. Dean J, Hailey H, Moore S, Lloyd D, Turnpenny P, Little J. Long term health and neurodevelopment in children exposed to antiepileptic drugs before birth. J Med Genetics. 2002;39:251-9.
11. Adab N, Jacoby A, Smith D, Chadwick D. Additional educational needs in children born to mothers with epilepsy. J Neurol Neurosurg Psychiatry. 2001;70:15-21.
12. Moore S, Turnpenny P, Quinn A, et al. A clinical study of 57 children with fetal anticonvulsant syndromes. J Med Genetics. 2000;37:489-97.
13. Clayton-Smith J, Donnai D. Fetal valproate syndrome. J Med Genetics. 1995;32:724-7.
14. Dean JC, Moore SJ, Turnpenny PD. Developing diagnostic criteria for the fetal anticonvulsant syndromes. Seizure. 2000;9:233-4.
15. Gaily E, Granström ML, Hiilesmaa V, Bardy A. Minor anomalies in offspring of epileptic mothers. J Pediatr. 1988;112:520-9.
16. Tomson T, Battino D, Bonizzoni E, et al. Collaborative EURAP Study Group 2004. EURAP: an international registry of antiepileptic drugs and pregnancy. Epilepsia. 2004;45(11):1463-4.

17. Nelson-Piercy C. Handbook of Obstetric Medicine (Third Edition). Informa Healthcare, London, UK; 2006.
18. Rang HP, Dale MM, Ritter JM, Flower RJ. Rang and Dale'âs Pharmacology (Sixth Edition). Elsevier Limited, Oxford, UK;2007.
19. Vajda FJE, Hitchcock A, Graham J, Solinas C, O'âBrien TJ, Lander CM, et al. Foetal malformations and seizure control: 52 months data of the Australian Pregnancy Registry. Eur J Neurology. 2006;13:645-54.
20. EURAP study group. Seizure control and treatment in pregnancy: observations from the EURAP epilepsy pregnancy registry. Neurology. 2006;66(3):354-60.
21. Petrenaite V, Sabers A, Hansen-Schwartz J. Individual changes in lamotrigine plasma concentrations during pregnancy. Epilepsy Res. 2005;65(3):185-8.
22. Stables D, Rankin J. Physiology in Childbearing with Anatomy and Related Biosciences (Third Edition). Elsevier Limited, Oxford, UK;2010.
23. Sabers A, Petrenaite V. Seizure frequency in pregnant women treated with lamotrigine monotherapy. Epilepsia. 2009;50(9):2163-6.
24. Patsalos PN, Berry DJ, Bourgeois BF, et al. Antiepileptic drugs—best practice guidelines for therapeutic drug monitoring: a position paper by the subcommission on therapeutic drug monitoring. ILAE Commission on Therapeutic Strategies. Epilepsia. 2008;49(7):1239-76.
25. Johannessan SI, Tomson T. Pharmacokinetic variability of newer antiepileptic drugs: when is monitoring needed? Clin Pharmacokinetics. 2006;45(11):1061-75.
26. Kanner AM, Frey M. Adding valproate to lamotrigine: a study of their pharmacokinetic interaction. Neurology. 2000;55:588-91.
27. Fotopoulou C. Prospectively assessed changes in lamotrigine-concentration in women with epilepsy during pregnancy, lactation and the neonatal period. Epilepsy Res. 2009;85(1):60-4.
28. Hiilesmaa VK, Bardy A, Teramo K. Obstetric outcome in women with epilepsy. Am J Obstet Gynecol. 1985;152:499-504.
29. Hiilesmaa VK. Pregnancy and birth in women with epilepsy. Neurology. 1992;42(Suppl):8-11.
30. Teramo K, Hiilesmaa V, Bardy A, Saarikoski S. Fetal heart rate during a maternal grand mal seizure. J Perinat Med. 1979;7:3.
31. Goetting MG, Davidson BN. Status epilepticus during labor: a case report. J Reprod Med. 1987;32:313.
32. McPherson JA, Harper LM, Odibo AO, et al. Maternal seizure disorder and risk of adverse pregnancy outcomes. Am J Obstet Gynecol. 2013;208:378.e1-5.
33. Adab N, Kini U, Vinten J, et al. The longer term outcome of children born to mothers with epilepsy. J Neurol Neurosurg. Psychiatry. 2004;75:1575-83.
34. Omtzigt JG, Los FJ, Grobbee DE, et al. The risk of spina bifida aperta after first-trimester exposure to valproate in a prenatal cohort. Neurology. 1992;42(4 Suppl. 5):119-25.
35. Samren EB, Van Duijn CM, Koch S, et al. Maternal use of antiepileptic drugs and the risk of major congenital malformations: a joint European prospective study of human teratogenesis associated with maternal epilepsy. Epilepsia. 1997;38:981-90.
36. Lindhout D, Omtzigt JG, Cornel MC. Spectrum of neural-tube defects in 34 infants prenatally exposed to antiepileptic drugs. Neurology. 1992;42(4 Suppl. 5):111-8.
37. Koch S, Losche G, Jager-Roman E, et al. Major and minor birth malformations and antiepileptic drugs. Neurology. 1992;42(4 Suppl. 5):83-8.

38. Morrow J, Russell A, Guthrie E, et al. Malformation risks of antiepileptic drugs in pregnancy: a prospective study from the UK Epilepsy and Pregnancy Register. J Neurol Neurosurg Psychiatry. 2006;77:193-8.
39. Tomson T, Battino D, Bonizzoni E, et al. Collaborative EURAP Study Group 2004. EURAP: an international registry of antiepileptic drugs and pregnancy. Epilepsia. 2004;45(11):1463-4.
40. Bromfield EB, Dworetzky BA, Wyszynski DF, Smith CR, Baldwin EJ, Holmes LB. Valproate teratogenicity and epilepsy syndrome. Epilepsia. 2008;49(12):2122-4.
41. Committee on safety of medicines. Sodium valproate and prescribing in pregnancy. Current problems in pharmacovigilence. 2003;29:6.
42. Wyszynski DF, Nambisan M, Surve T, Alsdorf RM, Smith CR, Holmes LB. Increased rate of major malformations in offspring exposed to valproate during pregnancy. Neurology. 2005;64:961-5.
43. Vajda FJ, O'âBrien TJ, Hitchcock A, et al. Critical relationship between sodium valproate dose and human teratogenicity: results of the Australian register of anti-epileptic drugs in pregnancy. J Clin Neurosci. 2004;11:8548.
44. Jentink J, Loane M, Dolk H et al. For the EUROCAT Antiepileptic Study Working Group. Valproic acid monotherapy in pregnancy and major congenital malformations. N Engl J Med. 2010;362(23):2185-93.
45. Tomson T, Battino D, Bonizzoni E, Craig J, Lindhout D, Sabers A, et al. For the EURAP study group. Lancet Neurol. 2011;10:609–17.
46. Dolk H, Jentink J, Loane M, Morris J, de Jong-van den Berg LTW. Does lamotrigine use in pregnancy increase orofacial cleft risk relative to other malformations? Neurology. 2008;(71):714-22.
47. Molgaard-Nielsen D, Hviid A. Newer generation antiepileptic drugs and the risk of major birth defects. JAMA. 2011;395(19):1996-2002.
48. Hunt S, Craig J, Russell A, et al. Levetiracetam in pregnancy: preliminary experience from the UK Epilepsy and Pregnancy Register. Neurology. 2006;67:1876-80.
49. Gaily E, Kantola-Sorsa E, Hiilesmaa V, et al. Normal intelligence in children with prenatal exposure to carbamazepine. Neurology. 2004;62:42(Suppl. 5):128-31.
50. Koch S, Jäger-Roman E, Lösche G, Nau H, Rating D, Helge H. Antiepileptic drug treatment in pregnancy: drug side effects in the neonate and neurological outcome. Acta Paediatr. 1996;85:739-46.
51. Ozyurek H, Bozkurt A, Bilge S, Ciftcioglu E, Ilkaya F, Bas DB. Effect of antiepileptic drugs on psychomotor development in offspring of epileptic mothers. Epilepsia. 1999;40(Suppl. 2):296.
52. Cummings C, Stewart M, Stevenson M, Morrow J, Nelson J. Neurodevelopment of children exposed in utero to lamotrigine, sodium valproate and carbamazepine. Arch Dis Child. 2011;96:643-7.
53. Shallcross R, Bromley RL, Irwin B, Bonnett LJ, Morrow J, Baker GA. Liverpool Manchester Neurodevelopment Group; UK Epilepsy and Pregnancy Register. Child development following in utero exposure: levetiracetam vs sodium valproate. Neurology. 2011;76(4):383-9.
54. Schachter C Steven, Management of epilepsy and pregnancy. www.uptodate.com (2013).
55. National Institute for clinical excellence. The epilepsies: the diagnosis and management of the epilepsies in adults and children in primary and secondary care. Royal College of General Practitioners, London, UK (2004).
56. Scottish Intercollegiate Guidelines Network. Diagnosis and management of epilepsy in adults. Scottish Intercollegiate Guidelines Network (SIGN). Edinburgh, UK (2003); Updated October 2005.

57. Ropper AH, Samuels MA, Adams and Victor'âs. Principles of Neurology (9th Edition). McGraw-Hill Companies, London, UK (2009).

58. Marson A, Jacoby A, Kim L, Gamble C, Chadwick D. On behalf of the Medical Research Council MESS Study Group. Immediate versus deferred antiepileptic drug treatment for early epilepsy and single seizures: a randomised controlled trial. Lancet. 2005;365(9476):2007-13.

59. MRC Vitamin Study Research Group. Prevention of neural tube defects: results of the Medical Research Council vitamin study. Lancet. 1991;338(8760):131-7.

60. Crawford P, Appelton R, Betts T, Duncan J, Gutherie E, Morrow J. Best practice guidelines for the management of women with epilepsy. Seizure. 1999;8:201-17.

61. Morrow J, Hunt S, Russell A, et al. Folic acid use and major congenital malformations in offspring of women with epilepsy: a prospective study from the UK Epilepsy and Pregnancy Register. J Neurol Neurosurg Psychiatry. 2009;80(5):506-11.

62. The neurological disorders. In: Bradley W, Daroff RB, Fenichel MG (Eds). Neurology in Clinical Practice, Volume Two, Second Edition. Butterworth-Heinemann, NY, USA. 1996;2538.

63. Pryl BJ, Greech H, Stoddard PA, et al. The toxicity of norpethidine in sickle cell crisis. BMJ. 1992;304:1478-9.

64. Meador KJ, Baker GA, Browning N, et al. Effects of breastfeeding in children of women taking antiepileptic drugs. Neurology. 2010;75(22):1954-60.

65. Brodtkorb E, Reimers A. Seizure control and pharmacokinetics of antiepileptic drugs in pregnant women with epilepsy. Seizure. 2008;17(2):160-5.

66. Guillebaud J. Contraception: Your questions answered 4th Edition. Edinburgh: Churchill Livingstone. 2004;294.

Management of Bronchial Asthma in Pregnancy

Deependra Kumar Rai

INTRODUCTION

Bronchial asthma is a chronic inflammatory disease of the airways that is characterized by increased responsiveness of the tracheobronchial tree to multiple stimuli. It is the most common chronic condition in pregnancy[1] complicating 4–8% of pregnancies.[2] This illness is becoming an increasing concern, as its prevalence has increased among all women over the past decade.[3,4] Studies have shown that pregnant asthmatic women have an increased risk of adverse perinatal outcome[5,6] whereas controlled asthma is associated with reduced risks.[7] The severity of asthma often varies during pregnancy. In approximately one-third of women asthma becomes worse, in another one-third becomes less severe and in the remaining one-third it remains unchanged during pregnancy.[8-10]

PATHOPHYSIOLOGY

The hormonal, immunological and physiological changes of pregnancy affect asthma symptoms. Values of FEV1 throughout pregnancy are not significantly different from the nonpregnant condition, and similarly the ratio of FEV1/VC or peak flow in patients with asthma; this stability means that criteria for diagnosis and monitoring of asthma do not change. The physiological changes such as increase in free cortisol levels may protect against inflammatory triggers, increase in the bronchodilator substance such as progesterone may improve airway responsiveness, increase in bronchoconstricting substance such as prostaglandin $F_2\alpha$ may promote airway constriction, and similarly decreased activity of placental 11 β-hydroxysteroid dehydrogenase type 2 is associated with an increase in placental cortisol concentration and low birth weight. The modification of cell mediated immunity may influence maternal response to infection and inflammation.

EFFECT OF ASTHMA ON PREGNANCY

Poorly controlled asthma can have adverse effects on both mother and fetus which may lead to increased risk of perinatal mortality, preterm delivery, cesarean delivery, intrauterine growth retardation, stillbirth etc.[11] But recent studies contradict this generalization. Indeed, recent data suggests that most women with asthma will have an uneventful pregnancy course. For women with well controlled asthma, pregnancy outcomes are similar to those of women without asthma.[12-15] Women with more severe or poorly controlled asthma are prone to adverse perinatal outcomes. The study showed statistically significant increase in gestational diabetes, small for gestational age newborns and caesarean delivery for women with moderate to severe asthma, even with optimal control.[16] Need for oral steroids for control of asthma was independently predictive of delivery prior to 37 weeks and low birth weight (less than 2500 g). Pulmonary function testing was also predictive of pregnancy outcomes: an FEV1 less than 80% of predicted values is associated with preterm delivery, pre-eclampsia, cesarean delivery and small for gestational age newborns.[16]

EFFECT OF PREGNANCY ON ASTHMA

Asthma improves during pregnancy in one-third of women, worsens in one-third of women, and remains unchanged in one-third of women. Large number of studies have demonstrated that severity of asthma pre-conceptionally and during early pregnancy is predictive of the clinical course during the remainder of the pregnancy.[17,18] Asthma symptoms tend to correlate with rhinitis symptoms, and women with significant symptoms during pregnancy experience asthma exacerbations as well.[19] Women pregnant with female fetuses experience more severe asthma symptoms than women pregnant with male fetuses.[20,21] It has been postulated that the surge in androgens at 12–16 weeks gestation produced by male fetuses has a protective effect on maternal asthma.

DIAGNOSIS OF ASTHMA

The diagnosis of asthma is based on history, physical examination and pulmonary function tests. The signs and symptoms of asthma differ from patient to patient, and their severity may also vary in any given patient at different times. The clinical diagnosis of asthma is often prompted by symptoms such as episodic breathlessness, wheezing cough and chest tightness.[22] Episodic symptoms after incidental allergen exposure, seasonal variability of symptoms and a positive family history of asthma and atopic disease are also helpful diagnostic guides.

The physical examination of respiratory system may be normal due to variable nature of asthma symptoms. The most usual abnormal physical finding is wheezing on auscultation. However, in some people with asthma wheezing may be absent or only detected when the person exhales forcibly, even in presence of significant airflow limitation.

A good history and clinical examination usually suffices to diagnose asthma in most patients. Pulmonary function tests like measurement of peak expiratory flow rate (PEFR) with help of a simple tool called peak flow meter can also aid in the diagnosis of asthma. PEFR is the easiest & most commonly performed test. It is the fastest rate at which air can move through the airways during a forced expiration starting with fully inflated lungs. The peak flow varies according to age, sex and height. Patients should be educated on how to perform accurate peak flow measurements. They should establish with their physician, the personal best baseline peak flow measurement which is used to compare future value: PEFR in pregnancy: 380–550 L/min, Green zone: >80% of personal best, Yellow zone: 50–80%, Red zone: <50%.

The spirometric evaluation of asthma in pregnant patients is similar to that of nonpregnant patients, as airway mechanics do not change significantly during pregnancy. Forced vital capacity (FVC), forced expiratory volume in one second (FEV_1), FEV_1/FVC ratio, and peak expiratory flow are stable to slightly increased in pregnancy.[11-15] As in nonpregnant patients, the diagnosis of asthma can be confirmed by demonstrating reversible airflow limitation before and after bronchodilator inhalation or before and after initiation of empiric treatment for asthma.[17]

DIFFERENTIAL DIAGNOSIS

- **Asthma:** Acute or progressive dyspnea with wheezing and cough, more often with a history of asthma and precipitating factors; diagnosis is confirmed by pulmonary function tests. Physiological dyspnea of pregnancy—hyperventilation is mainly due to increased progesterone; it may occur early in pregnancy and does not interfere with daily activities.
- **Pulmonary embolism:** Acute respiratory distress or gradually progressive dyspnea with or without tachycardia, cough, chest pain, hemoptysis, or signs of deep venous thrombosis; diagnosis is established by scintigraphic ventilation perfusion scan, computed tomographic angiography, or pulmonary angiography.
- **Pulmonary edema:** Acute or progressive respiratory distress in the presence of heart disease, hypertension, thromboembolic disease, tocolytic therapy, aggressive fluid replacement, or sepsis; diagnosis is confirmed by chest radiography.
- **Peripartum cardiomyopathy:** Dyspnea caused by dilated cardiomyopathy occurs during the final month of pregnancy to six months after delivery; signs and symptoms of heart failure are confirmed by echocardiographic evaluation.
- **Amniotic fluid embolism:** Acute respiratory distress occurring more often during the evacuation of the uterus and they may be complicated by hypotension, seizure, disseminated intravascular coagulation, and cardiac arrest.

MANAGEMENT OF ASTHMA

Management of asthma is divided into three broad headings: (1) Management of asthma during pregnancy, (2) Management of asthma during exacerbation and (3) Management of asthma during labor and delivery.

Management of Asthma During Pregnancy

General Principles

The general principles of management and treatment of asthma are same in pregnant women as in nonpregnant women and in men.[23,24] The ultimate goal of asthma therapy during pregnancy is to maintain adequate oxygenation of the fetus by prevention of hypoxic episodes in the mother. Other goals include: achievement of minimal or no maternal symptoms day or night, minimal or no exacerbations, no limitation of activities, maintenance of normal or near-normal pulmonary function, minimal use of short-acting beta 2-agonists, and minimal or no adverse effects from medications. As in other situations, the focus of asthma treatment should be control of symptoms and maintenance of normal lung function.[25]

A detailed history and physical examination should be performed to identify signs/symptoms of asthma during the initial encounter with the patient. Optimally, this assessment should occur prior to conception in order to establish a baseline.[26] Patients who have not had a baseline status established prior to pregnancy should have it established at their first obstetric visit.[27,28] A detailed history of disease status during prior pregnancies should be elicited because asthma symptoms experienced during prior pregnancies are generally predictive of symptoms experienced in subsequent pregnancies in any given patient.[29] Patients should be encouraged to take an active role in their disease management, paying close attention to factors which affect their disease status and the onset of exacerbations.[30] Management or co-management of these patients by a physician with sufficient experience in caring for pregnant asthmatics improves outcome.

Asthma management during pregnancy can be divided in to four basic component of therapy:
➲ Assessment and close monitoring of asthma
➲ Patients education
➲ Avoidance of triggers
➲ Pharmacotherapy.

Assessment and Monitoring

Normal lung function is important to a mother's health and to her baby's well-being. Objective assessment and monitoring should be performed on a monthly basis. Such assessment should include pulmonary function testing (ideally spirometry), detailed symptom history (symptom frequency, nocturnal asthma, interference with activities, exacerbations, and medication use), and physical examination with specific attention paid to auscultation of the lungs. Schatz and colleagues[31] observed that 30% of subjects whose asthma was classified as mild at entry "switched" categories during pregnancy to the moderate or severe groups. Thus, pregnant asthmatic patients, even those who have mild or well-controlled disease, need to be monitored closely during pregnancy.

The FEV1 after a maximal inspiration is the single best measure of pulmonary function. When adjusted for confounders, a mean FEV1 less than 80% has been found to be significantly associated with increased preterm delivery less than 32 weeks and less than 37 weeks, and birth weight less than 2,500 g.[32] However, measurement of FEV1 requires a spirometer. The PEFR correlates well with the FEV1, and has the advantages that it can be measured reliably with inexpensive, disposable, portable peak flow meters. Patient's self-monitoring of PEFR provides valuable insight to the course of asthma throughout the day, assesses circadian variation in pulmonary function, and helps detect early signs of deterioration so that timely therapy can be instituted. Patients with persistent asthma should be evaluated at least monthly and those with moderate to severe asthma should have daily PEFR monitoring.[33] The typical PEFR in pregnancy should be 380–550 L/min. Patient should establish her "personal best" PEFR, then calculate her individualized PEFR zone: Green Zone more than 80% of personal best, Yellow Zone—50 to 80% of personal best, and Red Zone—less than 50% of personal best PEFR.

A baby's well-being is monitored in a variety of ways during regular medical visits throughout pregnancy. These visits are particularly important for women who have asthma. Women should be aware of their baby's movements. If the baby is not moving normally, contact the obstetrical provider immediately. This is especially true for women who are also having asthma symptoms or an asthma attack. Non-stress test is sometimes recommended after 32 weeks of pregnancy for women who have frequent asthma symptoms or attacks. The test is performed to assess the baby's condition. It is done by monitoring the baby's heart rate with a small ultrasound device that is placed on the mother's abdomen. The baby's heart rate should increase when it moves. The test is considered reassuring if two or more fetal heart rate increases are seen within a 20-minute period. Further testing may be needed if these increases are not observed after monitoring for 40 minutes. Ultrasound examination to check the baby's growth and activity, and also the amount of amniotic fluid around the baby, is sometimes performed.

Education

Pregnancy is a good time to review the patient's basic understanding of asthma and its management, including trigger avoidance, asthma control, and adequate use of devices, medication, and personal action plans. The patient must understand the potential adverse effects of uncontrolled asthma on the well-being of the fetus, and that treating asthma with medications is safer than increased asthma symptoms that may lead to maternal and fetal hypoxia. The patients should be able to recognize symptoms of worsening asthma and be able to treat them appropriately. All this requires an individualized action plan that is based on a joint agreement between the patient and the clinician. Correct inhaler technique should be assured, and the patient also should understand how the exposure can be reduced, or control the factors that exacerbate her asthma. Useful information is available on the websites of

National Pulmonary Societies and International organizations, and patients can be referred to these if they seek additional information. (Global Initiative for Asthma: www.ginasthma.com).

Avoidance of Triggers

Avoidance of asthma triggers, such as animal dander, tobacco smoke, and pollutants, is important because exposure may lead to increased asthma symptoms and the potential need for more medication. Often, allergen immunotherapy is effective for those patients in whom symptoms persist, despite optimal environmental control and proper drug therapy. Allergen immunotherapy can be continued carefully during pregnancy in patients who are deriving benefit, who are not experiencing systemic reactions, and who are receiving maintenance doses. Benefit–risk considerations do not generally favour beginning immunotherapy during pregnancy for most patients because of: (1) the undefined propensity for systemic reactions, (2) the increased likelihood of systemic reactions during initiation of immunotherapy, (3) the latency of immunotherapy effect, and (4) the frequent difficulty in predicting which asthmatic patients will benefit from immunotherapy.[34] Smoking should be completely prohibited. Morbidity during pregnancy that is due to smoking may be independent of, and additive to, morbidity that is due to asthma.[35]

Pharmacological Treatment

Almost all anti-asthma drugs are safe to use in pregnancy and during breastfeeding (Table 1). In fact, under-treatment of the pregnant patient is a frequent occurrence, because such patients are worried about medication

Table 1: FDA categories of anti-asthma drug during pregnancy

Drug		*Categories*
Beta 2 agonist	Salbutamol	C
	Levosalbutamol	C
	Formoterol	C
	Salmeterol	C
Inhaled corticosteroid	Budesonide	B
	Beclomethasone	C
	Fluticasone	C
	Ciclesonide	C
	Mometasone	C
Leukotriene receptor antagonist	Montelukast	B
	Zafirlukast	B
Cromolyn		B
Theophylline		C

effects on the fetus. Appropriate monitored use of theophylline, inhaled glucorticosteroids, β_2-agonists and leukotriene modifiers (especially montelukast) is not associated with increase incidence of fetal abnormality.

Drugs for asthma are categorized in two groups:
- ⟳ Controller medication
  - Inhaled glucocorticosteroids
  - Leukotriene modifiers
  - Long-acting inhaled β_2-agonists in combination with inhaled glucocorticosteroids
  - Systemic glucocorticosteroids
  - Theophylline
  - Cromones
  - Anti-IgE
- ⟳ Reliever medication
  - Short-acting beta-agonists (SABA)
  - Short acting anticholinergic such as ipratropium bromide.

Table 2 shows the estimated daily doses for inhaled corticosteroids. The dose of anti-asthma drugs in pregnancy is shown in Table 3.

Table 2: Estimated comparative daily doses for ICS (Inhaled corticosteroid)

Drug	Low daily dose (µg) medium daily dose (µg) high daily (µg)		
Beclomethasone	200–500	>500–1000	>1000
Budesonide	200–600	>600–1000	>1000
Budesonide-Neb inhalation suspension	250–500	500–1000	>1000
Ciclesonide flunisolide	80–160	>160–320	>320–1280
Fluticasone	100–250	>250–500	>500
Mometasone furoate	200–400	400–800	>800–1200
Triamcinolone acetonide	400–1000	1000–2000	>2000

Table 3: Usual doses of anti-asthma drugs in pregnancy

Medication	Dosage form	Adult dose
LABA		
Salmeterol	MDI 21 µg/puff	2 puffs every 12 hours
	DPI 50 µg/blister	1 blister every 12 hours
Formoterol	DPI 12 µg/single-use capsule	1 capsule every 12 hours
Combined medication		
Fluticasone/Salmeterol	DPI 100 µg/50 µg, 250 µg/50 µg, or 500 µg/50 µg	1 inhalation bid; dose depends on level of severity or control

Contd...

Contd...

Medication	Dosage form	Adult dose
Budesonide/Formoterol	HFA 45 µg/21 µg 115 µg/21 µg 230 µg/21 µg	2 puffs bid; dose depends on level of severity or control
Formeterol/Fluticasone	HFA MDI 80 µg/4.5 µg 160 µg/4.5 µg 6, 12 µg/250 µg	2 puffs bid; dose depends on level of severity or control

Leukotriene Modifiers
1. Leukotriene receptor antagonists (LTRAs)
   Montelukast
   Zafirlukast
2. 5-Lipoxygenase inhibitor
   Zileuton
	
	Tab 10 mg
	Tab 10/20 mg
	
	Tab 600 mg
		
		1 tab OD
		20 mg bid
		
		1 Tab qid

Immunomodulators 1. Omalizumab (Anti IgE)	Subcutaneous injection, 150 mg/1.2 mL following reconstitution with 1.4 mL sterile water for injection	150–375 mg SC q 2–4 weeks, depending on body weight and pretreatment serum IgE level
Oral Systemic Corticosteroids 1. Methylprednisolone 2. Prednisolone 3. Prednisone	2, 4, 8, 16, 32 mg tablets 5, 10, 20, 40 mg 1, 2.5, 5, 10, 20, 50 mg tablets	7.5–60 mg daily in a single dose in am or qid as needed for control Short-course burst": to achieve control, 40–60 mg per day as single or 2 divided doses for 3–10 day

β_2-Agonist

β_2-agonists activate β_2-adrenergic receptors, which are widely expressed in the airways. β_2-receptors are coupled through a stimulatory G protein to adenyl cyclase, resulting in increased intracellular cyclic adenosine monophosphate (AMP), which relaxes smooth muscle cells and inhibits certain inflammatory cells, particularly mast cells. The primary action of β_2-agonists is to relax airway smooth muscle cells of all airways, where they act as functional antagonists, reversing and preventing contraction of airway smooth muscle cells by all known bronchoconstrictors. This generalized action is likely to account for their great efficacy as bronchodilators in asthma. There are also additional nonbronchodilator effects that may be clinically useful, including inhibition of mast cell mediator release, reduction in plasma exudation, and inhibition of sensory nerve activation. β_2-agonists are usually given by inhalation to reduce side effects. They can be further classified as short acting agents used for acute exacerbations, and long acting agents used for maintenance therapy in patients with moderate to severe persistent disease. Short acting β_2 agonist (SABAs) such as albuterol and terbutaline have duration of action of 3–6 hours. They have a rapid onset of bronchodilation and are, therefore, used for symptom relief. Increased use of SABAs indicate that asthma is not controlled. Short acting agents are considered first line therapy for the management of acute exacerbations as well as for patients with mild intermittent disease but not for maintenance therapy. Long acting β_2 agonist (LABAs) include salmeterol and formoterol, both of which have a duration of action over 12 hours and are given twice daily by inhalation. LABAs have replaced the regular use of SABAs, but LABAs should not be given in the absence of ICS therapy as they do not control the underlying inflammation. They do, however, improve asthma control and reduce exacerbations when added to ICS, which allows asthma to be controlled at lower doses of corticosteroids. This observation has led to the widespread use of fixed combination inhalers that contain a corticosteroid and a LABA, which have proved to be highly effective in the control of asthma. Although human data are scant, they lack evidence of an increased risk of congenital malformations. Risk–benefit considerations favor the use of LABA.

Inhaled Corticosteroids

Inhaled corticosteroids should be initiated as maintenance therapy in patients with persistent asthma symptoms. They are not contraindicated in pregnancy and have not been associated with an increased risk of congenital malformation or adverse pregnancy outcome. The risk of asthma exacerbations associated with pregnancy can be reduced and lung function (FEV1) improved with the use of inhaled corticosteroid therapy. Till date no study shows any increase in congenital malformation or adverse perinatal outcomes. Most of the studies were done on budesonide and recommended its use as inhaled corticosteroid.

Leukotriene Modifiers

Leukotriene modifiers include two compounds available as oral tablets (the receptor antagonists: montelukast and zafirlukast) and 5-lipoxygenase pathway inhibitors (e.g. zileuton). Minimal data is currently available on the use of leukotriene modifiers during pregnancy. Reassuring animal studies have been submitted to the Food and Drug Administration (FDA) for leukotriene receptor antagonists but not for the leukotriene lipoxygenase inhibitor.

Systemic Corticosteroids

Oral corticosteroid use, especially during the first trimester of pregnancy, is associated with an increased risk for isolated cleft lip with or without cleft palate (the risk in the general population is 0.1 percent; the risk in women on oral corticosteroids is 0.3 percent). Oral corticosteroid use during pregnancy in patients who have asthma is associated with an increased incidence of preeclampsia and the delivery of both preterm and low birth weight infants. However, the available data makes it difficult to separate the effects of the oral corticosteroids on these outcomes from the effects of severe or uncontrolled asthma, which has been associated with maternal and/or fetal mortality. If an oral corticosteroid is needed, it is better to use prednisone rather than prednisolone as it cannot be converted to the active prednisolone by the fetal liver, thus protecting the fetus from systemic effects of the corticosteroids.

Treatment of Asthma During Pregnancy

A. Each patient should be assessed to establish her current treatment regimen, adherence to the current regimen and level of asthma control (Table 4). This working scheme has been developed and is validated for various applications, including use by healthcare providers to assess the state of control of patient's asthma and patients, for self-assessment as part of a written action plan. Uncontrolled asthma may progress to exacerbation.
B. Assessment of future risk such as risk of exacerbation, rapid decline in lung function, side effects: These factors are poor clinical control, frequent exacerbation in past year, over admission to critical care for asthma, low FEV1, exposure to cigarette smoke.

Stepwise Approach to Pharmacologic Therapy

The patient's current level of asthma control and current treatment determine the selection of pharmacologic treatment. For example, if asthma is not controlled on the current treatment regimen, treatment should be stepped up until the control is achieved. If control has been maintained for at least three months, treatment can be stepped down with the aim of establishing

Table 4: Level of asthma control			
Assessment of current clinical control			
Characteristics	**Controlled (All of the following)**	**Partly controlled (Any measure present)**	**Uncontrolled**
Daytime symptoms	None (twice or less/week)	More than twice/week	Three or more features of partly controlled asthma and exacerbation in any week
Limitation of activities	None	Any	
Nocturnal symptoms/ awakening	None	Any	
Need for reliever/ rescue treatment	None (twice or less/week)	More than twice/week	
Lung Function (PEF or FEV1 (without bronchodilator)	None	< 80% predicted or personal best, if known	

the lowest step and dose of treatment that maintains control. If asthma is partly controlled, an increase in treatment should be considered, subject to whether more effective options are available (increase dose or an additional treatment), safety and cost of possible treatment and the patient's satisfaction with level of control achieved.

Key Features of Asthma Treatment

The stepwise approach is meant to assist, not replace, the clinical decision-making required to meet individual patient's needs. Stepwise care is shown in Table 5.

‑ Each patient should be assessed to establish her current treatment regimen, adherence to the current regimen and level of asthma control
‑ Minimize use of short-acting inhaled β_2-agonist

Table 5: Management approach based on control

Level of control	Reduce / Increase	Treatment action
Controlled		Maintain and find lowest controlling step
Partly controlled		Consider stepping up to gain control
Uncontrolled		Step up until controlled
Exacerbation		Treat as exacerbation

Step 1	Step 2	Step 3	step 4	Step 5
Asthma education, Environmental control If step-up treatment considered for poor symptom control, check inhaler technique, adherence and confirm that symptoms due to asthma				
SABA as on need basis	SABA as on need basis			
Controller option	Select one	Select one	Select one or more	To step four, add either
	Low dose ICS	Low dose ICS plus LABA	Medium or high dose ICS plus LABA	Oral Glucocorticoides (lowest dose)
	Leukotriene modifier	Medium or high dose ICS or Low dose ICS plus leukotriene modifier	Leukotriene modifier	Anti-IgE treatment
		Low dose ICS plus sustained release theophylline	Sustained release theophylline	

SABA: Short acting β_2-agonist
ICS: Inhaled corticosteroid
LABA: long-acting β_2-agonist, e.g. salmeterol, formoterol

- At each treatment step, a reliever medication (rapid onset bronchodilator, either short-acting or long-acting) should be provided for quick relief of symptoms
- Provide education on self-management and controlling environmental factors that make asthma worse (e.g. allergens, irritants)
- Refer to an asthma specialist if there are difficulties controlling asthma or if Step 4 care is required. Referral may be considered if Step 3 care is required.

The treatment Step 1 to 5 provides options of increasing efficacy, except for step 5 where availability and safety influence the selection of treatment. Step 2 is the initial treatment—naïve patients with persistent asthma symptoms. If symptoms at initial consultation suggest that asthma is severely uncontrolled, treatment should be commenced at step 3. At each treatment step, a reliever medication (rapid onset bronchodilator, either short-acting or long-acting) should be provided for quick relief of symptoms. However, regular use of reliever medication is one of the elements defining uncontrolled asthma and indicates that controller treatment should be increased. Thus reducing or eliminating the need of reliever treatment is both an important goal and measure of success of treatment.

Management of Asthma During Exacerbation

Exacerbations of asthma are episodes of progressive increase in shortness of breath, cough, wheezing, or chest tightness or some combination of these symptoms. An asthma exacerbation that causes minimal problems for mother may have severe sequelae for the fetus. A decrease in fetal movement may be an early manifestation of an asthma exacerbation. Indeed abnormal fetal heart rate tracing may be the initial manifestation of an asthmatic exacerbation. A maternal PO_2 less than 60 or Hb saturation less than 90% may be associated with profound fetal hypoxia. Therefore, asthma exacerbation during pregnancy should be managed aggressively. Exacerbations are most likely to occur between 24 to 36 weeks of pregnancy. Hence the most important part of managing such condition is prevention of exacerbation. The mechanisms that lead to asthma exacerbations during pregnancy are poorly understood, but viral infections and discontinuation of anti-inflammatory medications are likely to be important.[36,37] Exacerbation are characterized by decrease in expiratory airflow that can be quantified by measurement of Lung function (PEF or FEV1). Effective management of exacerbations incorporates the same four components of asthma management used in managing asthma long term: assessment and monitoring, patient education, avoidance of triggers, and medications. Management depends upon severity of exacerbation (Table 6). Asthma with mild to moderate exacerbation can be managed at home but all severe exacerbation and some cases of moderate exacerbation should be managed in emergency.

Table 6: Severity of asthma exacerbation			
Severity	*Symptoms and sign*	*PFT*	*Treatment*
Mild	Dyspnea only with activity	PEF over 80%	Home management
Moderate	Dyspnea interferes with or limits usual activities	PEF 60–80%	Home management
Severe	Dyspnea at rest, interfere with conversation	PEF <60% predicted	Require Hospitalization
Very severe (Life-threatening)	Too dyspneic to speak, perspiring		ICU management

Home Management for Asthma Exacerbation

Patients should be given an individualized guide for decision-making and rescue management, and educated to recognize signs and symptoms of early asthma exacerbations such as coughing, chest tightness, dyspnea, or wheezing, or by a 20% decrease in their PEFR. This is important so that prompt home rescue treatment may be instituted to avoid maternal and fetal hypoxia. For mild to moderate exacerbation, repeated administration of rapid acting inhaled β_2-agonist (2 to 4 puffs every 20 minutes for 1st hour) is usually best and most cost-effective approach for reversal of airflow obstruction. If there is poor response defined by PEFR—less than 50% predicted, or severe wheezing and shortness of breath, or decreased fetal movement, repeat inhaled β_2-agonist 2–4 puffs by MDI and obtain emergency care. If there is incomplete response, PEFR is 50–80% predicted or if persistent wheezing and shortness of breath, then repeat inhaled β_2-agonist treatment 2–4 puffs MDI at 20-minute intervals up to two more times. If repeat PEFR shows 50–80% predicted or if decreased foetal movements, contact doctor or go for emergency care. If there is good response, PEFR more than 80% predicted, no wheezing or shortness of breath, and fetus is moving normally, continue inhaled β_2-agonist 2–4 puffs MDI every 3–4 hours as needed.

Hospital and Emergency Management

The principal goal should be the prevention of hypoxia. Measurement of oxygenation by pulse oximetry is essential, arterial blood gases should be obtained if oxygen saturation remains less than 95 percent. Continuous electronic fetal monitoring should be initiated if gestation has advanced to the point of potential fetal viability. To achieve arterial oxygen saturation of 90 percent, oxygen should be administered by nasal cannulae, or by mask. Rapid acting inhaled β_2-agonist should be administered at regular interval. The most cost effective and efficient delivery is by metered dose inhaler and spacer but occasionally nebulization is used. Flow chart 1 shows the management of asthma with severe exacerbation.

Flow chart 1: Management of asthma with severe exacerbation

Initial assessment

History, physical examination (auscultation, use of accessory muscles, heart less and respiratory rate), PEF or FEV1, oxygen saturation, and other tests as indicated. Initiate fetal assessment (consider continuous electronic fetal monitoring and/or biophysical profile if pregnancy has reached fetal viability)

FEV1 or PEF >50%
- Rapid acting inhaled β_2-agonist by MDI or nebulizer, up to three doses in first hour
- Oxygen to achieve O_2 saturation $\geqslant$95%
- Oral systemic corticosteroids if no immediate response or if patient recently took oral systemic corticosteroids

FEV1 or PEF <50%
(Severe exacerbation)
- High-dose rapid acting inhaled β_2-agonist by nebulization every 20 minutes or continuously for 1 hour plus inhaled ipratropium bromide. Oxygen to achieve O_2 saturation >95%
- Oral systemic corticosteroids

Impending or actual respiratory arrest
- Intubation and mechanical ventilation with 100% O_2
- Nebulized rapid-acting inhaled β_2-agonist plus inhaled ipratropium bromide Intravenous corticosteroids
- Admit to Intensive care unit

Repeat assessment symptoms,
Physical examination, PEF, O_2 saturation, other tests as needed, Continue fetal assessment

Moderate exacerbation
FEV1 or PEF 50–80% predicted/personal best
Physical examination: moderate symptoms
- Short-acting inhaled β_2-agonist every 60 minutes
- Systemic corticosteroids β_2
- Oxygen to maintain O_2 saturation >95%
- Continue treatment 1–3 hours, provided there is improvement

Severe exacerbation
FEV1 or PEF <50% predicted/personal best
Physical examination: severe symptoms at rest, accessory muscle use, chest retraction
History: high-risk patient
No improvement after initial treatment
- Short-acting inhaled β_2-agonist hourly or continuously plus inhaled ipratropium bromide
- Oxygen
- Systemic corticosteroids

Good Response
- FEV1 or PEF $\geqslant$70%
- Response sustained 60 minutes after last treatment
- No distress
- Physical examination: normal
- Reassuring fetal status

Incomplete Response
- FEV1 or PEF $\geqslant$50% but <70%
- Mild or moderate symptoms
- Continue fetal assessment

Poor Response
- FEV1 or PEF <50%
- PCO_2>42 mm Hg
- Physical examination: symptoms severe, drowsiness,confusion
- Continue fetal assessment

Individualized decision, Re-hospitalization

Discharge Home
- Continue treatment with rapid-acting inhaled β_2-agonist
- Continue course of oral systemic corticosteroid
- Initiate or continue inhaled corticosteroid until review at medical follow-up
- Patient education
  - Review medicine use
  - Review/initiate action plan
  - Recommend close medical follow-up

Admit to Hospital Ward
- Rapid-acting inhaled β_2 agonist plus inhaled ipratropium bromide
- Systemic (oral or intravenous) corticosteroid
- Oxygen
- Monitor FEV1 or PEF, O_2 saturation, pulse
- Continue fetal assessment until patient stabilized

Admit to Hospital Intensive Care
- Rapid-acting inhaled β_2-agonist hourly or continuously plus inhaled ipratropium bromide
- Intravenous corticosteroids
- Oxygen
- Possible intubation and mechanical ventilation
- Continue fetal assessment until patient is stabilized

Contd...

Contd...

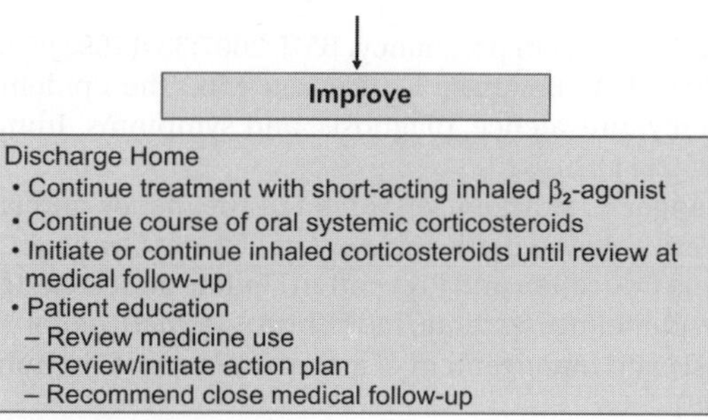

FEV1, Forced expiratory volume in 1 second
MDI : Metered-dose inhaler
PCO$_2$: Carbon dioxide partial pressure
PEF : Peak expiratory flow

Management of Asthma During Labor

Asthma exacerbation occurs in approximately 10–20% during labor and delivery.[38] Asthma medications should not be discontinued during labor and delivery. If systemic corticosteroids have been used in the previous four weeks, then intravenous corticosteroids (e.g. hydrocortisone 100 mg every 8 hours) should be administered during labor and for the 24-hour period after delivery to prevent adrenal crisis.[39] Asthma is usually quiescent during labor; consideration should be given to assess PEFRs upon admission and at 12-hour interval. The patient should be kept hydrated and should receive adequate analgesia to decrease the risk of bronchospasm. It is rarely necessary to perform a cesarean delivery for an acute asthma exacerbation. Usually, maternal and fetal compromise will respond to aggressive medical management. Occasionally, delivery may improve the respiratory status of a patient with unstable asthma who has a mature fetus. Prostaglandin E2 or E1 can be used for cervical ripening, the management of spontaneous or induced abortions, or postpartum hemorrhage, although the patient's respiratory status should be monitored.[40] Prostaglandin F$_2$-α and methylergonovine, used for postpartum hemorrhage, can induce bronchospasm.[41] Magnesium sulfate is a bronchodilator, but indomethacin can induce bronchospasm in the aspirin-sensitive patient. There are no reports of the use of calcium channel blockers for tocolysis among patients with asthma, although an association with bronchospasm has not been observed with wide clinical use. Lumbar anesthesia has the benefit of reducing oxygen consumption and minute ventilation during labor.[42] Fentanyl may be a better analgesic than meperidine, which causes histamine release, but meperidine is rarely associated with the onset of bronchospasm during labor. A 2% incidence of bronchospasm has been reported with regional anesthesia.[43] Ketamine is useful for induction of general anesthesia because it can prevent bronchospasm.

REFERENCES

1. Rey E, Boulet LP. Asthma in pregnancy. BMJ. 2007;334(7593):582-5.
2. Kwon HL, Triche EW, Belanger K, Bracken MB. The epidemiology of asthma during pregnancy: prevalence, diagnosis, and symptoms. Immunol Allergy Clin North Am. 2006;26(1):29–62.
3. Kwon HL, Belanger K, Bracken MB. Effect of pregnancy and stage of pregnancy on asthma severity: A systematic review. Am J Obstet Gynecol. 2004;190:1201-10.
4. National Asthma Education and Prevention Update on selected topics, 2002. www. nhlbi. nih.gov/guidelines/asthma/index.htm.) (Expert panel report. Guidelines for the diagnosis and management of asthma. J Allergy Clin Immunol. 2007;120(5 Suppl):S94-138).
5. Clark SL, National Asthma Education Program Working Group on Asthma and Pregnancy, National Institutes of Health, National Heart, Lung, and Blood Institute. Asthma in pregnancy. Obstet Gynecol. 1993;82:1036-40.
6. Schatz M. Asthma during pregnancy: interrelationships and management. Ann Allergy. 1992;68:123-32.
7. Derbes VJ. Reciprocal influences of bronchial asthma and pregnancy. Am J Med. 1946;1:367-75.
8. Schatz M, Harden K, Forsythe A, Chilingar L, Hoffman C, Sperling W, et al. The course of asthma during pregnancy, postpartum and with successive pregnancies: a prospective analysis. J Allergy Clin Immunol. 1988;81(3):509-17.
9. Schatz M. Interrelationships between asthma and pregnancy: a literature review. J Allergy Clin Immunol. 1999;103(2 Pt 2):S330-6.
10. Demissie K, Breckenridge MB, Rhoads GG. Infant and maternal outcomes in the pregnancies of asthmatic women. Am J Respir Crit Care Med. 1998;158(4):1091-5.
11. Schatz M, Harden K, Forsythe A, et al. The course of asthma during pregnancy, postpartum, and with successive pregnancies: A prospective analysis. J Allergy Clin Immunol. 1988;81:509-17.
12. Murphy VE, Gibson PG, Smith R, et al. Asthma during pregnancy: mechanisms and treatment implications. Eur Resp J. 2005;25(4):731-50.
13. Alexander S, Dodds L, Armson BA. Perinatal outcome in women with asthma during pregnancy. Obstet Gynecol. 1998;92:435-40.
14. Bracken MB, Triche EW, Belanger K, et al. Asthma symptoms, severity, and drug therapy: a prospective study of effects on 2205 pregnancies. Obstet Gynecol. 2003;102:739-52.
15. Dombrowski M. Outcomes of pregnancy in asthmatic women. Immunol Allergy Clin North Am. 2006;26:81-92.
16. Park-Wyllie, Mazzotta P, Pastuszak A, et al. Birth defects after maternal exposure to corticosteroids: prospective cohort study and meta-analysis of epidemiological studies. Teratology. 2000;62:385-92.
17. Nelson-Piercy C. Asthma in pregnancy. Thorax. 2001;56:325-8.
18. Schatz M, Dombrowski M, Wise R, et al. The relationship of asthma medication use to perinatal outcomes. J Allergy Clin Immunol. 2004;113:1040-5.
19. Kircher S, Schatz M, Long L. Variables affecting asthma course during pregnancy. Ann Allergy Immunol. 2002;89:463-6.
20. Beecroft N, Cochrane GM, Milburn HJ. Effect of sex of fetus on asthma during pregnancy: blind prospective study. BMJ. 1998;317:856-7.

21. Kwon HL, Belanger K, Holford TR, et al. Effect of fetal sex on airway lability in pregnant women with asthma. Am J Epidemiol. 2006;163:217-21.
22. Levy ML, Fletcher M, Price DB, Hausen T, Halber RJ, Yawn BP. International Primary Care Respiratory Group (IPCRG) Guidelines: diagnosis of respiratory diseases in primary care. Prim Care Respir J. 2006;15(1):20-34.
23. National Asthma Education and Prevention Program Working Group. Managing asthma during pregnancy: recommendations for pharmacologic treatment—2004 update. Expert panel report. J Allergy Clin Immunol. 2005;115:34-46. Global Initiative for Asthma (www.ginaasthma.com).
24. Murphy VE, Gibson PG, Smith R, Clifton VL. Asthma during pregnancy: mechanisms and treatment implications. Eur Rspir J. 2005;25(4):731-50.
25. Dombrowski MP, Schatz M, Wise R, et al. Asthma during pregnancy. Obstet Gynecol. 2004;103:5-12.
26. Blaiss MS. Management of asthma during pregnancy. Allergy Asthma Proc. 2004;25:375-9.
27. Bakhireva LN, Jones KL, Schatz M, et al. Asthma medication use in pregnancy and fetal growth. J Allergy Clin Immunol. 2005;116:503-9.
28. Schatz M, Harden K, Forsythe A, et al. The course of asthma during pregnancy, postpartum, and with successive pregnancies: A prospective analysis. J Allergy Clin Immunol. 1988;81:509-17.
29. Namazy JA, Schatz M. Pregnancy and asthma: recent developments. Curr Opin Pulmonary Med. 2005;11:56-60.
30. Schatz M, Dombrowski MP, Wise R, et al. Asthma morbidity during pregnancy can be predicted by severity classification. J Allergy Clin Immunol. 2003;112:283-8.
31. SchatzM, Dombrowski MP, Wise R, Momirova V, Landon M, Mabie W, et al. Spirometry is related to perinatal outcomes in pregnant women with asthma. Am J Obstet Gynecol. 2006;194:120-6.
32. National institutes of Health, National heart, Lung and Blood Institute, National Asthma Education and Prevention Program. Working group report on managing asthma during pregnancy: recommendations for pharmacologic treatment Update 2004. Available at: http://www.nhlbi.nih.gov/health/prof/lung/asthma/astpreg.htm. Retrieved June 28, 2006.
33. Asthma and pregnancy—update 2004. NAEPP Working Group Report on Managing Asthma During Pregnancy: recommendations for pharmacologic treatment-update 2004.
34. Schatz M, Zeiger RS, Hoffman CP. Intrauterine growth is related to gestational pulmonary function in pregnant asthmatic women. Chest. 1990;98:389-92.
35. Apter AJ, Greenberger PA, Patterson R. Outcomes of pregnancy in adolecents with severe asthma. Arch Intern Med. 1989;149(11):2571-5.
36. Hartert TV, Neuzil KM, Shintani AK, et al. Maternal morbidity and perinatal outcomes among pregnant women with respiratory hospitalizations during influenza season. Am J Obstet Gynecol. 2003;189(6):1705–12.
37. Schatz M, Dombrowski MP, Wise R, et al. Asthma morbidity during pregnancy can be predicted by severity classification. J Allergy Clin Immunol. 2003;112:283–8.
38. National Institutes of Health, National Heart, Lung, and Blood Institute, National Asthma Education and Prevention Program. Working group report on managing asthma during pregnancy: recommendations for pharmacologic treatment,

update 2004. Available at: ttp://www.nhlbi.nih.gov/health/prof/lung/asthma/astpreg.htm. Retrieved June 28, 2006.

39. Towers CV, Briggs GG, Rojas JA. The use of prostaglandin E2 in pregnant patients with asthma. Am J Obstet Gynecol. 2004;190:1777–80.

40. Crawford JS. Bronchospasm following ergometrine. Anesthesiology. 1980;35:397–8.

41. Hagerdal M, Morgan CW, Sumner AE, Gutsche BB. Minute ventilation and oxygen consumption during labor with epidural analgesia. Anesthesiology. 1983;59:425–7.

42. Fung DL. Emergency anaesthesia for asthma patients. Clin Rev Allergy. 1985;3:127–4.

Psychiatric Disturbances in Pregnancy

Alokananda Ray, Navneet Magon

INTRODUCTION

Pregnancy is generally considered to be a time of happiness and emotional well being for a woman. However, it is now well documented that pregnancy does not protect a woman from the persistence or emergence of psychiatric disorders.[1-3] Infact, pregnancy and motherhood can increase the vulnerability to psychiatric conditions such as depression, anxiety, eating disorders, and psychosis. Many psychiatric disorders in the reproductive years maybe chronic or recurrent in nature, requiring maintenance therapy and women often face difficult treatment decisions regarding psychotropic medications and pregnancy.

Needless to say, that treatment of psychiatric disorders during pregnancy involves a thoughtful weighing of the risks and benefits of the proposed interventions against the documented and theoretical risks associated with the disorders when left untreated.[4,5] Treatment options should be discussed and decided in collaboration with the women trying to conceive or who are pregnant.

There is increasing evidence of high rates of relapse following sudden discontinuation of psychotropic medications during pregnancy—a decision mostly taken, fearing fetal side effects.[6-9] Also the risks associated with untreated mental illness during pregnancy, both to the fetus and mother deserve attention and should be considered before discontinuation of any psychotropic medication.[5] It is, therefore, imperative that medications with adequate reproductive safety profiles should be used as first line agents, in women of reproductive age group for treatment of psychiatric illness even when they are not pregnant.

PERINATAL PSYCHIATRY—SCREENING AND TREATMENT

Several psychiatric conditions like depression, anxiety, panic disorder and bipolar disorder, can occur during pregnancy and should be considered when assessing the health of a pregnant woman. Obstetricians, therefore, should screen more aggressively for psychiatric disorders in women during pregnancy. Questions about psychiatric symptoms or previous treatment for psychiatric illness should be an integral part of obstetric history, with identification of women at risk.

Several screening tools have been validated for use in pregnancy and postnatal period such as:

⮞ Edinburgh Postpartum Depression Scale (EPDS)—It is a ten item questionnaire used to screen women during pregnancy and in the postpartum period for depression. Each symptom is scored 0–3 depending on the severity. A score of >9 needs further assessment using the Diagnostic and Statistical Manual IV (DSM-IV) of American Psychiatric Association.

⮞ The Two Question Test—This consists of asking the patient two simple questions[10,11]
  - Over the past 2 weeks, have you felt down, depressed or hopeless?
  - Over the past 2 weeks, have you little interest or pleasure doing things?

Screening should occur at least once in every trimester, and is also recommended at 2 weeks, 6 weeks and 6 months postpartum.[12]

DEPRESSION DURING PREGNANCY

Depression is the most common psychiatric disorder associated with pregnancy. Symptoms of depression such as changes in sleep pattern, appetite, fatigue and loss of libido are often difficult to distinguish from the normal experiences of pregnancy.[13] Almost 70% of women report some negative mood symptoms during pregnancy, however, the prevalence of women who meet the diagnostic criteria for depression has been shown to be between 5 to 30%.[14]

Major depressive disorder (MDD) is diagnosed by symptoms of—anhedonia, feeling of guilt and hopelessness, low self-esteem and thoughts of suicide (Table 1). A recent population-based survey of more than 15, 000 women found that the prevalence of MDD during pregnancy is 8.4% and 9.3% during the postpartum period.[15]

DSM-IV of American Psychiatric Association for diagnosing MMD[16] (Table 1).

Table 1: Diagnostic criteria for major depression
1. Depressed mood most of the days, nearly everyday.*
2. Markedly diminished interest or pleasure in activities.*
3. Major change in appetite or weight.
4. Decrease or increase in sleep.
5. Psychomotor agitation or retardation.
6. Fatigue or loss of energy.
7. Feeling of worthlessness or excessive or inappropriate guilt.
8. Diminished ability to think or concentrate: indecisiveness.
9. Recurrent thoughts of death or suicide.
*Must be present to establish diagnosis.

Five of the nine symptoms must be present over a time period of at least 2 weeks to meet the criteria for diagnosing MDD and one of them must be (1) or (2).

These symptoms must be present most of the days, nearly every day for 2 weeks.

These symptoms should interfere with everyday activities, work, and relationships at home.

As a general guiding principle, treatment of depression during pregnancy should be determined by the severity of the underlying disorder, history of previous treatment and response to it, as well as patient preferences.[13,17] Asking women for participation in decision making and their treatment preferences may lead to improved communication, decision making and quality of care.[18]

Fetal exposures to antidepressants are associated with risks—the full spectrum and relative severity of risks of prenatal exposure to psychotropic medications is incomplete. Some antidepressants however have favorable risk/benefit profile during pregnancy. Moreover, the risks of medication should be balanced against the risks associated with untreated psychiatric disorders in pregnancy both to the mother and the baby (e.g. poor nutrition, lack of antenatal care, inadequate weight gain, inability to care for oneself, substance abuse, termination of pregnancy, preterm delivery, postpartum depression, sudden neonatal death and suicides).[17] Most psychotropic drugs are classified as category C agents, for which human studies are lacking and risks cannot be ruled out. No psychotropic drug is classified as safe for use during pregnancy (i.e Category A).[13]

For women who present with new onset depressive symptoms during pregnancy, or mild to moderate major depression, nonpharmacological treatment should be tried first, that include supportive psychotherapy, cognitive behavioral therapy (CBT), or interpersonal therapy (IPT).[19-21] CBT focuses on the link between negative thoughts, behavior and feelings and how to break them. IPT focuses on interpersonal relationships in couples who are expecting a child and the significant role transition that take place during pregnancy and after delivery.

In women with less severe major depression, discontinuation of ongoing pharmacological therapy should be considered, ideally prior to pregnancy—with use of IPT and CBT. However, there is a high risk of relapse during pregnancy. In one study, women who discontinued their medication were 5 times more likely to relapse compared to women who continued with the antidepressants throughout their pregnancy.[3] Thus women with recurrent or refractory depressive illness may decide (in collaboration with their clinician) that the safest option would be to continue with the medication during pregnancy to minimize the risk of recurrence. In such a situation, the clinician should attempt to select medications that have a well characterized reproductive safety profile during pregnancy. Relapse may however occur in spite of continuing an antidepressant during pregnancy (Cohen et al reported a relapse of major depressive disorder (MDD) in 26% of women who continued with their medication during pregnancy).[3] Therefore, careful monitoring and regular assessment is required. A possible explanation to this could be that some women have lower plasma concentration of medication in late pregnancy and therefore may require higher doses of medication as the pregnancy progresses.

ANTIDEPRESSANT MEDICATION DURING PREGNANCY

The medication with the safest reproductive profile should be selected.

Selective serotonin reuptake inhibitors (SSRI) are safe during pregnancy. Fluoxetine and citalopram, with extensive data that support their reproductive safety, should be considered as first line choice. Cumulative reports describing the safety of SSRI as a group has been reassuring,[22,23] although some initial reports implicated paroxetine use in the first trimester to be associated with cardiovascular malformations in the fetus. In one study, sertraline was associated with omphalocele and septal defects, whereas paroxetine was associated with right ventricular outflow tract defects.[24] However two independent peer reviewed meta-analysis failed to prove the increased teratogenicity of paroxetine.[25,26]

The tricyclic antidepressants (TCA) can also be considered as reasonable treatment options during pregnancy. Desipramine and nortriptyline are cited as preferred because they are less anticholinergic and less likely to cause orthostatic hypotension during pregnancy.[13]

Newer SSRI like bupropion can be an attractive option for women who do not respond to fluoxetine and TCAs. Data so far have not indicated any increase in the risk of congenital malformations with its use during pregnancy.[27-29]

Limited data is available on the use of the serotonin-norepinephrine reuptake inhibitor (SNRI)—venlafaxine and duloxetine during pregnancy.[30] The data supporting the safety of venlafaxine during pregnancy is increasingly reassuring in small studies of medicine exposure.[31] It is however important to understand that large definitive trials are required to assess risks that might be rare and observed only with adequate sample size with these newer drugs.

During pregnancy, an increase in plasma volume and increase in hepatic metabolism and renal clearance may significantly affect drug levels.[32,33] Sub-therapeutic levels may be associated with depressive relapse, therefore an increase in the dosage of the SSRI or TCA may be required to sustain effective well being as pregnancy advances.[34]

Although there is a growing literature that supports the relative safety of fetal exposure to SSRIs with respect to teratogenicity, multiple studies have reported adverse neonatal outcome such as prematurity, Intrauterine growth restriction (IUGR) and poor neonatal adaptation or neonatal withdrawal syndrome following in utero exposure to these medications.[35,36] Late pregnancy exposure to SSRIs have been associated with jitteriness, tachypnea and tremulousness in the newborn, which are usually self-limiting and transient, not requiring clinical intervention.[37] There are also conflicting reports suggesting an association of SSRIs in late pregnancy with a serious but rare lung condition—persistent pulmonary hypertension of the newborn (PPHN).[38] Some physicians, therefore, suggest the discontinuation of antidepressants just prior to delivery to minimize the neonatal toxicity.[38] This may however increase the risk of recurrent depression in the mother as she is about to enter the postpartum period which is a time of increased risk for affective illness.

There is limited data regarding the long-term effects of fetal exposure to antidepressants as a class; but fluoxetine and TCAs are the best agents in this regard. Children exposed to fluoxetine, TCAs or no medicine, do not differ in behavioral or cognitive development in terms of IQ, language, behavior, reactivity, mood, learning and activity level.[39,40]

ELECTROCONVULSIVE THERAPY (ECT) DURING PREGNANCY

Safety of ECT in pregnancy has been well documented in the last five decades particularly when instituted in collaboration with a multidisciplinary team including anesthetists, psychiatrists and obstetricians. ECT during pregnancy is underused because of the concerns that treatment might harm the fetus. Considerable experience support that its safe in severely ill gravid patients.[41] Given its relative safety, it can also be used as an alternative to conventional pharmacotherapy for women who wish to avoid extended exposure to psychotropic drugs during pregnancy or women who fail to respond to the standard antidepressants.

BIPOLAR DISORDER (BPD) DURING PREGNANCY

The effect of pregnancy on the natural course of bipolar disorder is not well understood, studies do not suggest a protective effect of pregnancy on BPD and risk of relapses and chronicity following discontinuation of mood stabilizers is high during pregnancy.[42-44]

In the past, women with BPD requiring treatment with mood stabilizers have been counseled to defer pregnancy or to terminate the pregnancy following exposure to drugs such as, lithium or valproic acid. In recent years, the risk of lithium therapy has been reassessed and considered to be safer than it was previously thought to be. More recent studies suggest that the risk of cardiovascular malformations like Ebstein's anomaly following antenatal exposure to lithium is smaller than previously estimated (1/2000 versus 1/1000).[45] Women on lithium during the first trimester should be counseled regarding the small risk of organ dysgenesis (0.05–0.1%) and should undergo fetal echocardiography at about 16–18 weeks of gestation to screen for cardiac anomalies.

Lamotrigine can also be used in pregnancy for women with BPD requiring a mood stabilizer. Although previous studies have failed to show an increase in the risk of congenital anomalies in women receiving lamotrigine, more recent data indicate an increase in the risk of oral clefts in infants exposed to this drug in the first trimester (prevalence-9/1000).[46]

Other anticonvulsants used as a mood stabilizer in BPD like valproic acid and carbamazepine are associated with neural tube defects (3–8%) and spina bifida (1%).[47] Other side effects include—midface hypoplasia, cleft lip and palate, microcephaly and IUGR. The risk for teratogenesis increase with multiple drug regime and is dose dependent—thus the lowest effective dose should be used during pregnancy and treatment with valproic acid should be avoided in women of reproductive age group. The safety profile of the newer anticonvulsants sometime used to treat BPD (gabapentin, oxcarbazepine and topiramine) are not well documented. Prenatal assessment of women on anticonvulsants as mood stabilizers include—fetal anomaly scan at 18–22 weeks, coupled with the assessment of maternal alpha-fetoprotein to rule out the possibility of neural tube defects (NTD). Daily folic acid supplementation (4 mg) is recommended to attenuate the risk of neural tube defect (NTD), however, its role in the setting of anticonvulsant therapy has not been systematically reviewed.[13]

Newer atypical antipsychotics like olanzapine are best avoided, although they are not absolutely contraindicated in pregnancy. These drugs should be reserved for more challenging clinical situations not responding to the conventional therapy.

Women with a history of single episode of mania, full recovery, followed by sustained wellbeing can be advised to discontinue the mood stabilizer before attempting to conceive.[45,48] However, it may be associated with the risk of recurrence during pregnancy.

For women with BPD and history of frequent episodes of mania or bipolar depression, several options can be considered. Some patients may choose to stop the medication as mentioned in the previous group or an alternative would be to continue the medication till the pregnancy is confirmed. The uteroplacental circulation is not established for the first two weeks after conception and hence the risk for fetal exposure is minimal at this time. Most home pregnancy tests are reliable and can diagnose pregnancy as early as 10 days after conception; this coupled with the home ovulation predictor kit can enable a woman to accurately time the discontinuation of her treatment. However, a potential problem with this strategy is the abrupt discontinuation of the drug which can cause a relapse.

For women who tolerate discontinuation of medication, the decision of when to resume treatment is a matter of clinical judgment. Some patients and clinicians wish to wait till the reappearance of symptoms and others might want to limit the risk of a relapse by resuming medication after the first trimester of pregnancy.

In women with severe forms of BPD with multiple severe episodes, especially with psychosis and prominent thoughts of suicide, maintenance treatment with a mood stabilizer before and during pregnancy is the safest option. These women need to be counseled and will have to accept the small absolute increase in the risk of teratogenicity with first trimester exposure to lithium or lamotrigine.

POSTPARTUM MOOD AND ANXIETY DISORDERS

Historically, the postpartum period has been considered a time of risk for development of affective illness.[49] Almost 85% of women experience some mood disturbance—for most they are mild symptoms. About 10–15% experience clinically significant symptoms requiring some form of treatment. Postpartum depressive disorders are classified into three groups—(1) postpartum blues, (2) nonpsychotic major depression and (3) puerperal psychosis. There may be some overlap across these subtypes and it is not clear if they are three different entities or two extremes of a disease spectrum—with postpartum blues as the mildest and psychosis as the most severe form of psychiatric illness in the postpartum period.

Postpartum blues occur in 50–80% after delivery—with symptoms of irritability, tearfulness and reactivity of mood. Typically, it remits by the 10th postpartum day, is not associated with impairment of function and no specific treatment is required. Symptoms that persist beyond 2 weeks may evolve into depressive disorder and needs evaluation.[50]

The prevalence of postpartum MDD is between 10–15%, signs and symptoms usually appear within 2–3 months of delivery and are indistinguishable from the characteristics of MDD that occur during any other time of a women's life. Risk factors for postpartum MDD include—antenatal depression, antenatal anxiety and a history of depression.

Nonpharmacological treatment with CBT and IPT has been shown to be as effective as psychotropic agents like fluoxetine in women with mild to moderate postpartum depression.[51,52] These interventions may be particularly welcome to women who are breastfeeding and wish to avoid medication. Conventional antidepressants (e.g. fluoxetine, sertraline and venlafaxine) have shown efficacy in the treatment of postpartum depression.[51,53-56] The choice of drug largely depends on the patient's prior response to treatment and the side-effect profile of a given medication. SSRIs are ideal first line agents because they are anxiolytic, non-sedating and well tolerated. TCAs are also used frequently and because they are sedating may be more appropriate for women who have prominent sleep disturbances. Anxiety is commonly associated with depression and adjunctive use of benzodiazepines like clonazepam and lorazepam may be of help.

Several authors have explored the role of hormonal therapy in women who suffer from postpartum depression. The postpartum period is associated with a rapid and sudden change in the hormonal levels, specially estrogen and progesterone and this has been attributed to mood disturbances in women during the puerperium. Exogenous progesterone or estrogen alone or in conjunction with antidepressants has been shown to be of benefit,[57-59] however, estrogen can affect breast milk production and cause thromboembolic manifestations. Antidepressants are safe, effective and well tolerated and remain the first line of treatment in women with moderate and severe postpartum depression.

In severe postpartum depression, hospitalization may be required especially for those with thoughts of suicide. Women with severe postpartum depression are good candidates for ECT and this option should be considered early in treatment because it is safe and highly effective.

Postpartum psychosis is an emergency. Clinical picture is consistent with mania or a mixed state consistent with BPD and may include symptoms like restlessness, agitation, sleep disturbance, paranoia, delusions, disorganized thinking, impulsivity and behaviors that place mother and baby at risk.[60] The onset is usually within the first two weeks of delivery and may appear as early as 72 hours postpartum. Treatment options include hospitalization, use of mood stabilizers, antipsychotics, benzodiazepines and ECT.

Although it is difficult to predict which women will develop serious postpartum mood disturbances, it is possible to identify certain subgroups of women. Those with a history of BPD or puerperal psychosis in the past are more vulnerable to postpartum affective illness. These women may benefit from prophylactic treatment with lithium from 36 weeks of gestation or no later than 48 hours after delivery.[61,62] For women with previous history of postpartum depression, prophylactic antidepressants (TCA or SSRI) can be advised after delivery.[63]

SCHIZOPHRENIA

Schizophrenia usually affects young adults and the lifetime risk is about 1%. The diagnosis requires at least two of the following features over a period of one month—delusions, hallucinations, disorganized speech, grossly disorganized or catatonic behavior, affective flattening and markedly decreased volition. There should be marked social and occupational dysfunction of at least six months duration. Maternal fetal risks include—neglect of self, lack of antenatal care and substance abuse. Optimal dose of antipsychotic medication should be continued in pregnancy. Relapse or exacerbations of symptoms require hospitalization with administration of antipsychotics like haloperidol, chlorpromazine and trifluperazine. Adequate psychosocial support should be available and assessment of the mother regarding her ability to care for the new born is necessary.

PSYCHIATRIC MEDICATIONS AND BREASTFEEDING

Given the incidence of psychiatric illness during the puerperium, especially postpartum depression, a significant number of women may need to take psychiatric medications while nursing. The safety of infant exposure to medications through the mother's breast milk has been a reason for concern. Current research indicates that all medications are secreted into the breast milk but adverse events in nursing infants are rare. Whether or not the infant experiences toxicity depends on the medication, amount of exposure (dosage, frequency, rate of maternal drug metabolism), and how well the medicine is metabolized in the infant's liver.

Antidepressants: Data suggests that using tricyclic antidepressants, fluoxetine, paroxetine, and sertraline during breastfeeding exposes the infant to low amounts of the drug and complications in the infant are rare.[51,53,54] Accumulated data regarding the use of SSRIs have been reassuring, showing that the typical serum levels of the medication in the infant is either very low or undetectable.[23]

Mood stabilizers: There have been reports of toxicity in nursing infants related to exposure to several mood stabilizers. Lithium is excreted in high levels in the breast milk with large exposures to nursing infants. Signs of toxicity in the infant include cyanosis, poor muscle tone, and hypothermia.[14] The lowest possible effective dosage should be used along with close monitoring of the infant's condition.[61,62] Carbamazepine and valproic acid are associated with the risk of hepatotoxicity, which is greatest in children under the age of two. The American Academy of Pediatrics, however, has deemed both medications to be appropriate for use in lactating mothers.

Anti-anxiety agents: Data suggests that the use of benzodiazepines exposes the nursing infant to low levels of medication and associated with a relatively low incidence of adverse events. The studies conducted have been limited, however, and further research is needed in this area.

Anti-psychotic agents: Information regarding these medications is limited. The use of chlorpromazine has been associated with sedation and linked to developmental delay in the newborn. Less data is available on atypical anti-psychotic medications.

SUMMARY

- Pregnancy increases the vulnerability to psychiatric illness. Obstetricians should screen aggressively for psychiatric disorders in women during pregnancy. Questions about psychiatric symptoms or previous treatment for psychiatric illness should be an integral part of obstetric history, with identification of women at risk.

- Depression is the most common psychiatric disorder associated with pregnancy. As a general guiding principle, treatment of depression during pregnancy should be determined by the severity of the disorder, history of previous treatment and response to it, as well as patient preferences.

- Most psychotropic drugs are classified as category C agents. No psychotropic drug is classified as safe for use during pregnancy (i.e. Category A). For new onset and mild to moderate depression, nonpharmacological treatment should be tried first, that include supportive psychotherapy, cognitive behavioral therapy (CBT), or interpersonal therapy (IPT). For MDD, the medication with the safest reproductive profile should be selected. SSRIs are safe during pregnancy. Fluoxetine and citalopram should be considered as first line therapy. Tricyclic antidepressants and ECT are other treatment options with a good safety profile.

➲ A policy of discontinuation of mood stabilizers in pregnant women with BPD can be adopted in the first trimester of pregnancy wherever possible, to avoid teratogenicity. Lithium and lamotrigine are the safest options available. Prenatal assessment in women with BPD on mood stabilizers or anticonvulsants includes—fetal ultrasound between 18–22 weeks to rule out anomalies and estimation of maternal alpha-fetoprotein.

➲ Historically, the postpartum period has been considered as a time of risk for development of affective illness. Nonpharmacological treatment with CBT and IPT has been shown to be effective in women with mild to moderate postpartum depression. In the absence of response to nonpharmacological therapy, conventional antidepressants can be advised, which are safe, effective and well tolerated. SSRIs remain the first line of treatment in these women. In severe postpartum depression, and psychosis, hospitalization may be required specially for those with thoughts of suicide. Treatment options include ECT, mood stabilizers, antipsychotics and benzodiazepines.

➲ Pregnancy and motherhood can increase the vulnerability to psychiatric illness. Treatment of psychiatric disorders during pregnancy involves a thoughtful weighing of the risks and benefits of the proposed interventions. Whenever indicated, psychotropic medications with adequate reproductive safety profiles should be used as first line agents in women attempting to conceive, during pregnancy and postpartum period.

REFERENCES

1. Evans J, Heron J, Francomb H, et al. Cohort study of depressed mood during pregnancy and after child birth. Br MED J. 2001;323:257-60.
2. Cohen LS, Sichel DA, Dimmock JA, et al. Impact of pregnancy on panic disorder: A case series. J clin Psychiatry. 1994;55:284-8.
3. Cohen LS, Alshuler LL, Harlow BL, et al. Relapse of major depression during pregnancy in women who maintain or discontinue antidepressant treatment. JAMA. 2006;295:499-507.
4. Orr S, Miller C. Maternal depressive symptoms and the risk of poor pregnancy outcome. Review of the literature and preliminary finding. Epidiomol REV. 1995;17:165-71.
5. Wisner KL, Sit DK, Hanusa BH, et al. Major depression and antidepressant treatment: Impact on pregnancy and neonatal outcome. Am J Psychiatry. 2009;166(5):557-66.
6. Kupfer D, Frank E, Perel J, et al. Five year outcome for maintenance therapies in recurrent depression. Arcg Gen Psychiatry. 1992;49(10):769-73.
7. Suppes T, Baldessarini RJ, Faedda GL, et al. Risk of recurrence following discontinuation of lithium treatment in bipolar disorder. Arch Gen Psychiatry. 1991;48:1082-8.

8. Dencker SJ, Maim U, Lepp M. Schizophrenic relapse after drug withdrawl is predictable. Acta Psychiatry Scand. 1986;73:181-5.

9. Byrne R, Dager SR, Cowley DS, et al. Relapse and rebound following discontinuation of benzodiazepine treatment of panic attacks: Alprazolam versus diazepam Am J Psychiatry. 1989;146:860-5.

10. Whooley MA, Avins Al, Miranda J, et al. Case finding instruments for depression: Two questions are as good as many. J Gen Intern Med. 1997;12:439-45.

11. Kroenke K, Spitzer R, Williams JB, et al. The patient health questionnaire-2: Validity of a two-item depression screener. Med Care. 2003;41:1284-92.

12. American College of Obstetricians and Gynecologist. ACOG Committee Opinion No. 343. Obstet Gynecol. 2006;108:469-77.

13. Cohen LS, Wang B, Nonacs R, et al. Treatment of mood disorders during pregnancy and postpartum. Psychiatric Clinics of North America. 2010;33(2):273-93.

14. Pregnancy and mental health—Stanford school of medicine. Stanford center of Neuroscience. http://womensneuroscience.stanford.edu/wellness clinic/2013.

15. Vesga LO, Blanco C, Keyes K, et al. Psychiatric Disorders in Pregnant and postpartum women in the United States. Arch Gen Psychiatry. 2008;65(7): 805-15. [PubMed: 18606953].

16. American Psychiatry Association. Diagnostic and statistical manual of mental disorders: DSM-IV-TR, 4th Edition. Text version. Washington DC:APA, 2000.

17. Antenatal and postnatal mental health. Clinical management and service guidance Issued: February 2007, last modified: April 2007. NICE clinical guideline 45 guidance.nice.org.uk/cg45.

18. Patel SR, Wisner KL. Decision making for depression treatment during pregnancy and the postpartum period. NIH Public access Author manuscript. Depress Anxiety. 2011;28(7):589-95. doi:10.1002/da.20844.

19. Yonkers KA, Wisner KL, Stewart DE, et al. The management of depression during pregnancy: A report from the American Psychiatric Association and the American College of Obstetricians and Gynecologists. Gen Hosp Psychiatry. 2009;31:403-13.

20. Freeman M, Davis M, Sinha P, et al. Omega 3 fatty acids and supportive psychotherapy for perinatal depression: a randomized placebo controlled study. J Affect Disord. 2008;110(1-2):142-8.

21. Spinelli M. Interpersonal psychotherapy for depressed antepartum women: a pilot study. Am J Psychiatry. 1997;154:1028-30.

22. Einarson TR, Einarson A. Newer antidepressants in pregnancy and rates of major malformations: A meta-analysis of prospective comparative studies. Pharmacoepidemiol Drug Saf. 2005;14:823-7.

23. Halberg P, Sjobolm V. The use of selective serotonin reuptake inhibitors during pregnancy and breast feeding: A review and clinical aspects. J Clin Psychopharmacol. 2005;25:59-73.

24. Louik C, Lin AE, Werler MM, et al. First-trimester use of selective serotonin reuptake inhibitors in pregnancy and the risk of birth defects. N Engl J Med. 2007;356:2675-83.

25. Alwan S, Reefhuis J, Rasmussen Sa, et al. Use of selective serotonin reuptake inhibitors in pregnancy and the risk of birth defects. N Engl J Med. 2007;356:2684-92.

26. Einarson A, Pistelli A, DeSantis M, et al. Evaluation Dif the risk of congenital cardiovascular defects associated with use of paroxetine during pregnancy. Am J Psychiatry. 2008;165:749-52.

27. Updated preliminary report on bupropion and other antidepressants, including paroxetine, in pregnancy and the occurrence of cardiovascular and major con-

genital malformation 2005. Available at: http://www.gsk.com/media/paroxetine/ingerix_study.pdf. Accessed Feb 3, 2010.

28. Chun-Fai-Chan B, Koren G, Fayez I, et al. Pregnancy outcome of women exposed to bupropion during pregnancy: A prospective comparative study. Am J Obstet Gynecol. 2005;192:932-6.

29. Cole JA, Modell JG, Haight BR, et al.Bupropion in pregnancy and the prevalence of congenital malformations. Pharmacoepidemiol Drug Saf. 2007;16:474-84.

30. Einarson A, Fatoye B, Sarkar M, et al. Pregnancy outcome following gestational exposure to venlafaxine: A multicenter prospective controlled study. Am J Psychiatry. 2001;158:1728-30.

31. Henshaw S. Unintended pregnancy in the United States. Fam Plann Perspect. 1998;30:24-9.

32. Krauer B. Pharmacotherapy during pregnancy emphasis on pharmacokinetics In: Eskes TK, Finster M, editors. Drug therapy during pregnancy. London Butterworths. 1985. P. 9-31.

33. Jeffries WS, Bochner F. The effect of pregnancy on drug pharmacokinetics. Med J Aust. 1988;149:675-7.

34. Wisner K, Perel J, Wheeler S. Tricyclic dose requirements across pregnancy. Am J Psychiatry. 1993;150:1541-2.

35. Zeskind P, Stephens L, Maternal selective serotonin reuptake inhibitor use during pregnancy and new-born neurobehavior. Pediatrics. 2004;113:368-75.

36. Simon GE, Cunningham ML, Davis RL, et al. Outcomes of prenatal antidepressant exposure. Am J Psychiatry. 2002;159:2055-61.

37. Levinson-Castiel R, Merlob P, Linder N, et al. Neonatal abstinence syndrome after inutero exposure to selective serotonin reuptake inhibitors in term infants. Arch Pediatr Adolesc Med. 2006;160:173-6.

38. Chambers CD, Hernadez-Diaz S, Van Marter LJ, et al. Selective serotonin reuptake inhibitors and risk of persistant pulmonary hypertension in the new born. N Engl J Med. 2006;354:579-87.

39. Nulman I, Rovet J, Stewart D, et al. Neurodevelopment of children exposed in utero to antidepressant drugs. N Engl J Med. 1997;336:258-62.

40. Nulman I, Rovert J, Stewart DE, et al. Child development following exposure to tricyclic antidepressants or fluoxetine throughout fetal life—A prospective controlled study. Am J Psychiatry. 2002;159:1889-95.

41. Anderson El, Reti IM. ECT in pregnancy: A review of the literature from 1941 to 2007. Psychosom Med. 2009:235-42.

42. Faedda GL, Tondo L, Baldessarini RJ, et al. Outcome after rapid versus gradual discontinuation of lithium treatment in bipolar disorders. Arch Gen Psychiatry. 1993;50:448-55.

43. Suppes T, Baldessarini R, Faedda GL, et al. Discontinuation of maintenance treatment in bipolar disorder: Risks and implications. Harv Rev Psychiatry. 1993;1:131-44.

44. Newport DJ, Stowe ZN, Viguera AC, et al. Lamotrigine in bipolar disorder: Efficacy during pregnancy. Bipolar Disord. 2008;10:432-6.

45. Cohen LS, Friedman JM, Jefferson JW, et al. A re-evaluation of risk of in utero exposure to lithium. JAMA. 1994;271:146-50.

46. Holmes LB, Wyszynski DF, Baldwin EJ, et al. Increased risk for nonsyndromic cleft palate among infants exposed to lamotrigine during pregnancy. In: 46th Annual Meeting of the Teratology Society . Tucson (AZ). June 24-29. 2006.

47. Wyszynski D, Nambisan M, Surve T, et al. Increased rates of major malformations in offsprings exposed to valproate during pregnancy. Neurology. 2005;64:291-5.

48. Viguera AC, Cohen LS, Baldessarini RJ, et al. Managing bipolar disorder during pregnancy: weighing the risks and benefits. Can J Psychiatry. 2002;47:426-36.
49. Kendell RE, Chalmers JC, Platz C. Epidemiology of puerperal psychosis. Br J Psychiatry. 1987;150:662-73.
50. O Hara MW. Postpartum depression—causes and consequences. New York: Springer- Verlag: 1995.
51. Appleby L, Warner R, Whitton A, et al. A controlled study of fluoxetine and cognitive behavioural counselling in the treatment of postnatal depression. BMJ. 1997;314:932-6.
52. O Hara MW, Stuart S, Gormann LL, et al. Efficacy of interpersonal psychotherapy for postpartum depression. Arch Gen Psychiatry. 2000;57:1039-45.
53. Suri R, Burt VK, Altshuler LL, et al. Fluvoxamine for postpartum depression. Am J Psychiatry. 2001;158:1739-40.
54. Stowe ZN, Casarella J, et al. Sertraline in the treatment of women with postpartum major depression. Depression. 1995;3:49-55.
55. Cohen LS, Viguera AC, Bouffard SM, et al. Venlafaxine in the treatment of postpartum depression. J Clin Psychiatry. 2001;62:592-6.
56. Nonacs RM, Soares CN, Viguera AC, et al. Bupropion SR for the treatment of postpartum depression—a pilot study. Int J Neropsychopharmacol. 2005;8:445-9.
57. Dalton K. Progesterone prophylaxis used successfully in postnatal depression. Practitioner. 1985;229:507-8.
58. Gregoire AJ, Kumar R, Everitt B, et al. Transdermal estrogen for treatment of severe postnatal depression. Lancet. 1996;347:930-3.
59. Ashokas A, Kaukoranta J, Wahlbeck K, et al. Estogen deficiency in severe postpartum depression—successful treatment with sublingual physiologic 17 beta-estradiol: A preliminary study. J Clin Psychiatry. 2001;62:332-6.
60. Appleby L. Suicide during pregnancy and the first postnatal year. BMJ. 1991; 302:137-40.
61. Austin MP. Peurperal affective psychosis—Is there a case for lithium prophylaxis? Br J Psychiatry. 1992;161:692-4.
62. Stewart DE, Klompenhouwer JL, Kendal Re, et al. Prophylactic lithium in puerperal psychosis: The experience of three centers. Br J Psychiatry. 1991;158:393-7.
63. Wisner KL, Wheeler SB. Prevention of recurrent postpartum. Hosp Community Psychiatry. 1994;45:1191-6.

Thyroid Disorders in Pregnancy

Sujata Misra

Thyroid hormones have a significant impact on maternal metabolism and fetal development and its dysfunction is the second most common endocrine disorder in women of childbearing age. The net effect of pregnancy is an increased demand on the thyroid gland. As the changes in thyroid economy occurring early in pregnancy, it is imperative to advice women with longstanding thyroid diseases to plan their pregnancies and contact their health care professionals as soon as pregnancy is diagnosed. A team approach with close cooperation of the obstetrician, endocrinologist, pediatrician and anesthesiologist is best for optimal maternal and perinatal outcomes.

The thyroid gland synthesizes two related hormones, triiodothyronine (T3) and thyroxin (T4). Thyrotropin-releasing hormone (TRH), produced in a tonic fashion in the paraventricular nucleus of the hypothalamus, is responsible for stimulating the thyroid axis. It reaches the pituitary gland by way of the pituitary stalk and stimulates the production and release of thyrotropin (TSH—Thyroid-stimulating hormone). TSH consists of an alpha- and a beta-subunit; the beta subunit confers specificity. TRH also stimulates prolactin-secretion. In addition to the direct stimulatory effect that TRH has on TSH secretion, TSH secretion is regulated by negative feedback from circulating thyroid hormone, dopamine and somatostatin. TSH then stimulates the thyroid gland to produce as well as secrete thyroxin (T4) and triiodothyronine (T3).

PHYSIOLOGY

Thyroid hormone synthesis largely depends on an adequate supply of iodine in the diet. In the small intestine, iodine is absorbed as iodide, which is then transported to the thyroid gland. Plasma iodide enters the thyroid under the influence of TSH. Iodine supplementation is very essential for normal fetal thyroid function and deficiency causes severe neurological cretinism, which can be prevented by iodine supplementation during pre-pregnancy or up to the second trimester. The suggested total daily iodine ingestion for pregnant women is 229 μg a day and for lactating women 289 μg daily; prenatal vitamins should contain at least 150 μg of iodine.

Human chorionic gonadotropin (hCG) possesses intrinsic thyroid-stimulating activity, leading transiently to a partial TSH suppression near the end of the first trimester in about 20% pregnancies. In one-tenth of the latter cases, serum free T4 levels may become transiently elevated to exceed the normal range; in turn, these women develop the syndrome of gestational transient thyrotoxicosis or GTT.

Hyperemesis gravidarum (HG) is often present during the first months of gestation. Women with HG may have biochemical features suggesting hyperthyroidism that results from excessive hCG-induced thyroid stimulation. Iodides, thiomides, TRH and T4 are transferred by the placenta but TSH is not transferred. Placental transfer of T4 occurs in the first trimester, when it is required for fetal brain development. Euthyroid women with a hypothyroid fetus have placental adaptation allowing T4 transfer beyond the first trimester to protect the fetal brain. Biochemical assessment of thyroid function must be with reference to pregnancy-specific ranges.

Pre-pregnancy Counseling

- It is advisable for a patient with hyperthyroidism and under antithyroid medication to wait for 6 months after the therapeutic dose is administered before contemplating pregnancy (GPP). It is important for the patient to be euthyroid for three months before conception (IVC).
- Women on treatment for hypothyroidism should be well monitored.
- Pregnancy does not affect the natural history of patients treated with radioactive iodine for thyroid carcinoma. In these cases, it is reasonable to wait for four months after completion of treatment before contemplating pregnancy.

Thyroid Function Tests in Pregnancy

Measurement of serum thyroid stimulating hormone (TSH) is the most practical, simple and economic screening test for thyroid dysfunction. A value of 2.5 mIU/L is presently accepted as the upper limit of serum TSH for the first trimester of pregnancy. In the presence of an abnormal serum TSH value, the determination of free thyroxine (FT4) or its equivalent free thyroxine index (FT4I) may be done. A suppressed TSH value and high concentrations of FT4 or FT4I are diagnostic of hyperthyroidism.

The determination of TSH receptor antibodies (TSHRBab or TRAb) are indicated only in special circumstances in order to predict the possibility of fetal or neonatal thyroid dysfunction (e.g. in Grave's disease; fetal/neonatal hypothyroidism in previous pregnancies; Active disease on treatment with antithyroid drugs).

The detection of goiter in pregnancy is an abnormal finding and is most commonly caused by chronic autoimmune thyroiditis or Hashimoto's thyroiditis. Most patients are euthyroid and diagnosis is made by determination of thyroid antibodies, mainly thyroid peroxidise (TPO) Antibody concentration decreases during pregnancy and increases in the postpartum period. High values in the first trimester of pregnancy are a predictor of the syndrome of postpartum thyroid dysfunction.

The values of thyroid hormones during pregnancy are trimester specific, which is shown in Table 1.

Maternal-Placental-Fetal Interactions

- Maternal TSH and TRH do not cross the placental barrier.
- Maternal thyroxine crosses the placenta in the first half of pregnancy, at a time when the fetal thyroid is not functional. This has a positive effect on the intellectual development of the fetus.
- Methimazole (MM) and propylthiouracil (PPU) used for treatment of hyperthyroidism cross the placental barrier.

HYPERTHYROIDISM IN PREGNANCY

Hyperthyroidism affects 0.2% of all pregnant women. Inappropriate production of human chorionic gonadotropin (hCG) is a leading cause of hyperthyroidism during first trimester of pregnancy (Table 2).

Transient hyperthyroidism is the most common cause of hyperthyroxinemia in pregnancy and is caused due to high or inappropriate levels of hCG. It is also known as gestational thyrotoxicosis. This condition is suspected in women who present at 4–8 weeks of gestation with sudden onset of severe nausea and vomiting and the thyroid tests are in the hyperthyroid range. They have no clinical manifestations of Grave's disease. Common findings are weight loss of at least 5 kg, ketonuria, abnormal liver function tests, and hypokalemia.

Table 1: Values of thyroid hormones during pregnancy

Test	Non Pregnant	First Trimester	Second Trimester	Third Trimester
Free T4 (pmol/L)	11–23	10–24	9–19	7–17
Free T3 (pmol/L)	4–9	4–8	4–7	3–5
TSH (pmol/L)	<4	0–1.6	1–1.8	7–7.5

Table 2: Etiology of hyperthyroidism in pregnancy

Transient hyperthyroidism due to inappropriate production of hCG	
Transient hyperthyroidism of hyperemesis gravidarum	
Graves' disease	Subacute thyroiditis
Hydatidiform mole	Iatrogenic thyrotoxicosis
Multinodular goitre	Thyrotoxicosis factitia
Toxic adenoma	TSH-producing pituitary tumor
Struma ovarii	

The FT4 levels are elevated up to four to six times. FT3 too is elevated in 40% of patients. The T4/T3 ratio is less than 20 in HG while it is higher than 20 in Grave's hyperthyroidism. This disorder resolves spontaneously between 14–20 weeks and anti-thyroid drugs are usually not needed.

Graves' Disease

Overt hyperthyroidism affects 0.2% of pregnant women; 95% of these have Grave's disease (autoimmune disorder). The natural course of hyperthyroidism due to Grave's disease in pregnancy is characterized by an exacerbation of symptoms in the first trimester and in the postpartum period while there is an amelioration of symptoms in the second half of pregnancy.

Thyroid tests in the hyperthyroid range with or without clinical hyperthyroidism may be found in first half of pregnancy. History of hypermetabolic symptoms before pregnancy, presence of goiter and exophthalmopathy, and positive antithyroid peroxidase (TPO) titer support the diagnosis of hyperthyroidism caused by Graves. One should be cautious in interpreting the results of thyroid function tests in early pregnancy as TSH levels decrease as a result of increasing levels of hCG (II A/B). Usually the symptoms antedate conception.

The diagnostic clinical clues in favor of hyperthyroidism are—presence of goiter, ophthalmopathy, proximal muscle weakness, tachycardia (> 100 beats per minute), hyperdynamic circulation with a loud systolic murmur and weight loss or inability to gain weight in spite of a good appetite.

Pregnancy specific reference ranges should be used when interpreting the results of thyroid function tests. A suppressed TSH value in presence of a high FT4 or FT4 index confirms the diagnosis. If FT4 is at the upper limit of normal or slightly elevated, the determination of FT3 or FT3I will confirm the diagnosis of hyperthyroidism. Thyroid peroxidase antibodies (anti-TPO) are indicated in cases where the etiology of hyperthyroidism is in doubt.

Fetal ultrasound helps to monitor fetal growth, tachycardia, or goiter. The size of the fetal thyroid gland is an indicator to guide maternal therapy in women with Grave's disease.

The goal of treatment is normalization of thyroid tests as soon as possible and to maintain euthyroidism with the minimal amount of antithyroid medication.

The initial recommended dose of PTU (propylthiouracil) is 100–450 mg/day in divided doses (half-life is 8 hours) and for MM (Methimazole), 10–40 mg/day divided in two daily doses. In patients with minimal symptoms, an initial dose of 10 mg MM daily or PTU 50 mg two to three times per day is initiated.

Clinical improvement is evident in 2–6 weeks and improvement in the thyroid function tests are seen within the first 2 weeks of therapy, with normalization to chemical euthyroidism in 3 to 7 weeks.

The dose is adjusted every few weeks according to the clinical response and the result of thyroid function tests.

Normalization of serum TSH is an indicator to reduce the dose of medication.

Common side effects of antithyroid drugs are pruritus and skin rash. Very few cases of "Methimazole embryopathy" have been reported in infants of mothers treated with MM in the first trimester. This includes choanal atresia, esophageal atresia and minor developmental delay. This is not seen with the use of PTU.

Beta adrenergic blocking agents (Propranolol 20-40 mg 6 hourly or Atenolol 25 to 50 mg/day) are very effective in controlling the hyperdynamic patients and may be used in the first few weeks in symptomatic patients. They are used in patients with symptoms like tremors, tachycardia and palpitations. Dose is adjusted to keep resting the pulse within 70–90 bpm. Not used for long term as there is risk of IUGR. Iodine *131* therapy is contraindicated in pregnancy.

Surgery is indicated in a few selected cases like those with allergy to ATDs. Non-responders to ATDs or unusually large goiter needing high dose of ATD. Surgery is best done in the second trimester of pregnancy.

Breastfeeding is permitted if the daily dose of PTU or MM is less than 200 or 20 mg/day, respectively. The total dose should be distributed in divided doses after each feeding.

The infant should be screened for neonatal thyrotoxicosis on days 3–4 and 7–10 days of delivery, if the TSH receptor antibody titer is high late in pregnancy (III/B).

Special Situations

If serum FT4 levels or FT4I are within normal limits, the amount of antithyroid drugs (ATD) should be minimized to achieve FT4 value in the upper one-third of the normal. If TSH is in normal limits, ATD may be discontinued. Monitoring with thyroid tests should be done. There is no need to switch from carbimazole to propylthiouracil (PTU).

Hyperthyroidism in Remission Following ATD Therapy

Hyperthyroidism may recur in early pregnancy due to increased TSI titers and hCG. ATD therapy may be needed for a few weeks.

History of Ablation Therapy for Graves' Disease

Following ablation therapy, thyroid replacement therapy is needed in almost every patient; after conception, the dose of thyroid hormone needs to be increased. Serum TSH should be kept within normal limits and determined at the time of diagnosis of pregnancy between 20 and 24 weeks gestation and again between 28 and 32 weeks gestation. In some patients, TSI levels remain high despite ablation therapy. This IgG immunoglobulin can cross placenta and stimulate fetal thyroid gland producing fetal hyperthyroidism. The obstetrician should be aware of early signs of fetal hyperthyroidism such as fetal tachycardia, fetal growth restriction, or occasional fetal goiter on ultrasound.

Previous Birth of an Infant with Thyroid Dysfunction

Fetal and neonatal hyperthyroidisms are reported in 1–2% of pregnancies with Graves' disease. Recurrences in subsequent pregnancies are not unusual. Morbidity and mortality are significant, and early detection and prompt treatment are mandatory.

Recurrence of Hyperthyroidism in the Postpartum Period

Hyperthyroidism often recurs in the postpartum period in women with a previous history of Graves' disease or may present for the first time within 1 year following delivery.

Subclinical Hyperthyroidism

Subclinical hyperthyroidism is characterized by normal FT4 and suppressed TSH. It is associated with the following:
- Normal pregnancy (up to 15%)
- Mild nausea/vomiting
- Multiple gestation
- Hyperreactio luteinalis—luteoma of pregnancy (later in pregnancy)—a rare condition in which hCG levels are higher than in normal pregnancy and hyperthyroidism in second trimester of pregnancy and resolution after delivery.

THYROID STORM

Thyroid crisis or "storm" is a rapid worsening of the thyrotoxicosis brought about by stress, e.g. infection, labor, or surgery. This usually occurs in uncontrolled thyrotoxicosis. Fever is a prominent feature and may exceed 40°C. Mental status is altered, ranging from extreme nervousness and restlessness, confusion to psychosis, seizures and coma. There may be diarrhea, nausea and vomiting, and nonspecific abdominal pain. Tachycardia and atrial fibrillation may be present. As thyroid storm is a life-threatening condition with mortality rates as high as 10% immediate treatment should be instituted. The goals of treatment are to decrease the production of thyroid hormone, decrease the effect of circulating hormone, provide supportive therapy, and treat the underlying cause. Propylthiouracil 300–400 mg every 8 hourly orally, by nasogastric tube or rectally, is the drug of choice. It inhibits thyroid hormone synthesis and helps in restoring the electrolyte balance. Aspirin should not be used as an antipyretic agent since it displaces thyroid hormone from TBG and thus increases the free-hormone concentrations. Heart failure due to rapid atrial fibrillation should be treated with digoxin and diuretics, though the dose of digoxin needs to be higher than normal in the thyrotoxic patient, since the rate of degradation is increased.

HYPOTHYROIDISM IN PREGNANCY

Subclinical Hypothyroidism (SCH)

Subclinical hypothyroidism is a form of mild thyroid dysfunction where there is an elevated levels of thyroid stimulating hormone (TSH) accompanied with normal free thyroxine levels. This entity is assuming clinical importance as it indicates the inability of the thyroid gland to increase its output in response to increased demand such as pregnancy. Serum TSH is one of the most sensitive tools in the diagnosis of thyroid disorders. It is also the most economical and hence, is most frequently employed for screening and follow-up in subclinical hypothyroidism.

Points to Remember

- TSH levels are also subject to circadian variation, rising several hours before the onset of sleep, and reaching peak levels between 11 PM and 6 AM. Nadir concentrations are observed during the afternoon. Diurnal variation of TSH levels could account for up to ± 50% of the TSH value. Hence, measuring TSH levels at the same time of the day is recommended.
- In subjects with a normal hypothalamic pituitary axis there is an inverse correlation between the free thyroxine and TSH concentrations in the serum but, in central hypothalamic defects, the TSH as well as the thyroxine concentrations will be low.
- TSH levels may be transiently elevated following strenuous exercise, like a morning jog or after sleep deprivation.
- TSH levels may be falsely elevated in any autoimmune disease due to the presence of heterophile antibodies.
- TSH levels may be unreliable during the first trimester of pregnancy as rising concentrations of human chorionic gonadotrofin (hCG) have an intrinsic thyroid stimulating activity. This will suppress the TSH secretion during the first trimester which recovers and remains normal during the other two trimesters.
  Due to these variations, it is better to evaluate TSH and free T4 levels rather than TSH alone.
- Normal serum TSH levels in disease free individuals are 0.45–4.5 mU/L.

Screen or Not to Screen?

The cost effectiveness of routine screening of all pregnant women was evaluated by Thung et al. from New Haven and he concluded that screening for subclinical hypothyroidism in pregnancy will be a cost-effective strategy under a wide range of circumstances, the American College of Obstetricians and Gynecologists has stated that routine screening and treatment of subclinical hypothyroidism cannot be recommended. However, other authors have stated that screening of all pregnant patients is a cost effective strategy. Pregnant women should be screened at booking visit.

Indian data: Orissa study: A prospective study on Prevalence of subclinical hypothyroidism in pregnancy and its impact on fetomaternal outcome was done in Obstetrics and Gynecology Department of SCB Medical College, Cuttack, Odisha by A Misra, Sujata Misra, et al. they reported a 5.3% prevalence of SCH. Out of total 566 cases screened, 30 cases had subclinical hypothyroidism. Both euthyroid and hypothyroid group were compared in terms of age, parity, gestational age, socioeconomic status and geographical area distribution and pregnancy outcome. The mean age for SCH in pregnancy was 28 years. About 60% of SCH patients belong to rural area and 23% cases were more than 30 year age. Abruptio placentae was present in 17% of cases of SCH, which was 2% in euthyroid group (p < 0.001, odds ratio 9). About 20% of SCH cases had preterm delivery (p<0.001, odds ratio 6). Low birth weight was prevalent in 17.5% cases of SCH, which was 2.5% in euthyroid control group. About 30% cases of SCH were delivered by LSCS, the most common indication being fetal distress (43%). APGAR score was ≤ 3 in 5 min in 6% cases of SCH. Admission to NICU was 30% in SCH which was 3.5% in euthyroid group. Cord blood TSH was >20 mIU/dL in 6% cases of SCH. This strongly supports the need for screening for SCH in pregnancy.

Hypothyroidism and Pregnancy Complications

Both overt and subclinical hypothyroidism were associated with increased risk of eclampsia, preeclampsia, and pregnancy induced hypertension.

The incidence of postpartum depression may also be increased in these patients, necessitating the need for initiating therapy with selective serotonin uptake inhibitors. Delayed neurological problems are seen in the affected fetus.

Management

Levothyroxine sodium is the drug of choice for treatment of subclinical hypothyroidism and is started in an initial dose of 25–50 μg daily, empty stomach prior to breakfast. Usually the dose required is 1.5 μg/lb body weight. Dosage may be increased in steps of 25–50 μg at intervals of 4 weeks till the TSH levels falls in the lower half of the normal range.

Evaluation of Therapy

The goal of therapy is to maintain the TSH levels in the lower half of the range 0.3–2.0 mU/L. The full response of TSH to T4 therapy is relatively slow. A minimum of 8 weeks is necessary between changes in dosage and assessment of therapy. Once the dose is stabilized, follow-up should be yearly with ultrasensitive TSH assay.

Overt Hypothyroidism (OH)

Overt hypothyroidism during pregnancy is uncommon because many women are anovulatory leading to subsequent infertility, and an increased rate of early spontaneous abortion, if conception occurs. The two most common etiology of primary hypothyroidism is autoimmune thyroiditis (Hashimoto's thyroiditis) and post-thyroid ablation therapy, either surgical or Iodine 131 induced.

Pregnant women with pre-existing hypothyroidism carry an increased risk of abortion, anemia, gestation hypertension (including severe forms of eclampsia and preeclampsia), abruptio placentae, and postpartum hemorrhage. The likelihood of complications depends upon the severity of the hypothyroidism and the adequacy of maternal treatment.

Diagnosis

The diagnosis of hypothyroidism is confirmed by the determination of serum TSH and FT4 or FT4I. Regardless of etiology, primary hypothyroidism is classified into subclinical hypothyroidism (normal FT4 and elevated TSH) and overt hypothyroidism (low FT4 and elevated TSH). Those with positive anti-TPO antibodies and a serum TSH > 2.5 mU/L should be treated with L-thyroxine, to keep the serum level between 0.3 and 2.0 mU/L.

Patients on thyroid therapy before conception should have their TSH checked at 4–6 weeks of gestation and dose of L-thyroxine should be adjusted accordingly. Routine increase in thyroxine dose is not indicated.

The serum TSH should be repeated every 4–6 weeks during the first 20 weeks, at 24 to 28 weeks and at 32 to 34 weeks gestation. Immediately after delivery, it should return to pre-pregnancy level.

If hypothyroidism has been diagnosed before pregnancy, it is recommend to adjust the preconception L-T4 dose to maintain a TSH level not higher than 2.5 mU/L (ideally lower than 2.0), prior to conception.

The L-T4 dose usually needs to be increased by 4–6 weeks gestation, and may require a 20–50% increase in dosage (or even more). Patients should separate L-T4 ingestion and the ingestion of iron supplements vitamins containing iron, calcium supplements, and soy-based food by at least 4 hours.

If OH is diagnosed during pregnancy, TFTs should be normalized as rapidly as possible. L-T4 dosage should be titrated rapidly to reach and thereafter maintain serum TSH concentration lower than 2.5 mU/L (ideally lower than 2.0) or trimester-specific normal TSH ranges. TFTs should be readministered within 30–40 days.

SCH has been shown to be associated with an adverse outcome for both the mother and the offspring. L-T4 treatment has been shown to improve obstetric outcome, but has not been proved to modify long-term neurological development in the offspring.

After delivery, most hypothyroid women need the L-T4 dosage they received during pregnancy to be decreased to the preconception dosage. TSH level should be rechecked at 6 weeks postpartum, and it is important to continue monitoring TFTs for at least 6 months after delivery.

SINGLE NODULE OF THYROID GLAND

Nodular thyroid disease is detectable in 10% of pregnant women and the chance of the nodule being malignant is between 5–10%.

Recommended Approach

- A suppressed serum TSH indicates the presence of an autonomic nodule.
- Ultrasonography distinguishes a solid from a cystic lesion.
- A solid lesion is < 2 cm, or a cystic lesion is < 4 cm requires observation with or without thyroxine suppression therapy. If size increases during pregnancy, fine needle aspiration biopsy (FNAB) is indicated.
- In patients with a solid or mixed lesion > 2 cm, or cystic lesion > 4 cm, diagnostic approach depends on the gestational age:
  a. Before 20 weeks gestation—FNAB done
  b. For lesions diagnosed after 24 weeks—FNAB postponed until after delivery, unless there is a strong suspicion of malignancy.
  c. For lesions diagnosed between 20–24 weeks—the decision to wait until delivery or to complete the workup is made by the patient and her physician.
- If the lesion is a papillary carcinoma, surgery is recommended prior to 24 weeks.
- For follicular lesions, the decision about surgery is a personal one, as the chance of malignancy is only between 15–20%.
- General principles of care include:
  a. Determination of the serum thyroglobulin level, a good indicator of tumor activity, before surgery and at regular intervals thereafter
  b. Decision to use radioactive iodine, which is indicated for completeness of thyroid ablation
  c. Importance of thyroid suppression therapy to keep the serum TSH suppressed in order to prevent possible recurrence of the lesion.

POSTPARTUM THYROID DYSFUNCTION (PPT)

Thyroid dysfunction, either hyper or hypothyroidism, has been recognized with increasing frequency in the first 13 months following delivery, and after abortions. Postpartum thyroiditis is prevalent in 1.1–16.7% of all women and is the most common cause of thyroid dysfunction in the postpartum period. Most of the cases are due to intrinsic thyroid disease, while a few may be the result of hypothalamic or pituitary lesions. Patients with pre-existing auto-immune thyroid disease, chronic thyroiditis, and Graves' disease are most frequently affected. The disease is three-fold higher in those with type 1 diabetes mellitus with the incidence being close to 30% in those with a family history of the disease or thyroid peroxidase antibodies. The propensity for thyroiditis antedates pregnancy and is directly related to increasing serum levels of thyroid autoantibodies. Women with high antibody titres in early pregnancy are commonly affected.

The symptoms are usually non-specific and include tiredness, fatigue, depressions, palpitations and irritability.

Two forms of PPT are generally encountered:

1. An autoimmune form, which is more common and eventually develops into chronic hypothyroidism.

2. A nonautoimmune form, without antibodies, that appears to be transient without progressing to permanent hypothyroidism.

Predictability

Features which predict the development of PPT in pregnant women are:
1. Hypothyroidism antedating pregnancy
2. Episodes of PPT in previous pregnancies
3. Presence of goiter and high titers of thyroid antibodies in the first half of pregnancy
4. A strong family history of autoimmune thyroid disease. Women with type 1 diabetes mellitus are at a high-risk of developing PPT. PPT may recur in subsequent pregnancies, with a recurrence rate between 30% and 70%. It may be associated with other auto-immune endocrine disorders, such as adrenal insufficiency and lymphocytic hypophysitis.

The clinical course is not uniform. It may present in four forms:
1. An episode of hyperthyroidism (2–4 months), followed by hypothyroidism (4–6 months) and reverting to euthyroidism after the seventh month.
2. An episode of hyperthyroidism (3–4 months) reverting to euthyroidism.
3. An episode of hypothyroidism (4–6 months) reverting to euthyroid state.
4. Permanent hypothyroidism after the hypothyroid phase.

Management

Most recover spontaneously. For hypothyroid symptoms, small dose of L-thyroxine (0.05 mg/day) will control symptoms allowing a spontaneous recovery of thyroid function following the discontinuation of the drug.

In the presence of hyperthyroid symptoms, β-adrenergic blocking agents (Propranolol 20–40 mg 6 hourly or Atenolol 25 to 50 mg/day) are very effective in controlling the symptoms. Antithyroid medication is not effective as the hyperthyroxinemia is secondary to release of thyroid hormones due to acute injury of the gland (destructive hypothyroidism).

Differential Diagnosis

The differential diagnosis of postpartum hyperthyroidism includes:
- Postpartum painless thyroiditis (commonest)
- Postpartum Graves' disease
- Postpartum toxic multinodular goiter.

Contraception

Oral contraceptives are known to affect serum concentration of various endocrine parameters, which under normal conditions are not involved in the regulation of ovarian activity. The thyroid status essentially remains normal in women taking oral contraceptive pills. As the conventional thyroid tests may be misleading when patients are taking steroidal contraceptives, the free thyroxine level should be measured in women with thyroid dysfunction desirous of using oral contraceptives.

Administration of estrogen or combined oral contraceptive pills possessing estrogenic activity, increases protein binding iodine and thyroxine (T4) in serum and decreases triiodothyronine uptake (T3U) to sephadex, resin, or erythrocytes. However, the free thyroxine level is unchanged and this provides an accurate assessment of the patient's thyroid status.

There is a good correlation between the percentage of free thyroxine and weight gain in contraceptive users. In addition, there is significant reduction in the 24-hour uptake by the thyroid gland in combination contraceptive users. This is due to a decrease in renal clearance of iodine and an increase in plasma inorganic iodine concentration thereby decreasing the thyroid clearance of iodine. The effect of progestational agents without estrogen component on protein binding of thyroxine has been reported as slight increase, no change or decrease. Hence, these agents do not significantly alter the thyroid status.

The non-hormonal contraceptive methods like IUCD, barrier methods, spermicidal creams, etc. do not influence thyroid status.

SUGGESTED READING

1. Bouillon R, Naesens M, Van Assche FA, et al. Thyroid function in patients with hyperemesis gravidarum. Am J Obstet Gynecol. 1982;143:922-6.
2. Brent GA, Mestman JH. Physiology and tests of thyroid function. In: Sciarra J (ed). Gynecology and Obstetrics, Vol 5. Phladelphia, Lippincot-Raven. 1999. p. 1.
3. Bruun T, Kristoffersen K. Thyroid function during pregnancy with special reference to hydatidiform mole and hyperemesis. Acta Endocrinol. 1978;88:383.
4. Clinical Gynecologic Endocrinology and Infertility, 5th ed. USA; Williams and Wilkins. 1994;715-64.
5. Davis LE, Lucas MJ, Hankins GDV, et al. Thyrotoxicosis complicating pregnancy. Am J Obstet Gynecol. 1989;160:63-70.
6. Demers LM, Spencer CA. Laboratory medicine practice guidelines: Laboratory support for the diagnosis and monitoring of thyroid disease. Clin Endocrinol (Oxford). 2003;58:138.
7. Easterling TR, Schnocker BC, Carlson KL, et al. Maternal hemodynamics in pregnancy complicated by hyperthyroidism. Obstet Gynecol. 1991;78:348-52.
8. Goodwin TM, Montoro MN, Mestman JH. Transient hyperthyroidism and hyperemesis gravidarum: clinical aspects. Obstet Gynecol. 1992;167:848-52.
9. Leon Speroff, Robert H, Glass Nathan G, Kase. Oral Contraception.
10. Mandel SJ, Spencer CA, Hollowell JG: Are detection and treatment of thyroid insufficiency in pregnancy feasible? Thyroid. 2005;15:44.
11. Mestman JH. Endocrine diseases in pregnancy. In: Sciarra JJ (ed). Gynecology and Obstetrics. Philadelphia, Lippincott-Raven. 1997. p. 27.
12. Mestman JH. Hyperthyroidism in pregnancy. Clin Ostet Gynecol. 1998;39:45-64.
13. Mestman JH. Thyroid and parathyroid diseases in pregnancy. Obstetrics – Normal and Problem pregnancies by SG Gabbe. 5th edition. 1011-37.
14. Mitsuda N, Tamaki H, Amino N, et al. Risk factors for developmental disorders in infants born to women with Graves' disease. Obstet Gynecol. 1992;80:359-4.

15. Penttila IM, Makkonen M, Castren O. Thyroid function during treatment with a new oral contraceptive combination containing desogestrel. Eur J Obstet Gynecol Reprod Biol. 1983;26:269-74.
16. Sriram U, Raut VS, Chauhan AR, Tank PD. FOGSI Focus: Thyroid womb to tomb. 2006;14:32-6, 39.
17. Thanawala U, Bhagat K, Divakar H. Clinical Pathways in Medical Disorders in Pregnancy. A FOGSI Publication.
18. Tisne L, Barzelano J, Stevenson S. Study of thyroid function during pregnancy and the postpartum period with radioactive iodine. Bol Soc Chile Obstet Gynecol. 1955;20:246-51.

Chapter 8

Bacterial Vaginosis in Pregnancy

Manju Gita Mishra, Mamta Singh

INTRODUCTION

Bacterial vaginosis (BV) is the most common cause of vaginal discharge in women of childbearing age (pregnant and non pregnant) accounting for 40 to 50 percent of cases.[1] In the United States, the national health and nutrition examination survey (NHANES), which included results from self collected vaginal swabs from over 3700 women, estimated the prevalence of BV was 29 percent in the general population of women aged 14 to 49 years and 50 percent in African-American women.[2] This included both symptomatic and asymptomatic infection.

In Obstetrics, bacterial vaginosis (BV) and its related organisms have been implicated in higher rates of late miscarriage, preterm premature rupture of membranes (PPROM), chorioamnionitis, spontaneous preterm labor (SPTL), preterm birth (PTB) and postpartum endometritis. BV has also been implicated with conditions in gynecology such as early miscarriage, pelvic inflammatory disease (PID), cervical intraepithelial neoplasia (CIN), postabortal sepsis, urethral syndrome, sexual acquisition of HIV and post hysterectomy vaginal cuff infection.

RISK FACTORS

There are several risk factors for acquisition of BV, some of which are still disputed. The trigger for the change from lactobacillus-dominated flora to BV-associated flora has been linked to many possible factors including age at first sexual intercourse, change in sexual partners, greater number of life time sexual partners and concurrent sexually transmitted diseases. Cigarette smoking and the use of intrauterine contraceptive device are both linked to an increased risk of acquiring BV. Vaginal douching also been implicated as a risk factor for BV by aiding in the ascent of microorganisms into the upper genital tract. Other research has also shown that black women have a high prevalence of BV compared to white women. Higher prevalence has been found in lesbian population when compared to heterosexual women.

PATHOGENESIS AND MICROBIOLOGY

The normal vaginal flora is dominated by *Lactobacillus* species, which plays a major part in maintaining the dynamic ecosystem in the vagina. By metabolizing glycogen in the vagina, *lactobacilli* produce lactic acid which lowers the vaginal pH to below 4.5. This creates a hostile environment which prevents the growth of potentially pathogenic bacteria, particularly *Gardnerella vaginalis* and anaerobes. The low pH generated by the production of lactic acid also reduces the adherence of bacteria to the vaginal epithelium. Other compounds produced by the *lactobacilli* such as lactacin B, acidolin and hydrogen peroxide inhibit the growth of other bacteria.

BV represents a complex change in the vaginal flora characterized by a reduction in concentration of the lactobacilli and an increase in the concentration of other organisms especially anaerobic Gram-negative rods.[3] While 5–15 species of bacteria may be cultured from normal vaginal secretions, the total bacterial count of normal flora is $<10^6$ organisms/mL, whereas women with BV have up to 10^9 organisms/mL. Anaerobic bacteria numbers increase 1000-fold and BV related organisms such as *Gardnerella vaginalis, Bacteroides* species, *Mobiluncus* species, *Mycoplasma hominis, Ureaplasma urealyticum, Porphyromonas* species, etc. dominate the flora with a reduction in quantity and quality of lactobacilli. These anaerobes are capable of producing large amounts of proteolytic carboxylase enzymes, which breakdown vaginal peptides into a variety of amines that are volatile, malodorous and associated with increased vaginal transudation and squamous epithelial cell exfoliation resulting in the typical clinical features observed in patients with BV. The rise in pH also facilitates adherence of *G. vaginalis* to the exfoliating epithelial cells.

The mechanism by which the floral imbalance occurs and the role of sexual activity in the pathogenesis of BV is not clear, but formation of an epithelial biofilm containing *G. vaginalis* appears to play an important role.[4]

CLINICAL FEATURES

Upto half the women diagnosed with BV are asymptomatic. Symptomatic women typically present with vaginal discharge and/or vaginal odor. The discharge is off white, thin and homogeneous. The odor is an unpleasant "fishy smell" that may be more noticeable after sexual intercourse and during menstruation. Pruritus and vulvovaginitis are uncommon symptoms and another cause should be sought if these are present.

DIAGNOSIS

In 1983, Amsel developed a set of composite clinical criteria, which are simple and useful in an office practice where microscopy is available. The diagnosis is made by finding three of the following four signs (the same for pregnant and nonpregnant women): (i) homogeneous, thin, grayish white discharge that smoothly coats the vaginal walls, (ii) an elevated vaginal pH > 4.5, (iii) Positive whiff-amine test, defined as the presence of a fishy odor when a drop of 10% KOH is added to the sample of vaginal discharge. (iv) Presence of clue cells on saline wet mount. For a positive result, at least 20 percent of the epithelial cells on wet mount should be clue cells. [Clue cells are vaginal epithelial cells studded with adherent coco bacilli that are best appreciated at the edge of the cell.]

The sensitivity of Amsel criteria for diagnosis of BV is over 90 percent and specificity is 77 percent.

Gram's stain: Gram's staining of the vaginal discharge is the gold standard for diagnosis of BV but is mostly performed in research settings. The most commonly used system is the Nugent score. The criterion for bacterial vaginosis is a score of seven or higher. A score of four to six is considered intermediate, and a score of zero to three is considered normal.

Cytology: The Papanicolaou smear is not reliable for diagnosis of BV (sensitivity-49 percent, specificity-93 percent).

Culture: As BV represents complex changes in the vaginal flora, there is no role of vaginal culture in diagnosis.

Commercial tests: These are not widely used, given the excellent performance of Amsel criteria, but can be useful where microscopy is not available.

Affirm VP III test: It is an automated DNS probe assay for detecting *G. vaginalis* when present at a high concentration. It takes less than one hour to perform the test.

The OSOM BV blue system: It is a chromogenic diagnostic test based on the presence of elevated sialidase enzyme activity in vaginal fluid samples. This enzyme is produced by bacterial pathogens associated with BV including *Gardnerella, Bacteroides, Prevotella* and *Mobiluncus*. The results are obtained in 10 minutes. Sensitivity ranging from 88 to 94 % and specificity ranging from 91 to 98 % has been reported.

Investigational test:
  i. Quantitative polymerase chain reaction (PCR)—based assays are based upon molecular quantification of *G. vaginalis* and *Atopobium vaginae,* and other bacteria. Although these tests have high sensitivity and specificity, they are expensive and of questionable advantage.
  ii. Urine test—It is also under investigation and it uses fluorescence in situ hybridization (FISH) to identify BV biofilm on desquamated vaginal epithelial in urine sediment and appears promising.

OBSTETRIC COMPLICATIONS ASSOCIATED WITH BACTERIAL VAGINOSIS

Spontaneous Preterm Labor (SPTL) and Preterm Birth (PTB)

The etiology of PTB is multifactorial, but there is now well-accepted evidence to implicate infection as a cause in up to 40% of cases. Abnormal genital tract colonization has been found to be associated with PTB. The total number of vaginal microbial flora increase as pregnancy progresses, with the concentration of *lactobacilli* increasing 10-fold. The concentration of anaerobes decreases while the number of aerobes remains constant. With increasing gestation, the vaginal flora becomes more benign and at term, the microbiological make-up of the vagina generally poses no significant threat to the fetus with the exception of group *B Streptococcus*.

The mechanism by which BV can induce PTB is linked to ascending genital tract infection with an immune response resulting in the production of pro-inflammatory cytokines such as interleukin-1alpha, interleukin-1beta and tumor necrosis factor alpha.[6] Women with polymorphism of genes regulating cytokine production have a greater pro-inflammatory immune response to infectious stimuli, such as BV. Enhanced induction of cytokines in these women could then lead to preterm labor (PTL) or PPROM. Other aspects of host response (e.g. low level of IgA to *Gardnerella vaginalis*) or the specific types of BV associated bacteria involved (e.g. bacteria that produce high levels of sialidase or protease) may also play a role in placing some women with BV at high risk of PTB.

Late Miscarriage

The incidence of late miscarriage (13-23 weeks gestation) has been demonstrated to be significantly higher in women who have BV than those who do not.

Postpartum Endometritis

It is relatively common complication.

Although the incidence is higher in women undergoing caesarean section, it may also occur following a vaginal delivery. Risk factors include PROM, prolonged labor and increased number of vaginal examinations. Early endometritis occurs with 2 days following a caesarean section and late endometritis can occur upto 6 weeks postnatal following vaginal delivery. Facultative anaerobes linked to BV are commonly isolated in cases of endometritis.

TREATMENT

The polymicrobial nature of BV poses a problem to clinicians in attempting to find the most appropriate drug therapy. Currently, treatment recommendations worldwide advocate that BV may be treated with metronidazole or clindamycin orally or vaginally. Oral metronidazole is generally well-tolerated, but may cause nausea and metallic taste. Alcohol can exacerbate this effect as well as cause a disulfiram-like reaction, so it should be avoided. Both oral and vaginal preparations of clindamycin have been linked to the development of pseudomembranous colitis.

BV resolves spontaneously in up to one-third of nonpregnant and one-half of pregnant women. Treatment is indicated for relief of symptoms in women with symptomatic infection and to prevent post operative infection in those with asymptomatic infection prior to abortion.

Treatment in Symptomatic BV Infection in Pregnant Women

All women with symptomatic BV should be treated to relieve symptoms. Oral treatment is effective and has not been associated with adverse fetal or obstetrical effect.[5] The therapeutic options include metronidazole 500 mg orally twice daily for 7 days or metronidazole 250 mg orally thrice daily for 7 days and clindamycin 300 mg orally twice daily for 7 days.

Some clinicians avoid use of metronidazole in the first trimester because it crosses the placenta, and has a potential for teratogenecity. However, meta-analysis has not found any relationship between metronidazole exposure during the first trimester of pregnancy and birth defects, and the center for disease control and prevention (CDC) no longer discourages the use of metronidazole in the first trimester. Some experts avoid topical therapy in pregnant women because they believe oral treatment is more effective against potential subclinical upper genital tract infections.

Treatment in Asymptomatic Infection in Pregnant Women

One-third of pregnant women in the United States have BV. Despite the association between BV and adverse outcome, screening and treatment of asymptomatic BV during pregnancy is controversial. Meta-analysis of randomized trials performed in general obstetric population have found that treatment of asymptomatic infection does not reduce the incidence of preterm labor or delivery.

The American College of Obstetricians and Gynecologists (ACOG), United States preventive services task force (USPSTF) and CDC recommendation are to not routinely screen and treat all pregnant women with asymptomatic BV to prevent preterm birth and its consequences.

Also, treatment is required in asymptomatic pregnant women who have to undergo pregnancy termination (grade 2B) to prevent postoperative infectious complications.

CONCLUSION

Bacterial vaginosis is common and may affect majority of women at some point in their life. There is good evidence that BV is associated with PTL and PTD, late miscarriage, postpartum endometritis. So, obstetricians should be aware of the potential adverse sequelae of BV and familiarize themselves with its diagnosis and treatment.

REFERENCES

1. Mooris M, Nicolli A, Simms 1, et al. Bacterial vaginosis: A public health review. BJOG. 2001;108:439.
2. Alisworth JE, Peipert JF. Prevalence of bacterial vaginosis: 2001–2004: National Health and Nutrition Examination survey data. Obstet Gynecol. 2007;109:114.
3. Hill GB. The microbiology of bacterial vaginosis. AmJ obstet Gynecol. 1993;169:450.
4. Suidsinki A, Mendling W, Locning-Baucke V, et al. Adherent biofilms in bacterial vaginosis. Obstet Gynecol. 2005;106:1013.
5. Caro-Paton T, Carvajal A, Martin de Diego 1, et al. Is metronidazole teratogenic ? A meta-analysis. BrJ Clin Pharmacol. 1997;44:179.
6. Hillier SL, Witkin S, Krohn M, Watts D, Kiviat N, Eschenbach DA. The relationship of amniotic fluid cytokines and preterm delivery, amniotic fluid infection, histological chorioamnionitis and chorioamnion infection. Obstet Gynecol. 1993;81:941-8.

Meena Samant, Esa Bose

Chapter 9
Chlamydia Infection in Pregnancy

INTRODUCTION

Chlamydia trachomatis is one of the most common organism causing pelvic inflammatory disease, which is a major cause of tubal factor infertility. However, *Chlamydia* infection do occur in pregnancy causing maternal complications—preterm parturition syndrome (preterm labor, prelabor rupture of membrane), meconium stained liquor, chorioamnionitis and postpartum endometritis. It also affects the neonate causing—conjunctivitis and pneumonia.[1]

Chlamydia trachomatis (CT) is the most common sexually transmitted pathogen in the United States and the Western world. Approximately, 3 million cases are diagnosed annually in the United States at a cost of greater than 2 billion dollars. Patients at risk are usually young (15 to early 20s), non-white, single, have multiple sexual partners, and use non barrier contraception methods.[1]

In a study conducted by All India Institute of Medical Sciences (AIIMS), the prevalence of *Chlamydia trachomatis* infection in mid-pregnancy and at labor was 17% and 18.6%, respectively. Women with infection were relatively older than those without it and incidence of low birth-weight [18.7% vs 20.7%] as well as prematurity [9.4% vs 10.7%] were similar among neonates born to women with or without infection. Neonates born to infected mothers experienced purulent conjunctivitis more frequently than those born to non-infected mothers [12.5% vs 2.8%, p = 0.04].[2]

PATHOGENESIS

Chlamydia trachomatis is an obligate intracellular parasite. Fifteen serotypes exist; serotypes D, E, F, G, H, I, J, and K are responsible for genital tract and perinatal infections.

It preferentially infects the columnar epithelium of the upper and lower genital tract, urethra, and anus. Although in many patients, *Chlamydia trachomatis* infection is "silent", common clinical manifestations include cervicitis, urethritis, vaginitis, and pelvic inflammatory disease (PID). Untreated infection can spread into the uterus or fallopian tubes and cause PID. This happens in up to 40% of women with untreated *Chlamydia trachomatis*. PID can cause permanent damage to the fallopian tubes, uterus, and surrounding tissues, which can lead to chronic pelvic pain, infertility, and ectopic pregnancy.[1]

CLINICAL FEATURES

About 75 percent of infected women have no symptoms. If they do not have symptoms, they are likely to show up about one to three weeks after exposure. These symptoms may include burning or discomfort during micturition, increased vaginal discharge or possibly spotting.

Before and after pregnancy, *Chlamydia* can travel up from cervix to infect uterus or fallopian tubes, causing pelvic inflammatory disease (PID). Infact, upto 15 percent of women who are not pregnant, have untreated *Chlamydia* infections develop PID.

Symptoms of PID include pain in lower abdomen or back, dyspareunia, vaginal bleeding, fever, and nausea. PID can result in permanent damage to fallopian tubes and lead to chronic pelvic pain and infertility, as well as an increased risk of ectopic pregnancy.[1]

During pregnancy, *Chlamydia* causes abortion, meconium stained liquor, pyrexia, pelvic inflammatory disease.

It is classically believed that in pregnant patients, cervical mucus and pregnancy itself prevent spread of infection from lower genital tract to the uterus and fallopian tubes. Nevertheless, some case reports and serologic work suggest that *Chlamydia* can possibly infect the placenta and thus harm the fetus. This, however, remains controversial. Whereas some studies found no correlation between *Chlamydia* infection and spontaneous abortion, others have found an increased risk of spontaneous first trimester abortion in patients infected with *Chlamydia*. Although the mechanism of pregnancy loss secondary to the infection is unclear, two models are proposed for the pathogenesis of *Chlamydia* related early abortions:[3] direct zygote infection, and[4] immune response to heat shock proteins expressed by the zygote and triggered by previous *Chlamydia* infections. In patients with PPROM, CT infection interferes with collagen maintenance and degradation.

There is no reported evidence of *Chlamydia trachomatis* causing direct harm to the developing fetus. Infact, up to half of the babies born vaginally to mothers with untreated *Chlamydia* (and even some babies born by c-section) contract the infection. Between 25 and 50 percent of these babies develop an eye infection (conjunctivitis) a few days to a few weeks after birth. The medicated drops or ointments put in the newborn's eyes soon after birth to prevent gonorrheal conjunctivitis, do not prevent *Chlamydia* eye infection. About 5 to 30 percent of babies who contract *Chlamydia* during delivery develop pneumonia a few weeks to several months after birth. Infact *Chlamydia trachomatis* is a leading cause of early infant pneumonia and conjunctivitis in newborns.

Although these infections can be very serious, babies who are treated promptly with antibiotics generally do well. The best time to treat is before delivery to prevent the baby from becoming infected in the first place.[1]

INVESTIGATIONS[4]

There are now a number of different techniques for detecting chlamydial infection:

- Cell culture
- Antigen detection or enzyme immunoassays (EIAs)
- Nucleic acid amplification tests (NAATs)
- Antibodies for *Chlamydia*, enzyme linked immunosorbent assay (ELISA)
- With reactive arthritis, paired serology may detect rising titers

    NAATs have largely superseded other methods due to higher sensitivity (in general, NAATs have a sensitivity of 90–95%, increased by increasing the number of patient sites sampled or the number of different NAATs used to test a sample) and the fact that testing can also be done on urine samples, reducing the need for invasive tests. Where NAATs are not available, it may be prudent to discuss with the patient the lower sensitivity of EIA tests (usually between 40–70%) and the risk of a false-negative result
- Follow local protocols for taking, storing and transporting swabs
- In women undergoing a vaginal examination, an endocervical swab is preferred. Clean the cervix and rotate the swab 360° inside the os
- In those who are not undergoing vaginal examination, a first-void urine sample (having held urine for at least 1–2 hours previously) or self-administered vaginal swab may be used
- There is interest in the use of rapid point-of-care testing that could allow a test-and-treat in a single visit approach. However, a recent review suggests that NAATs are still the most accurate and cost-effective method for diagnosing *Chlamydia* infection and concludes that there is little evidence as yet guiding the use of rapid point-of-care methods.

THE ENGLISH NATIONAL *CHLAMYDIA* SCREENING PROGRAM[5]

- Offers *Chlamydia* testing to all patients (male and female) aged 25 years or under, who are, or have previously been, sexually active
- These should be offered opportunistically when they visit general practice, community pharmacies and community sexual and reproductive health clinics. Simply relying on opportunistic testing within general practice will fail to reach a substantial minority of the at-risk population, due to low consultation rates in the teenager/young adult age range; thus, it is only one component of the overall screening strategy. Testing should be repeated annually or after a change in sexual partner
- Testing does not require an examination—for men, a first-void urine sample and for women, a self-taken vaginal swab or urine sample.

GENERAL ADVICE

- It is important to test for other sexually transmitted infections including human immunodeficiency virus (HIV) and hepatitis B
- Advice on safer sexual practices, contraception and condom use.

COMPLICATIONS

During pregnancy: Abortion, preterm labor, prelabor rupture of membranes, chorioamnionitis, fetal growth restriction, meconium stained liquor, stillbirth, neonatal conjunctivitis and pneumonia.

Neonatal complications: Neonatal conjunctivitis, pneumonia, neonatal ear infection.

Gynecological complications: pelvic inflammatory disease (PID), infertility, ectopic pregnancy, perihepatitis as part of Fitz-Hugh and Curtis syndrome, Reiter's syndrome.

TREATMENT [6,7]

First choice: Azithromycin 1 gram orally as a single dose or Amoxicillin 500 mg orally thrice a day for 7 days.

Alternative treatment: Erythromycin 500 mg four times a day for 7 days or Erythromycin 250 mg four times a day for 14 days.

Treatment reduces the number of pregnant woman with positive antibody by 90% and helps prevent pregnancy and neonatal complications (Level 1A evidence).

Centers for Disease Control and Prevention recommendations for testing include:[4] Annual screening for *Chlamydia trachomatis* for all sexually active women aged 25 years and younger; older women with risk factors for *Chlamydia trachomatis* (a new sex partner or multiple sex partners); and all pregnant women should have a screening test for *Chlamydia trachomatis*.

PROGNOSIS

- Untreated *Chlamydia* will either persist or spontaneously resolve. 46% of infections clear spontaneously within a year. Factors determining which course an infection takes are not fully understood; neither is the period of time over which asymptomatic infection can persist
- The natural history of Chlamydia infection remains elusive. There is much debate as to the rates of progression to pelvic inflammatory disease (PID) and infertility. One systematic review estimated incidence of PID as 0–30% in women with untreated *Chlamydia*. Another review estimated that 10–20% of women with PID develop tubal infertility and that women with *Chlamydia* have 0.1–6% risk of developing tubal infertility

- Antibiotic treatment is effective in at least 95% of cases if the full course is taken. Outlook is generally good if treated early with full compliance
- About two-thirds of the sexual partners of an individual with *Chlamydia* will also test positive for *Chlamydia*, emphasising the need for contact tracing and synchronized treatment of partners to prevent reinfection. Consider recurrence and repeat testing in those who remain symptomatic. A Dutch study looking at home-based screening in 15–29 years olds found that 10.4% of those who initially screened positive for *Chlamydia* remained positive a year later. Looking at subtypes, approximately half were new infections and half persisting infections (or reinfection with the same organism).

In conclusion, the recommendations are to test every pregnant women at the first prenatal visit using DNA probe. Tetracycline and Doxycycline show the greatest activity against CT; however, these agents are contraindicated in pregnancy. Thus, patients who test positive should be treated with Azithromycin 1 g orally in a single dose. There is 5% to 10% failure rate to initial treatment; therefore, a test of cure should be done 2 to 3 weeks after the initial treatment. These patients should also be screened for other sexually transmitted infections. In addition, the patient's partner should always be treated as well.

REFERENCES

1. Cunningham, Leveno, Bloom, Hauth, Rouse, Spong. Williams Obstetrics. 23rd edition.
2. Paul VK, Singh M, Gupta U, Buckshee K, Bhargava VL, Takkar D, et al. *Chlamydia trachomatis* infection among pregnant women: Prevalence and prenatal importance. Natl Med J India. 1999;12(1):11-4.
3. Brocklehurst P, Rsorey G. Interventions for treating genital *Chlamydia trachomatis* infection in pregnancy (Cochrane Review). In the Cochrane Library, Issue 1, 2002, oxford: Update software.
4. Centers for disease control and prevention: Sexually Transmitted Diseases Treatment Guidelines 2006: MMWR. 2002:55:1.2006b.
5. Sexually Transmitted Infections in Primary Care, Royal College of General Practitioners (RCGP), 2006.
6. http://www.cdc.gov/std/treatment/2010/chlamydial-infections.htm.
7. http://www.ncbi.nlm.nih.gov/pmc/articles/PMC3115062/.

HIV Infection and AIDS in Pregnancy

Alokendu Chatterjee, Sebanti Goswami

Starting from the inception of HIV into the human race in 1981, we have come a long way in our journey of tackling the nuisance of HIV. The total number of people living with HIV (PLHIV) in the world is 34 million out of which 50% are women.[1] There are an estimated 2.39 million PLHIV in India with National adult HIV prevalence of 0.31%. Of these, women constitute 39% of all PLHIV while 4.4% are children.[2] The main implication of HIV/AIDS in pregnancy is the transmission to the newborn. This transmission can occur during pregnancy, labor, delivery and through breastfeeding. Maximum transmission occurs in the intranatal period.

Prevention of parent to child transmission (PPTCT) is a program which was implemented to reduce the mother-to-child transmission. The transmission of HIV from infected mother to child is one of the modality of transmission that can be minimized with adequate and appropriate medical intervention as a health sector response. In the absence of any intervention, a substantial proportion of children born to women living with HIV will acquire the virus from their mother. Without any intervention, the risk of transmission from parent-to-child is estimated to be 15–45%.[2] With specific intervention this can be brought down to 2%.[2] The program aims towards reduction of new HIV infections in pediatric age group through this route.

The HIV positive pregnant women can be divided into two groups:

1. **Those who require antiretroviral therapy (ART) for their own health** (Pregnant women with CD4<350 cells/mm^3 or WHO clinical stage III & IV irrespective of CD4 count)
2. **Those who do not require ART for their own health but require antiretroviral prophylaxis (ARV) for PPTCT** (Pregnant women with CD4>350 cells/mm^3 and WHO clinical stage I & II.

The first line ART for women in group 1 is Tenofovir + Lamivudine + Efavirenz (TDF + 3TC + EFV), to be started as soon as the eligibility criteria for ART is met and continued lifelong. A small number of HIV infected pregnant women require lifelong ART for their own health and who have had previous exposure to single dose nevirapine (SdNVP) or EFV for PPTCT prophylaxis in prior pregnancies. Because of the risk of resistance to non-nucleoside reverse transcriptase inhibitor (NNRTI) drugs in this population, due to archived mutation, an NNRTI-based ART regimen such as TDF/3TC/EFV may not be fully effective. Thus, these women will require a protease inhibitor-based ART regimen viz: TDF + 3TC + LPV/r (Lopinavir/Ritonavir)

The endeavor of antiretroviral (ARV) prophylaxis started from PACTG 076 trial which was designed for the developed countries. This was followed by the HIVNET012 trial specially conforming to the economic structure of developing countries. The WHO guideline has changed its ingredients since 2005 and has skewed down to option A and option B. World Health Organization (WHO) guidelines in 2010 gave birth to the option A and option B of ARV prophylaxis.[3] The choice of the option depends on the socioeconomic structure and the diplomatic decision of the country.

PPTCT program was scaled up in the country in NACP (National AIDs Control Program) III, with nevirapine as the regimen of choice. This regimen has now been revised in view of higher efficacy of combination antiretroviral and utility of extended NVP prophylaxis amongst children who are breastfed. Exclusive breastfeeding is recommended for 6 months in India.

The NACO (National AIDS Control Organization) has adopted the option B, which recommends starting Tenofovir + Lamivudine + Efavirenz (TDF + 3TC + EFV) from 14 weeks of gestation (or as soon as possible thereafter) but not before 14 weeks and continuing same regimen throughout pregnancy and delivery. In case of exclusive breastfeeding, mothers continue regimen up to one week after breastfeeding has been stopped with 7 days tail of TDF + 3TC and infants are given daily Nevirapine (NVP) from birth for 6 weeks. In case of exclusive replacement feeding, mother is given a TDF + 3TC tail for 7 days after delivery and infants are given daily NVP from birth for 6 weeks.

The advantage of option B is the effectiveness of three drug regimen over monotherapy in option A, it is easier to execute avoiding the changes in the component in various stages of pregnancy and delivery as in option A. The main disadvantage is the cost factor. However, with the adoption of option B in the national PPTCT program this factor will be solved as it will be available free of cost.

Looking forward to expand the frontier of option B, the concept of option B plus is now being considered. It consists of the option B with continuation of the same lifelong once it is started in pregnancy. Advantages are easy execution.

Disadvantage is the probability of developing resistance to the first line drugs unnecessarily in those who would have not otherwise required it.

Antiretroviral prophylaxis is one of the components of PPTCT. Another vital part is proper conduction of delivery and choosing the right mode of delivery. Though the guidelines of the developed countries recommend elective cesarean section as the mode of delivery in HIV positive women, the NACO guideline in our country recommends vaginal delivery in all HIV positive women unless otherwise obstetrically indicated. Cesarean section is not recommended for prevention of mother-to-child transmission, particularly where women are taking ART for their own health or have had adequate duration of ARV prophylaxis for PPTCT.

Mother-to-child transmission risk is increased by the prolonged rupture of membranes, repeated P/V examination, assisted instrumental delivery (vacuum or forceps), invasive fetal monitoring procedures (scalp/fetal blood monitoring), episiotomy and prematurity. Thus, when delivering HIV-infected women, observation of the following is intended:

STANDARD/UNIVERSAL WORK PRECAUTIONS (UWP)

Not to rupture membranes artificially (keep membranes intact for as long as possible).

The membranes should be left intact as long as possible and artificial rupture of membranes reserved for cases of fetal distress or delay in progress of labor.

To minimize vaginal examination and use aseptic techniques

To avoid invasive procedures like fetal blood sampling, fetal scalp electrodes.

To avoid instrumental delivery as much as possible

To avoid routine episiotomy as far as possible

Suctioning the newborn with a nasogastric tube should be avoided unless there is meconium staining of the liquor.

When expanded ARV prophylaxis is the recommended regimen today, breastfeeding is no more an absolute contraindication in these mothers. Exclusive breastfeeding should be continued for six months and supplementary feeding started thereafter. Exclusive artificial feeding should be considered only when the mother has died or is too sick to feed or does not want to feed even after repeated counseling.

There has been a significant scale up of HIV counseling and testing, prevention of parent-to-child transmission (PPTCT) and ART services across the country over last five years. Between 2004 and 2011, the number of pregnant women tested annually under the prevention of parent-to-child transmission (PPTCT) program increased from 0.8 million to 6.6 million and reach of the services has expanded to the rural areas to a large extent.[4]

The care of pregnancy in HIV positive women has changed greatly down the years. The preventive programs have been revised from time to time and have changed their implementation and directives down the years. The spectrum of antiretroviral therapy in pregnancy has widened appreciably from the single dose nevirapine to multidrug ARV with expanded prophylaxis during breastfeeding. This helps in slashing down the rates of transmission of infection to the newborn and aims at giving the world a HIV free generation.

REFERENCES

1. www.avert.org: worldwide HIV/AIDS statistics.
2. National guidelines for PPTCT 2012, NACO.
3. WHO guidelines PPTCT 2010.
4. NACP IV Strategy document PPTCT.

Chapter 11

Rubella in Pregnancy

Manila Jain, Navneet Magon

ABSTRACT

Rubella infection of a pregnant woman may have devastating effects on the developing fetus. The best strategy of prevention is the universal immunization of all infants and identification and immunization of women at risk. The diagnosis of infection should be made as soon as possible. Contact with rubella should be avoided throughout the first two trimesters of pregnancy, even in IgG-positive pregnant women. Women should be counseled about the possible risk of vertical transmission if primary infection occurs prior to 16 weeks gestation. As there is no in utero treatment available for infected fetuses, prevention remains the mainstay action to eliminate all cases of congenital rubella syndrome (CRS).

INTRODUCTION

Rubella meaning 'Little Red' is a mild, febrile rash illness in children and adults that is generally subclinical and inconsequential. It is also known as German measles because the disease was first described by German physicians in the mid-eighteenth century.[1] Infection by Rubella virus during pregnancy can result in miscarriage, stillbirth, or an infant born with birth defect known as congenital rubella syndrome (CRS), which entails a range of serious incurable illnesses.[2]

Maternal rubella in the first eight weeks of pregnancy result in fetal damage in upto 85 percent of infants and multiple defects are common. The risk of damage declines to 10–20 percent by about 16 week's gestation, and after this stage of pregnancy, fetal abnormalities are rare.[2] Infants born with the congenital rubella syndrome (CRS) may have cataracts, nerve deafness, cardiac malformations, microcephaly, mental retardation and behavioral problems. Inflammatory changes may also be found in the liver, lungs and bone marrow. Many children born with CRS will demonstrate persistent neuromotor deficits later in life. Pneumonitis, diabetes mellitus, thyroid dysfunctions, and progressive panencephalitis are other late expressions of CRS.

In a nonpregnant woman, rubella is usually an infection of minor impact characterized by a mild, self-limited disease associated with a rash. The disease has an incubation period of 2 to 3 weeks and infectivity is from seven days before until seven days after the onset of the rash. It is transmitted via airborne droplet emission from the upper respiratory tract of active cases. The virus may also be present in the urine, feces and on the skin. In most people, the virus is rapidly eliminated. However, it may persist for some months postpartum in infants surviving the CRS. These children are a significant source of infection to other infants and more importantly, to pregnant female contacts.[3]

EPIDEMIOLOGY

In 1960, a rubella epidemic swept throughout the world, thousands of babies either died or developed birth defects from rubella. It is over 50 years since a triple vaccine containing attenuated measles, mumps and rubella (MMR) viruses was introduced.[4] Rubella is a vaccine preventable disease and the primary purpose of rubella vaccination is to prevent the occurrence of congenital rubella infections.

Following large-scale rubella vaccination during the last decades, rubella and CRS have almost disappeared from many countries.[5] However, cases of CRS continue to occur in many parts of the world. WHO estimates that worldwide more than 100,000 children are born with CRS each year, more in developing countries.[6] The Indian Union Health Ministry estimates that around 30,000 abnormal children born annually have rubella and thus CRS remains a concern.

RUBELLA SEROLOGY

The evaluation of immunity to rubella virus relies on the presence of specific antibodies and its titers in blood. When a woman is infected with the rubella virus, the body produces both immunoglobulin G (IgG) and immunoglobulin M (IgM) antibodies to fight against infection.[7] Once IgG exists, it persists for life, but IgM antibody usually wanes over six months. If rubella IgG is present, it confirms that a patient has immunity to rubella. Rubella immunoglobulin G (IgG) test is done to evaluate whether a woman is immune to rubella as a result of childhood exposure or immunization, or she may be presently infected with the disease. The rubella IgG test is regarded as a more reliable indicator of the patient immune status than her history, because re-infection with rubella is possible even after immunization.[8,9] Specific IgG determination is performed through enzyme linked fluorescent assay (ELFA) techniques. The results are expressed in IU/mL.

ANTENATAL SCREENING

It is recommended that all women should be screened for rubella antibody in their early reproductive years before pregnancy and in the antenatal period of every pregnancy. Rubella serology must be checked in all pregnant women even if they were seropositive during a previous pregnancy. Although it has been considered that a rubella antibody level of greater than 10 IU/mL indicates that protection is likely, reinfection with rubella can occur even with antibody levels are above 15 IU/mL and the risk is expected to be greater with rubella antibody levels of 10–15 IU/mL or lower.[10] However, CRS is less likely after reinfection with rubella in pregnancy compared with a primary infection. It is estimated that the incidence of CRS is 5% after reinfection with rubella in the first trimester, compared to 85% in primary infection, and negligible later in pregnancy.[11] It is, therefore, recommended that pregnant women with a rubella antibody level below 15 IU/mL be counseled to avoid contact with known cases of rubella. If the antibody level is below 15 IU/mL, the woman should be offered MMR after delivery if she has not already received two doses of a rubella-containing vaccine.

A pregnant woman with low anti-rubella antibody levels should have her serology repeated if she comes into contact with someone with a rash. If a rise in titer is detected, the results should be discussed further.[12] Reinfection with rubella is associated with a rise in immunoglobulin G (IgG), but not a rise in immunoglobulin M (IgM).

DIAGNOSIS OF RUBELLA INFECTION

Diagnosis of Maternal Infection

Asymptomatic infection is common. Clinical diagnosis is unreliable because the symptoms are often fleeting and can be mimicked by other viruses. A history of rubella should never be accepted without having confirmation by positive serology. The presence of a rubella infection is diagnosed either by a four-fold rise in rubella IgG antibody titer between acute and convalescent serum specimens or positive serologic test for rubella-specific IgM antibody or isolation of rubella virus in a clinical specimen from the patient.[10] Serologic studies are best performed within 7 to 10 days after the onset of the rash and should be repeated two to three weeks later.

Diagnosis of Fetal Infection

Rubella PCR, rubella culture and fetal IgM can be performed following chorionic villus sampling (CVS) amniocentesis or cordocentesis.[13] PCR is not widely available and sensitivity is generally not well validated.[14] Ultrasound diagnosis of CRS is extremely difficult, although any fetus presenting with growth restriction should be evaluated for congenital viral infections, including rubella.

Management of Maternal Rubella Infection

If a pregnant woman develop signs or symptoms of a rubella-like illness or has recently been exposed to rubella, gestational age as well as her state of immunity should be determined. Acute infection is diagnosed when IgM antibodies are positive. If a known immune is of more than 12 weeks of gestation, no further testing is necessary. CRS has not been reported after maternal reinfection beyond 12 weeks' gestation. But if she has less than 12 weeks of gestation and demonstrate a significant rise in rubella IgG antibody titer without detection of IgM antibody, she should be informed that reinfection is likely to have occurred.[15] Fetal risk for congenital infection after maternal reinfection during the first trimester has been estimated at 8%.[10]

For pregnant non-immune woman or whose immunity is unknown and gestational age is < 16 weeks, risk of CRS is high and needs counseling regarding CRS.[16]

A pregnant woman presenting late after exposure to a rash illness presents a diagnostic dilemma. If IgG antibodies are negative, the patient is clearly susceptible to rubella and but has no evidence of a recent infection. If IgG is positive, there is evidence of a previous infection. It is then difficult to determine the date of infection and the risk to the fetus, although a low level of antibody suggests more remote infection.[17] Testing for IgM antibody or repeating the test for IgG antibody levels to determine whether there is a significant rise or decline may be considered.

The routine use of immunoglobulin (Ig) for postexposure prophylaxis of rubella in early pregnancy is not recommended. It may be considered if termination of the pregnancy is not an option, but termination must be discussed for documented maternal infection. Although Ig has been shown to reduce clinically apparent infection in the mother, there is no guarantee that fetal infection will be prevented.

Risks of Rubella Infection

Serosurvey is frequently used to assess epidemiologic pattern of rubella in a community. There is dearth of information on the immune status of Indian women against rubella infection. Serosurveys in different parts of India have found that 6–47% of women are susceptible for rubella infection.

In a study conducted in North India among teenage girls, seronegativity to rubella has been reported from 10 to 36%,[18,19] whereas seronegativity among women of child-bearing age group has been reported to be 10–15%. However, these women were referred for rubella screening either due to bad obstetric history or possible infection during pregnancy or immunity to rubella. Therefore, seronegativity in this study is likely to be underreported than general population.

In a study conducted in five districts of Tamil Nadu among subjects aged 1–5 years and 10–16 years to assess susceptibility to rubella, overall, 48.3% of the study population was found to be seronegative.[20] Another study from South India, Tamil Nadu, conducted among female hospital staff of three eye hospitals, aged 18-40 years reported seronegativity to rubella in the range of 11.7–20.8%.[21]

Rubella Immunization

According to WHO, Immunization programs must achieve a higher level of population immunity than natural infection or there is a risk that more pregnant women will be infected (leading to more CRS cases) than happened in the pre-vaccine era. This means that rubella immunization is only recommended for countries that can achieve and maintain high immunization coverage (>80%).[22]

Experience from developed countries have shown that aiming for the individual protection of pregnant women is less effective as a control strategy than the prevention of rubella circulation by immunizing both male and female children. This is because of the failure of many women to be vaccinated, as well as occasional vaccine failure.[23]

Thus, vaccination should aim to prevent rubella outbreaks by insuring high rubella immunity across all age groups (both males and females) that can be achieved primarily through uniformly high vaccination coverage. A mass immunization campaign for all aged 1 to 14 years (or older) is recommended when introducing rubella vaccine so as to prevent ongoing infection, including epidemics, among older children and young adults.[24]

Rubella vaccination is not yet included in National Immunization Schedule in India.

It is available in private sector in the country and is commonly administered as MMR vaccine at 15 months of age. Only few states are using MMR vaccine for giving second dose of measles in their routine immunization program.

Rubella vaccine is available on its own or in combination as measles-mumps-rubella vaccine (MMR). The rubella vaccine strain that is most often used is the Wistar RA 27/3 strain is available in single-dose vials that were stored at 4–8ºC.[25]

Two doses of MMR vaccine administered on or after the first birthday are recommended for all children. The first dose is generally given at 12 to 15 months of age, and the second dose is generally given at four to six years of age. There must be a gap of minimum four weeks between doses. The second dose of MMR provides an added safeguard against all three diseases, but is recommended primarily to prevent outbreaks of measles.

If an individual has no documented history of immunization with MMR, they should be given a dose of MMR rather than performing serology. There are no undue adverse effects from vaccinating individuals who are already immune to measles, mumps and/or rubella. MMR vaccine should not be given to women who are pregnant, and pregnancy should be avoided for four weeks after immunization. However, inadvertent immunization with a rubella-containing vaccine in early pregnancy is no longer considered an indication for termination of pregnancy. There have been no cases of teratogenic damage from vaccine virus despite intensive surveillance in the US, the UK and Germany.[26]

The vaccine can be given safely to postpartum women who are breastfeeding and to the children of pregnant women, since infection is not transmitted from recently immunized individuals. Breastfeeding is not contraindicated. The vaccine can be administered in conjunction with other immune globulin preparations such as Rh-immune globulin.[27]

To conclude, large sero-surveillance of rubella among adolescent girls and women of childbearing age before conception for the assessment and analysis of the situation should be made. Looking at available data of serosurveys and incidence of rubella in India, like many other countries, important vaccination strategies should be made to prevent congenital rubella syndrome by insuring that all women are immune to rubella prior to pregnancy by eliminating the circulation of rubella in the population. An action revamping the national immunization policy should be considered.

REFERENCES

1. Siegel M, Fuerst HT, Guinee VF. "Rubella epidemicity and embryopathy. Results of a long-term prospective study". Am J Dis Child. 1971;121(6):469-73.
2. Edlich RF, Winters KL, Long WB 3rd, Gubler KD. Rubella and congenital rubella (German measles). J Long Term Eff Med Implants. 2005;15(3):319-28.
3. Richardson M, Elliman D, Maguire H, Simpson J, Nicoll A. "Evidence base of incubation periods, periods of infectiousness and exclusion policies for the control of communicable diseases in schools and preschools". Pediatr Infect Dis J. 2001;20(4):380-91.
4. Banatvala JE, Brown DWG. Rubella. The Lancet. 2004;363:1127-37.
5. Centers for Disease Control. Control and prevention of rubella: Evaluation and management of suspected outbreaks, rubella in pregnant women, and surveillance for congenital rubella syndrome. MMWR Recomm Rep. 2001;50(RR12):1-23.
6. Cutts FT, Vynnycky E. Modelling the incidence of congenital rubella syndrome in developing countries.Int J Epidemiol. 1999;28(6):1176-84.
7. Katow S, Umino Y. The present situation and limitation of antibody assays for diagnosis of rubella virus infection in pregnant women. Rinsho Byori. 2003;51(3):263-7.
8. Banerji A, Ford-Jones EL, Kelly E, Robinson JL. Congenital rubella syndrome despite maternal antibodies. CMAJ. 2005;21;172(13):1678-9.
9. Stegmann BJ, Carey JC. "TORCH Infections. Toxoplasmosis, Other (syphilis, varicella-zoster, parvovirus B19), Rubella, Cytomegalovirus (CMV), and Herpes infections". Curr Women's Health Rep. 2002;2(4):253-8.
10. Best JM, S O'Shea, Tipples, Davies, et al. Interpretation of rubella serology in pregnancy—pitfalls and problems. BMJ. 2002;325:147-8.
11. Bullens D, Smets K, Vanhaesebrouck P. Congenital rubella syndrome after maternal reinfection. Clin Pediatr (Phila). 2000;39:113-6.
12. Bar-Oz B, Ford-Jones L, Koren G. Congenital rubella syndrome. How can we do better? Can Fam Physician. 1999;45:1865-9.
13. Cradock-Watson JE, Ridehalgh MK, Anderson MJ, Pattison JR, Kangro HO. Fetal infection resulting from maternal rubella after the first trimester of pregnancy. J Hyg (Lond). 1980;85(3):381-91.
14. Bosma TJ, Corbett KM, Eckstein MB, O'Shea S, Vijayalakshmi P, Banatvala JE, et al. Use of PCR for prenatal and postnatal diagnosis of congenital rubella. J Clin Microbiol. 1995;33(11):2881-7.

15. Hofmann J, Liebert UG. Significance of avidity and immunoblot analysis for rubella IgM-positive serum samples in pregnant women. J Virol Methods. 2005;130(1–2):66-71.
16. Marret H, Golfier F, Di Maio M, Champion F, Attia-Sobol J, Raudrant D. Rubella in pregnancy. Management and prevention. Presse Med. 1999;4;28(38):2117-22.
17. Centers for Disease Control. Rubella prevention. Recommendations of the Immunization Practices Advisory Committee (ACIP). MMWR Recomm Rep. 1990;39(RR-15):1-18.
18. Yadav S, Wadhwa V, Chakarvarti A. Prevalence of rubella antibody in school going girls. Indian Pediatr. 2001;38:280-3.
19. Sharma H, Chowdhari S, Raina TR, Bhardwaj S, Namjoshi G, Parekh S. Serosurveillance to assess immunity to rubella and assessment of immunogenicity and safety of a single dose of rubella vaccine in school girls. Indian J Community Med. 2010;35:134-7.
20. Ramamurty N, Murugan S, Raja D, Elango V, Mohana, Dhanagaran D. Serosurvey of rubella in five blocks of Tamil Nadu. Indian J Med Res. 2006;123:51-4.
21. Vijayalakshmi P, Anuradha R, Prakash K, Narendran K, Ravindran M, Prajna L, et al. Rubella serosurveys at three Aravind Eye Hospitals in Tamil Nadu, India. Bull World Health Organ. 2004;82:259-64.
22. Rubella vaccines: WHO position paper. Wkly Epidemiol Rec. 2011;86:301-16.
23. Demicheli V, Rivetti A, Debalini MG, Di Pietrantonj C (2012). "Vaccines for measles, mumps and rubella in children". Cochrane Database Syst Rev. 2012;2: CD004407.
24. Best JM. Rubella vaccines: past, present and future. Epidemiol Infect. 1991;107–17
25. Immunization Practices Advisory Committee (ACIP). MMWR Recomm Rep. 1990;39(RR-15):1-18.
26. Badilla X, Morice A, Avila-Aguero ML, Saenz E, Cerda I, et al. Fetal risk associated with rubella vaccination during pregnancy. Pediatr Infect Dis J. 2007;26(9):830-5.
27. Böttiger M, Forsgren M. Twenty years' experience of rubella vaccination in Sweden: 10 years of selective vaccination (of 12-year-old girls and of women postpartum) and 13 years of a general two-dose vaccination. Vaccine. 1997;15(14):1538-44.

Dengue in Pregnancy

Suneeta Singh, Navneet Magon

INTRODUCTION

Dengue is a mosquito-borne viral infectious disease with outbreaks occurring in many parts of the world.[1] It is also known as 'break bone fever'. It is potentially fatal disease for which treatment is limited to supportive care only. It is caused by a flavivirus and spread by vector mosquito *Aedes aegypti*.[2]

EPIDEMIOLOGY

The first reported outbreak of dengue fever (DF) occurred in Africa, Asia, South America concurrently in 1780s.[3]

The first outbreak of dengue fever in India was recorded in 1812.[4] New Delhi has experienced eight major outbreaks between 1967and 2008. Over last two decades, DF has become the major cause of hospitalization and mortality after acute respiratory and diarrheal infections among children.[5]

In the last 50 years, incidence has increased 30-fold with increasing geographic expansion to new countries and, in the present decade, from urban to rural settings.

CAUSATIVE ORGANISM

Arbovirus from the genus flavivirus is the causative agent of dengue fever. It is a single stranded RNA genome surrounded by icosahedral nucleocapsid and covered by lipid envelop. Four subtypes are known DEN 1 to 4. Infection with one subtype provides lifelong immunity to that virus but not to other subtypes.[6,7] Vector for all subtypes is mosquito *Aedes aegypti*.

COURSE OF ILLNESS

After an incubation period of 4–10 days, infection by any of the four virus serotypes can produce a wide spectrum of illness, as shown in Figure 1 although most infections are asymptomatic or subclinical.[8] Others who develop febrile illness could be one of the following:

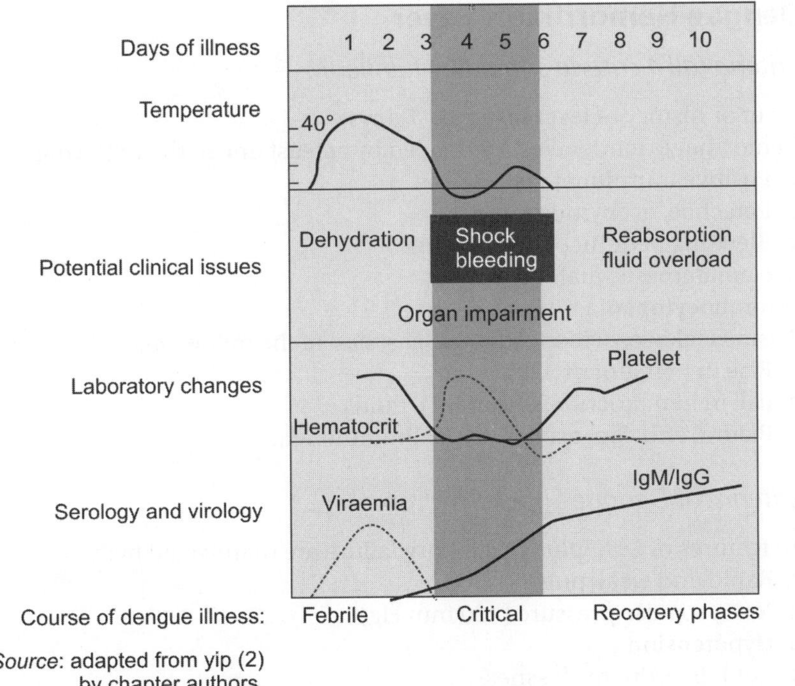

Fig. 1: Course of dengue illness

- Dengue fever
- Dengue hemorrhagic fever
- Dengue shock syndrome

CLINICAL FEATURES

Classic Dengue Fever ('Break Bone Fever')

Fever: Acute onset, typically 39–40°C, may be associated with chills, generally lasts for 5–7 days.
- Headache
- Retro-orbital pain
- Backache, myalgia
- Anorexia, nausea, vomiting
- Typical morbiliform rash appearing on trunk and spreading centripetally to face, trunk and limbs lasting for 1–5 days may be seen.

Clinical examination: Relative bradycardia, lymphadenopathy.

Investigation: Marked leucopenia, neutropenia.

Thrombocytopenia may occur between 3rd and 8th days.

Dengue Hemorrhagic Fever

Criteria (all 4 criteria should be fulfilled)

Fever or history of fever lasting 2–7 days
Hemorrhagic tendencies, evidenced by at least one of the following:
- Positive tourniquet test
- Petechae, ecchymosis, purpura
- Bleeding per mucosa, GIT, other
- Hematemesis, malena.
Thrombocytopenia
Plasma leakage, evidenced by at least one of the following:
- Rise in hematocrit >20%
- Fall in hematocrit >20% after IV fluids
- Pleural effusion, ascites, hypoalbuminemia.

Criteria for Dengue Shock Syndrome

All features of DHF plus circulatory failure are manifested by:
- Rapid and weak pulse
- Narrow pulse pressure (<20 mm Hg)
- Hypotension
- Cold dry skin, restlessness.

WHO Case Definition of Dengue Fever[9] (Fig. 2)

Probable Case

An acute febrile illness with two or more of the following:
- Headache
- Retro-orbital pain
- Backache, myalgia, arthralgia
- Anorexia, nausea, vomiting
- Skin rash
- Hemorrhagic manifestation
AND
Supportive serology
OR
Occurrence at the same location and time as other confirmed cases of dengue fever.

Confirmed Case

Virus isolation from serum or tissue samples
OR
Demonstration of four-fold or more rise in IgG and IgM titers to dengue antigens in paired serum samples
OR
Demonstration of dengue antigen in tissue CSF by immunocytochemistry or detection of genomic sequence by PCR.

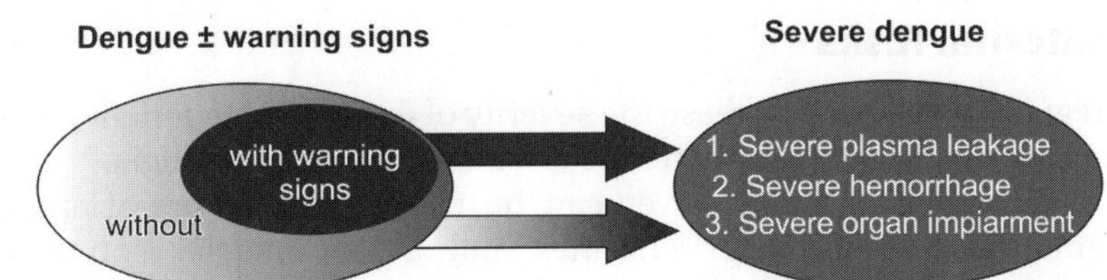

Fig. 2: Diagnosis of dengue

DIAGNOSIS

It is based on following investigations interpreted along with clinical picture:[6]

➲ Leukopenia (one of the earliest abnormality)

➲ Hemoconcentration (Suggestive of DHF)

➲ Thrombocytopenia — Platelet <100000/m^3 (Suggestive of DHF).

➲ Deranged LFT, RFT (in severe cases of DHF)

➲ Serological diagnosis (Table 1)

➲ Hemagglutination inhibition, complement fixation

➲ MAC-ELISA (Sensitivity- 95%, specificity-100%)

➲ RT-PCR—The gold standard, reverse transcriptase PCR using type-specific primers is highly sensitive and specific. It is only positive during the acute phase and becomes negative shortly after defervescence, so the detection window in the clinical setup to confirm infection is relatively narrow.[14]

Table 1: Interpretation of dengue diagnostic tests

Highly suggestive	*Confirmed*
One of the following: 1. IgM+ in a single serum sample 2. IgG+ in a single serum sample with a HI titer of 1280 or greater	One of the following: 1. PCR + 2. Virus culture + 3. IgM seroconversion in paired sera 4. IgG seroconversion in paired sera or four-fold IgG titer increase in paired sera

Maternal Risks

Pregnancy does not increase the severity of dengue infection. In general, the most common symptoms include fever, myalgia and arthralgia.[15]

Dengue hemorrhagic fever can be confused with pre-eclampsia and hemolysis elevated liver enzymes and a low platelet count (HELLP) syndrome as there is lot of similarity between the two clinical conditions such as thrombocytopenia, impaired liver function, edema, ascites.[10] Mortality rate can be almost 40% in untreated cases of DHF. The management of these two conditions is totally different, therefore DHF should be suspected in any pregnant women with fever during epidemics in endemic area and dengue serology should be done in such cases.

There is higher rate of caesarean deliveries and pre-eclampsia among women with dengue infection in pregnancy.[11]

Another possible effect of DF and DHF in pregnancy is bleeding due to severe thrombocytopenia especially in high-risk cases, such as placenta previa.[12]

Case report of multiorgan failure with maternal death is also reported.[13]

Dengue myocarditis has also been reported.[13]

Fetal Risks

Regarding the effect of DF and DHF in pregnancy, DF hardly causes any infant abnormality, but DHF might be responsible for fetal death.

Dengue infection in pregnancy carries the risk of hemorrhage for both the mother and the newborn. In addition, there is a risk of premature birth and fetal death and vertical transmission causing neonatal thrombocytopenia that necessitates platelet transfusion.[16-19]

If the mother acquires dengue infection close to term, there is a risk of vertical transmission to the newborn. The rate of vertical transmission varies between 1.6–10.5%. This may also be dependent upon the severity of maternal dengue infection.[12,20-22] Perinatal infection should be ruled out with serological studies and platelet count even if the newborn is asymptomatic.

➲ IUFD, miscarriage has also been reported.[13]

➲ Risk of preterm delivery is as high as 22%

➲ Sharma et al reported an increase in the incidence of fetal neural tube malformation in women who had dengue in the first quarter of pregnancy,[23] but such an association has been demonstrated following other febrile illnesses, due to pyrexia rather than to any teratogenic effect of the virus *per se.*[24]

TREATMENT

Prioritize patients according to the clinical picture and then treat patient accordingly.

Dengue fever in pregnancy most often is treated conservatively.[11] Hydration and supportive care that includes antipyretics, platelet transfusions, and management in an intensive care unit reduce the mortality rate.

REFERENCES

1. Halstead SB. Dengue. Lancet. 2007;370:1644-52.
2. Bancroft TL. On the etiology of Dengue fever. Australas Med Gaz. 1906;25:17-18.
3. Mairuhu ATA, Wagenaar J, Brandjes DPM, van Gorp ECM. Dengue: An arthropod-borne disease of global importance. Eur J Clin Microbiol Infect Dis. 2004;23: 425-33.
4. Jatanasen S and Thongcharoen P. Dengue hemorrhagic fever in South East-Asian countries. Monograph on dengue/dengue hemorrhagic fever. New Delhi: WHO. 1993;23-30.
5. Park K. The dengue syndrome. In Park's Textbook of Preventive and Social Medicine. Jabalpur: Banarasidas Bhanot. 1979;16:186-8.
6. Yeolekar ME. Chapter Dengue API Textbook of Medicine, 8th edition. 113-5.
7. Halstead SB. Etiologies of the experimental dengue of Siler and Simmons. American Journal of Tropical Medicine and Hygiene. 1974;23:974-82.
8. Rigau-Perez JG, et al. Dengue and dengue hemorrhagic fever. Lancet. 1998; 352:971-7.
9. World Heath Organization. Dengue Hemorrhagic fever—Diagnosis, treatment, prevention and control. Geneva. 1997;5-7,34.
10. Malhotra N, Chanana C, Kumar S. Dengue infection in pregnancy. Int J Gynaecol Obstet. 2006;94:131-2.
11. Pouliot SH, Xiong X, et al. Maternal Dengue and pregnancy outcomes: A systemic review. Obstet Gynaecol Surv. 2010 Feb;65.(2)107-18.
12. Carles G, Peiffer H, Talarmin A. Effects of dengue fever during pregnancy in French Guiana. Clin Infect Dis. 1999;28:637-40.
13. Kariyawasam, Senanayake SH. Dengue infections during pregnancy: Case series from a tertiary care hospital in Sri Lanka. Journal of infections in developing countries. 2010;4(11):767-75.
14. Sa-ngasang A, Wibulwattanakij S, Chanama S, O-rapinpatipat A, A-nuegoonpipat A, Anantapreecha S, et al. Evaluation of RT-PCR as a tool for diagnosis of secondary dengue virus infection. Jpn J Infect Dis. 2003;56:205-9.
15. Malavige GN, Velathanthiri VG, Wijewickrama ES, Fernando S, Jayaratne SD, Aaskov J, et al. Patterns of disease among adults hospitalized with dengue infections. QJM. 2006;99:299-305.
16. Chotigeat U, Kalayanrooj S, Nisalak A. Vertical transmission of dengue infection in Thai infants: Two case reports. J Med Assoc Thai. 2003;86: 628-32.
17. Chye JK, Lim CT, Ng KB, Lim JM, George R, Lam SK. Vertical transmission of dengue. Clin Infect Dis. 1997;25:1374-7.
18. Maroun SL, Marliere RC, Barcellus RC, Barbosa CN, Ramos JR, Moreira ME. Case report: Vertical dengue infection. J Pediatr (Rio J). 2008;84:556-9.
19. Fatimil LE, Mollah AH, Ahmed S, Rahman M. Vertical transmission of dengue: First case report from Bangladesh. Asian J Trop Med Public Health. 2003;34:800-3.
20. Tan PC, Rajasingam G, Devi S, Omar SZ. Dengue infection in pregnancy. Prevalence, vertical transmission and pregnancy outcome. Obstet Gynecol. 2008; 111:1111-7.

21. Basurko C, Carles G, Youssef M,Guindi WE. Maternal and fetal consequences of dengue fever during pregnancy. Eur J Obstet Gynecol Reprod Biol. 2009;147: 29-32.

22. Fernández R, Rodríguez T, Borbonet F, Vázquez S, Guzmán MG, Kouri G. Study of the relationship dengue-pregnancy in a group of cuban-mothers. Rev Cubana Med Trop. 1994;46:76-8.

23. Sharma JB, Gulati N. Potential relationship between dengue fever and neural tube defects in a northern district of India. Int J Gynaecol Obstet. 1992;39:291-5.

24. Moretti ME, Bar-Oz B, Fried S, Koren G. Maternal hyperthermia and the risk for neural tube defects in offspring: Systematic review and meta-analysis. Epidemiology. 2005;16:216-9.

Tuberculosis in Pregnancy

Sindhu Nandini Tripathy, SN Tripathy

INTRODUCTION

Mycobacterium tuberculosis infects about 32 % of the world's population. Tuberculosis has been a major cause of illness and death worldwide for ages and still continues to be so as a major health problem. In 2011, there were an estimated 8.7 million new cases of TB (13% co-infected with HIV) and 1.4 million people died from the disease. TB is one of the top killers of women, with 500000 deaths annually.[1] The greatest disease burden is during the childbearing years, which are between 15–49 years with 80% of all deaths from TB occurring in this group.

India is one of the highest TB burden countries of the world and it accounts for one-fifth of the diseased population (Fig. 1). Though it mostly affects the lungs, it can affect all the organs of the body including genital organs (Fig. 2).

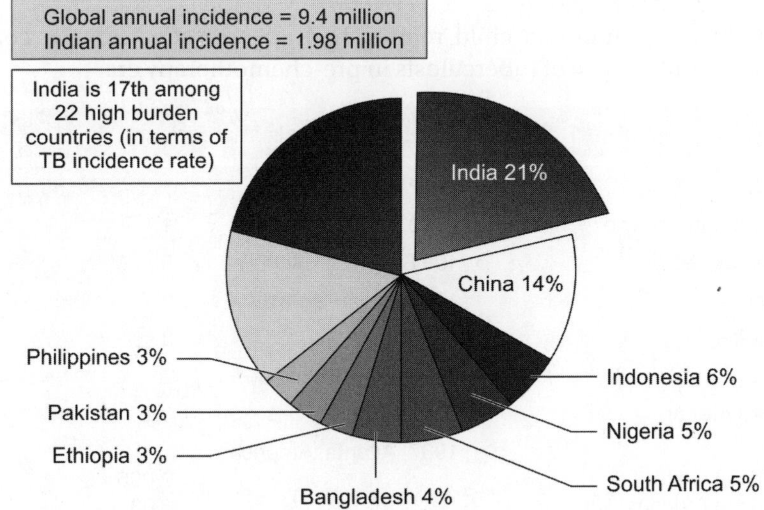

Fig. 1: World's TB burden WHO data, 2009[2]

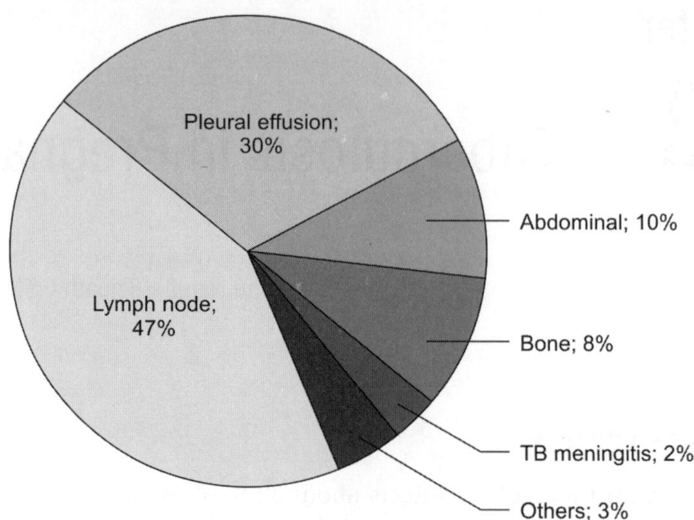

Fig. 2: Shows the EPTB incidences

There are very few studies about the incidence of tuberculosis in pregnant women. The prevalence rate in pregnant population varies between 2 and 5%. It is not much different from the general population of that country (Table 1).[3-9]

Though tuberculosis is a prehistoric disease, it is no older than pregnancy. Over the millennia, investigators have studied the interaction between the two, and in myriad of ways how the two interact, has been examined extensively and its for and against views,[10-17] even leading to the development of the dictum: For the virgin no marriage, for the married no pregnancy, for the pregnant no confinement and for the mother no suckling. Abortion was considered a viable option.

Childbearing, more so child rearing had adverse effect on the course, prognosis and relapse of tuberculosis in pre-chemotherapy era.

Table 1: Prevalence of tuberculosis in pregnancy		
Authors	*Year*	*%*
Browne and Browne	1960	1
Deshmukh et al[3]	1964 (Bombay, India)	5
Sikand[4]	1964 (Delhi, India)	2
Schaeffer[2]	1975	2
Tripathy and Tripathy[5]	1993 (Odisha, India)	2
Kothari A,et al	2006 (UK)	0.25
CDC American white American Africans American Asians	1987, Atlanta, America	 0.006 0.03 0.05

But presently with good chemotherapy, there is no difference between a pregnant woman and a nonpregnant woman, as regards the course, prognosis and relapse of tuberculosis. From different studies and from our study, it is conclusively proved that, if the patient takes adequate treatment for tuberculosis, pregnancy does not predispose the patient to a greater risk than the nonpregnant population. The relapse rate is not increased even if they become pregnant 3 to 4 times.[6]

Similarly, tuberculosis also does not have a deleterious effect on the outcome of pregnancy if treated early. There is no statistical difference in duration of gestation, preterm labor, and other complication of pregnancy labor and puerperium between the control and treated group.[6,19-21] There is also no increased risk of congenital anomalies in the treated group. However, the effect depends on factors like stage of pregnancy when management starts, nutritional status of mother, presence of concomitant disease, immune status and coexistence of HIV infection, availability of facilities for early diagnosis and treatment and the primary site of the tuberculosis. The results are good with pulmonary tuberculosis. Among the extrapulmonary tuberculosis, lymphadenitis is the most common form and has no adverse effect on the maternal and fetal outcome. The adverse perinatal outcomes are more pronounced in women with advanced disease, late diagnosis, and incomplete or irregular drug treatment. Intestinal, spinal, genital and meningeal tuberculosis are associated with an increased frequency of maternal disability, fetal growth retardation and infants with low Apgar scores.[22-25] Jana et al in an extensive nonrandomized review expressed the same view, though they highlighted the difficulties of diagnosing tuberculosis during pregnancy, especially extrapulmonary tuberculosis.[26]

CLINICAL PRESENTATION

Similar symptoms and signs between TB and pregnancy like tachycardia, anemia, raised ESR and low serum albumin level, as well as dissimilar parameters (like increase in weight during pregnancy and decrease due to TB, hypertension in the former and hypotension in the latter) confuse the clinical presentation of tuberculosis in pregnancy. Usually, the clinical presentation of tuberculosis in the pregnant women is similar to that in the nonpregnant patients. Cough, weight loss, fever, fatigue and hemoptysis are the usual features, but may be asymptomatic in up to 20% of women. A good history taking is a must as these women will not volunteer to tell that they are or might be suffering from tuberculosis even if they are taking the treatment as tuberculosis is a social taboo and stigma is still attached.[27] Other features like lethargy, abdominal distension, and irritability and skin lesions may also be seen. Extrapulmonary tuberculosis is also fairly common and has been observed in 20% of cases. Lymphadenitis is the most common form of extrapulmonary tuberculosis. Other forms of extrapulmonary tuberculosis such as intestinal, spinal and meningeal tuberculosis are associated with an increased frequency of maternal disability, fetal growth retardation and infants with low Apgar scores. Patients coinfected with HIV have a greater incidence of extrapulmonary tuberculosis. Multidrug resistant tuberculosis (MDR-TB) should be as common during pregnancy as in the nonpregnant patients, although this is not documented. However, pregnant mothers with MDR-TB have increased risk of maternal and neonatal complications.

DIAGNOSIS

A high degree of suspicion complete with relevant investigations is necessary for correct diagnosis. If the PPD is positive Flow chart 1, a careful history should be taken focusing on signs and symptoms of tuberculosis, any past or present contacts, history of a negative PPD in the past 2 years, and risk factors for immunosuppression. If there are no symptoms suspicious for active TB and no evidence of immunosuppression, a shielded chest radiograph (CXR) can be done in the second trimester. If symptoms or immunosuppression are present, a shielded CXR should be done immediately, even in the first trimester.

If the CXR is read as suspicious or positive for active TB, two sputum samples must be collected on two separate occasions to send for smear and culture to identify acid fast bacilli.

Histopathological examination of biopsy material also clinches the diagnosis. Fine needle aspiration cytology/biopsy (FNAC/FNAB), helps in diagnosis, but negative findings do not exclude tuberculosis.

Flow chart 1: Algorithm for investigation and treatment of tuberculosis

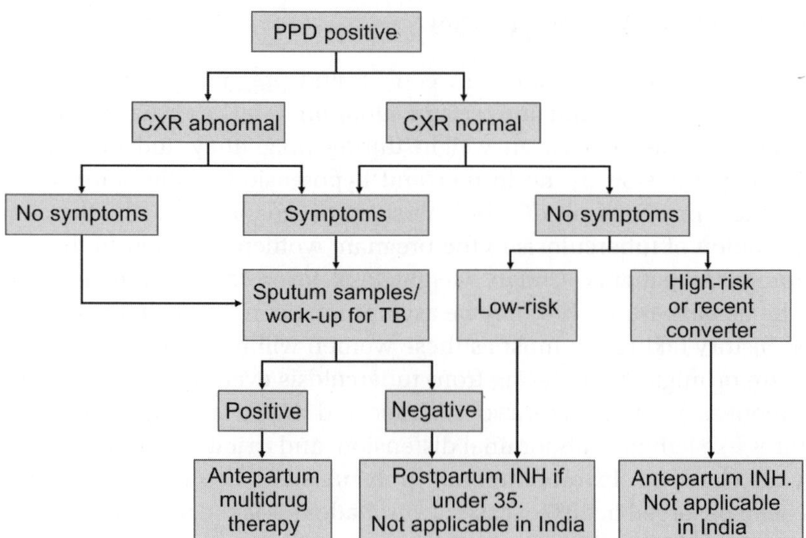

MANAGEMENT

In 1944, first drug that could kill the bacilli in the body of the patient without damaging normal tissues was discovered. The discovery of streptomycin changed the outlook of tuberculosis. A number of drugs have been discovered thereafter PAS (1949), Isoniazid (1952), Pyrazinamide (1954), Cycloserine (1950,) Ethambutol (1962) and Rifampicin in late 1960's. With the use of pyrazinamide and rifampicin, the treatment of tuberculosis could be shortened to six months, so called short course chemotherapy as opposed to conventional treatment using streptomycin and isoniazid, thiacetazone or ethambutol where the duration had to be for minimum of one-year duration. The introduction of rifampicin containing regimens of chemotherapy has had a great impact on the tuberculosis situation as a whole. Not only there is increased cure rate; it also makes the patient noninfectious early.

For 40 years, there were no significant advances in antituberculosis drug development, now few drugs are coming out. The new drugs are rifampicin derivatives (rifabutin and rifapentine), linezolid, and β-lactam antibiotics. Sudoterb LL 3858 is another new molecule which has a great promise. The nitroimidazopyrans are structurally similar to the antibiotic metronidazole. The lead compound, PA-824, is bactericidal against *Mycobacterium tuberculosis* including multidrug resistant strains. But their safety in pregnancy is not known.

A number of drugs are used in the treatment of tuberculosis. Some of them kill the bacilli (bactericidal drugs) while others do not allow the bacilli to multiply in vitro (bacteriostatic drugs), however, a bactericidal drug may become bacteriostatic on a lesser dose.[28]

Treatment must be multidisciplinary, which consists of a chest physician, general practitioner, pediatricians, health visitors, social workers, and of course the gynecologist and obstetrician. The ideal time to give advice concerning the risk and benefit of drug use during pregnancy is at a preconception counseling clinic. But unfortunately, most requests for information come after the pregnancy has began, usually after the exposure has occurred. Chemotherapy is the hallmark and short course chemotherapy is the treatment of choice. The maternal mortality, the neonatal mortality and morbidity is very less if the treatment starts earlier. No harmful effect is observed even if the drugs are given in first trimester.

Pulmonary and extrapulmonary diseases are treated with the same regimens. Some experts recommend 9–12 months of treatment for TB meningitis given the serious risk of disability and mortality and 9 months of treatment for TB bones or joints because of the difficulties in assessing treatment response. The WHO regimen to treat tuberculosis is given in Table 2.

The ideal chemotherapy of tuberculosis consists of two phases:

- Initial intensive phase to achieve a rapid reduction in bacterial population by use of at least two bactericidal drugs, preferably three or four. Rapid killing of bacilli reduces the chances of emergence of drug resistant mutants and also persistence, thus avoiding relapse after complete treatment
- Continuation phase that is aimed at sterilization of the lesions. Two or three drugs are usually continued.

Table 2: WHO, recommended doses of antitubercular drugs			
Drugs	**Daily doses (mg/kg)**	**Route**	**Thrice weekly dosage (mg/kg/dose)**
Isoniazid (H)	5 (4–6)	Oral	10 (8–12)
Rifampicin (R)	10 (8–12)	Oral	10 (8–12)
Pyrazinamide (Z)	25 (25–30)	Oral	35 (30–40)
Ethambutol (E)	15 (15–20)	Oral	30 (25–35)
Streptomycin (S)	15 (12–18)	IM	15 (12–18)

REVISED NATIONAL TB CONTROL PROGRAM (RNTCP) AND DIRECTLY OBSERVED TREATMENT, SHORT COURSE (DOTS)

Revised National TB Control Program (RNTCP) is based on the internationally recommended Directly Observed Treatment. The patient takes the drug under the supervision of a health worker to insure regularity of consumption of drugs.

We give daily DOTS, because if the patient misses one dose of the regimen, it will be more harmful than a single day regimen missing one dose, as it is very difficult to diagnose as well as monitor a case of MDR tuberculosis. This type of therapy can be easily accomplished in the case of pregnancy, with patients coming in regularly for routine prenatal care. The WHO now opines daily dosing under supervision. The rates of acquired drug resistance were higher among patients receiving three times weekly dosing than among patients who received daily drug administration throughout treatment.

A Fixed dose combination (FDC) is to be administered and all drugs should be administered in single daily doses (Tables 3 and 4). Rifampicin must be given in empty stomach followed by meals 1–2 hours after drug intake. It is well known that many of the toxicities of SCC drugs are dose related. Dose adjusted for pretreatment body weight is an important feature of antituberculous therapy. The three most important drugs HRZ are hepatotoxic. It has been shown that the risk of hepatotoxicity was only 2 % if drugs were accurately adjusted for body weight. Quality assurance is essential to insure adequate bioavailability of the component drugs of FDCs. Using them does not obviate the need for separate drugs for patients who develop drug toxicity or intolerance or for those with contraindications to specific component drugs.

Pyridoxine supplementation is recommended for all pregnant or breast-feeding women taking isoniazid.

Although all these drugs have been shown to cross the placenta, reaching 10–15 percent of maternal levels in utero, INH, RIF, and ETH, PZA have not been shown to have teratogenic effec . Streptomycin is the only first-line drug generally contraindicated in pregnancy. Maternal and fetal effects of anti TB Therapy are given in Table 5.

Table 3: Fixed dose formulation

Fixed dose formulation	Each tablet for 15 kg body weight
Isoniazid (H)	75 mg
Rifampicin (R)	150 mg
Ethambutol(E)	275 mg
Pyrazinamide (Z)	400 mg

Table 4: Recommended doses

<15 kg	1 tablet
15–30 kg	2 tablets
30–45 kg	3 tablets
45–60 kg	4 tablets
>60 kg	5 tablets

FOLLOW-UP

During treatment of patients with pulmonary TB, a sputum specimen for microscopic examination should be done at completion of the intensive phase of treatment. If smear is positive at month two, sputum sample should be obtained again at month three. In previously treated patients, if the specimen obtained at the end of the intensive phase (month 3) is smear positive, sputum culture and DST should be performed. In extrapulmonary tuberculosis, clinical monitoring is the usual way of assessing the response to treatment. As in the pulmonary smear negative disease, the weight of the patient is a useful indicator.[29] In addition, it is essential that patients have clinical evaluation at least monthly to identify possible adverse effects of the anti-tuberculosis medication and to assess adherence.

MDR TUBERCULOSIS

Though the incidence of single and multiple drug resistant TB is increasing throughout the world, the real incidence of MDR tuberculosis in pregnancy is not known, as also the effect of pregnancy on the disease and the *vice versa*. Literature available is very scanty and whatever is available are case reports or study of few cases from which no definite conclusion can be drawn.[30-32] Pregnant patients should be carefully evaluated taking into account gestational age and severity of the DR-TB. The risks and benefits of treatment should be carefully considered, with the primary goal of smear conversion to protect the health of the mother and the child. Management of drug resistant tuberculosis is done as recommended by WHO (PMDT). Drug susceptibility testing (DST) is a must for both first line and second line drugs.[33]

Table 5: Effect of anti-TB drugs on the fetus and newborn

Drug	Teratogenic effect	Pregnancy data	safety	Breastfeeding
Isoniazid (H)	NIL	Present in fetal blood	Yes	Pyridoxine 10mg/day to decrease peripheral neuropathy, yes
Rifampicin (R)	NIL	Present in fetal blood	Yes	Yes
Ethambutol (E)	NIL	-	Yes	Monthly visit for eye testing. Yes
Pyrazinamide (Z)	NIL	-	Yes	Yes
Streptomycin (S)		Present in fetal blood, Ototoxicity	No	
Thiacetazone (T)	NIL	-	Yes	
Kanamycin	Unknown	Category D Ototoxicity	No	Yes
Capreomycin	Wavy ribs in rats	Category C -	No	Concentration in breast milk –Unknown
Cycloserine	Unknown	Category C -	No	Yes, with B_6 supplementation
Ethionamide, Prothionamide	Teratogenic	Category C -	No	No
Amikacin		Ototoxicity, Category D	No	Alteration in bowel flora
Ciprofloxacin		Category C -	No	No, for arthropathy
Para-aminosalicylic acid (PAS)	Congenital defect	Category C -	No	Yes
Moxifloxacin	No adequate Study	Category C -	At present No	No
Colfazimine	Teratogenic	Category C -	No	No
Levofloxacin	Teratogenic	Category C -	No	No
Ofloxacin	No adequate Study	Category C -	No	Yes

When therapy is started, three or four oral drugs which are sensitive to the infecting strain should be used and then reinforced with an injectable agent and other drugs immediately post partum. The treatment lasts from 18 to 24 months. The drugs used are given in Table 6.

Formula food is preferred to breastfeeding. Till the mother is sputum positive, the baby should be taken care of by others. Whenever the mother and child are together, they should be in a well ventilated room and the mother must use a mask.

The obstetrician should suggest termination of pregnancy. If the patient still insists on continuing the pregnancy, all the risks and benefits of giving second line drugs should be explained and a written consent taken from the patient that she wants to continue the pregnancy. A case with MDR TB having resistance to any one of the second line injectable (Kanamycin, Capreomycin and Amikacin) and any one of the fluroquinolones will be considered as Extensively drug resistant (XDR) TB. In this type of tuberculosis, pregnancy is contraindicated and if it occurs, medical termination of pregnancy (MTP) is a mandatory.

HIV, Pregnancy and Tuberculosis

Most of the data regarding the pulmonary complications of HIV infection come from studies in nonpregnant patients. Apart from routine antenatal

Table 6: Groups of drugs to treat MDR TB

Group	Drugs with abbreviations
Group I First line Oral agents	Pyrazinamide (Z) Ethambutol (E) Rifabutin (Rfb)
Group II Injectable agents	Kanamycin (Km) Amikacin (Am) Capreomycin (Cm) Streptomycin (S)
Group III Fluroquinolones	Levofloxacin (Lfx) Moxifloxacin (Mfx) Ofloxacin (Ofx)
Group IV Oral Bacteriostatic second line drugs	Para Amino Salicylic Acid (PAS) Cycloserine (Cs) Terizidone (Trd) Ethionamide (Eto) Protionamide (Pto)
Group V Agents with unclear role in MDR TB	Colfazimine (Cfz) Linezolid (Lzd) Amoxicillin/clavunate (Amx/Clv) Thiacetazone (Thz) Imipenem/cilastatin (Ipm/Cin) High dose Isoniazid (high dose H) Clarithromycin (Clr)

Table 7: Antiretroviral drugs		
Drug class	**Name**	**Abbreviation**
Non-nucleoside reverse transcriptase inhibitors (NNRTI)	Efavirenz	EFV
	Nevirapine	NVP
Nucleoside reverse transcriptase inhibitor (NRTIs)	Zidovudine	AZT
	Lamivudine	3TC
	Stavudine	D4T
	Didanosine	Ddl
	Zalcitabine	ddC
	Abacavir	ABC
	Tenofovir	TDP
Protease inhibitors	Indinavir	IDV
	Ritonavir	RTV
	Saquinavir	SQV
	Nelfinavir	NFV
	Lopinavir/ritonavir	LPV/RTV

tests, screening for other sexually transmitted diseases should be done. As chest X-ray does not give a classical picture of pulmonary tuberculosis, the gold standard of diagnosis of pulmonary tuberculosis in HIV is sputum examination, that too repeatedly, as direct smear for acid-fast bacilli (AFB) is often negative, extrapulmonary tuberculosis is more common in HIV positive cases. No invasive procedure like cordocentesis should be done as it increases the vertical transmission rate. A high degree of suspicion coupled with relevant investigation is necessary for correct diagnosis.[34-37]

Treatment for tuberculosis, the short course chemotherapy like, 2 EHRZ + 7HR should to be given as soon as the disease is detected along with the antiretroviral therapy (Table 7). Now NACO and RNTCP are collaborating together to treat these cases.

LABOR AND DELIVERY IN TUBERCULOSIS WITH PREGNANCY

Close monitoring of labor and delivery should be done. Pulse and respiratory rate should be checked frequently. Prophylactic forceps or prophylactic vacuum delivery should be used wherever necessary. Lower segment cesarean section (LSCS) is done for obstetrics reasons, not for tuberculosis.

The Neonate

There is no statistically significant increase in congenital malformation in children born to mothers with tuberculosis. True congenital tuberculosis is rare, the risk to neonate being the acquisition of the same shortly after birth.[38] Delay in diagnosis contributes to high-risk of mortality. As usual, the treatment is chemotherapy for 6 months. They should be given INH prophylaxis for 3 months. If they become Mantoux positive after 3 months, continue prophylaxis for 9–12 months.

If negative, BCG vaccination is given. Other immunization is given as usual.

PREVENTION

Since Pulmonary TB is responsible for the spread of the disease, curing patients with sputum positive pulmonary form of the disease is the most effective form of prevention. It stops the disease at the source of infection.

In developing countries, preventive therapy is not recommended except in HIV positive patients, recent contact with patient with active tuberculosis, PPD skin test converting from negative to positive over the last two years, anyone at increased risk for progression to active disease (controversial).

In conditions where prophylaxis is considered, the management schedule is INH for 9 months (single drug regimen is used very rarely now a days), INH and Rifampicin for 6 months, INH, rifampicin, pyrazinamide for 3 to 6 months, BCG the anti TB vaccination has got limited effectiveness. It is not proven to be effective in preventing TB in adults or controlling TB in community.[39]

Usually the CDC Guidelines are followed. They are, infants and children in areas of high tuberculin positivity (greater than 1 %) and where surveillance is not feasible (India and other developing countries), PPD negative infants and children at high-risk of exposure to patients with persistently untreated or partially treated tuberculosis, PPD negative infants or children exposed to INH or rifampicin resistant tuberculosis.

There is no role for BCG vaccination in children who are tuberculin positive, since their cell mediated immunity has been sensitized to tuberculosis infection already due to prior exposure to the bacterium.

CONCLUSION

Tuberculosis is treatable, preventable, and a curable disease, neither the diagnosis nor the management poses much of a challenge. However, the challenge is still there. We are not able to control tuberculosis, though the tuberculosis control program has started from a long time the advent of HIV has a warning that the disease may reach epidemic proportions. In the new millennium, the vision of the Government of India is a 'TB Free India, works are going on in this respect to achieve the goal by 2015. For patients with pregnancy having active tuberculosis, therapy should be initiated as soon as the diagnosis is established. Irrespective of the duration of pregnancy, the treatment of choice is short course chemotherapy, 2 EHRZ+4HR in mg/kg body weight on daily regimen basis and preferably in fixed dose combinations.

REFERENCES

1. Global Tuberculosis Control: Surveillance, planning, financing: WHO report 2012.
2. Global Tuberculosis Control: A short update to the 2009 report: WHO/HTM/TB/2009;426.

3. Schaefer G, Zcrvoudakis lA, Tucks FF, David S, et al. Pregnancy and pulmonary Tuberculosis. Obstet Gynecol. 1975;46:706-15.
4. Deshmukha MD, Master TB, Kulkarni KG, Bahulkar HV. Pregnancy and Tuberculosis, Ind J of Tuberculosis, II. 1964;7:71.
5. Sikhand BK. Pregnancy and tuberculosis, Ind J Tuberculosis II, 1964.
6. Tripathy SN, Tripathy SN. Tuberculosis and pregnancy, Int.J of OB/GYN. 2003;80,3:247-53.
7. Kothari A, Mahadevan N, Girling J. Tuberculosis and pregnancy—results of a study in the high prevalence area in London, Eur J Obst, Gynae Reproductive Biology. 2006;126:48-55.
8. Centers for Disease Control (CDC) Leads from the MMWR, Tuberculosis in minorities- United States, JAMA. 1987;257:1291-2.
9. Ormerod P. Tuberculosis in pregnancy and the puerperium. Thorax. 2001;56: 494-9.
10. Snider DE. Pregnancy and Tuberculosis, Chest. 1984;86:S10-3.
11. Grisolle A. De L influence que la grossesse et la phthisis excercent receproquement l'une sur L'autre Arch Genre de Med. 1850;22-41.
12. Drolet G. Clinical Tuberculosis, Philadelphia, FA Davis company, 1939.
13. Rich AR. Pathogenesis of Tuberculosis. 2nd Edition, Springfield, Illinois, Charles C. Thomas. 1951;72.
14. Meheta BR. Pregnancy and Tuberculosis. Dis Chest. 1961;39:505-11.
15. Cohen RC. TB and pregnancy. Br J TB. 1946;40:10.
16. Hedvall E. Pregnancy and Tuberculosis. Acta Med Scand. 1953;147:1-101.
17. Stewart CJ and Simmonds FAH. Prognosis of tuberculosis in married women. Tubercle. 1954;35:28-30.
18. Crombie JB. Pregnancy and Pulmonary Tuberculosis. Br J of Tuberculosis. 1954;48:97-101.
19. Armstrong L, Garay S. Tuberculosis and pregnancy. In: Rom WN, Garay S (eds). Tuberculosis, Lippincott New York, NY. 1996;694-5.
20. Figueroa-Damian R, Arredondo-Garcia JL. Pregnancy and tuberculosis: Influence of treatment on perinatal outcome: American Journal of Perinatology. 1998;15(5):303-6.
21. Kovganko PA. The course of pregnancy, labor and perinatal outcomes in females with extrapulmonary tuberculosis Probl Tuberk Bolezn Legk. 2004;(2);38-41.
22. Jana N, Vasist K, Saha SC, Ghosh K. Obstetrical Outcomes among women with extrapulmonary tuberculosis. N Eng J Med. 1999;341:645-9.
23. Tripathy SN, Tripathy SN. Infertility and pregnancy outcome in female genital tuberculosis. International J of OB/Gyn. 2002;76:159-63.
24. Tripathy SN, Tripathy SN. Genital Tuberculosis and fertility Outcome. Book of Abstracts, 53 All India Congress of OB/GYN. 2010;129.
25. Tripathy SN, Tripathy SN. Perinatal outcome in Extrapulmonary Tuberculosis. Paper presented in 56th All India Congress of Obstretics and Gynecology, Bombay, 2013.
26. Jana N, Barik S, Arora N and Singh AK, Tuberculosis in pregnancy: The challenges for South Asian countries. J Obstet Gynaecol Res September 2012;38(9):1125-36.
27. Das P, Basu M, Dutta S, Das D. Perception of tuberculosis among general patients of tertiary care hospitals of Bengal. Lung India. 2012;4,29,319-24.
28. Zhang Y. The magic bullets and tuberculosis drug targets. Annu Rev Pharmacol Toxicol. 2005;45:529-64.
29. Treatment of Tuberculosis, Guidelines, Fourth Edition, 2010, WHO.

30. Shin S, Guerra D, Rich M, Seung KJ, Mukherjee J, Joseph K, et al. Treatment of multidrug-resistant tuberculosis during pregnancy: A report of 7 cases, Clinical infectious disease. 2003;3p,8:996-1003.
31. Palacios E, Dallman R, Muñoz M, Hurtado R, Chalco K, Guerra D, et al. Drug-resistant tuberculosis and pregnancy: Treatment outcomes of 38 cases in Lima, Peru, Clinical infectious diseases. 2009;1413-9.
32. Takashima T, Danno K, Tamura Y, Nagai T, Matsumoto T, Han Y, et al. Treatment outcome of patients with multidrug-resistant pulmonary tuberculosis during pregnancy, Kekkaku. 2006;81:413-8.
33. The programmatic management of drug resistant tuberculosis emergency update 2008,Geneva, WHO, 2008. WHO/HTM/TB/2008.402.
34. Espinal M, Reingold AL. The role of Pregnancy and puerperium in Tuberculosis development in HIV infected women. Int Con On AIDs. 1994;7-12,10:311.
35. Dalerio DlG, Mahamad AY, Leulseged TCl, Lopiso EK, Lindetjam B. The rate of TB HIV co infection depend on the prevalence of HIV infection in a Community BBC public Health. 2008;8:266.
36. Rapid advice for antiretroviral therapy for HIV infection in adults and adolescents, Geneva, WHO, 2009 (available at http/www.who.cdc.gov/tb/pub.arv/rapid_art_pdf).
37. Managing drug interactions in the treatment of HIV related Tuberculosis, Atlanta, GA, Centers for disease control and prevention 2007 (available at http/www.cdc.gov/tb/publications/guidelines/TB_HIV_Drugs/PDF/tbhiv.pdf).
38. Cantwell MF, Shehab ZM, Costello AM. Brief Report, Congenital tuberculosis. N Eng J Med. 1994;330:1051.
39. Young T, Hershfield E. A case control study to evaluate effectiveness of mass neonatal BCG Vaccination among Canadian Indians, AM J of Public Health. 1986;76:783-6.

Malaria in Pregnancy

Hiralal Konar, Picklu Chaudhuri

OVERVIEW

Malaria is a febrile illness caused by an intraerythrocytic parasite of the genus *Plasmodium* which is transmitted by the bite of female anopheles mosquito. It is estimated to affect between 350 to 500 million people annually and accounts for 1 to 3 million deaths per year.[1,2] Sub-Saharan Africa has the largest burden of malarial disease, with over 90% of the world's malaria-related deaths occurring in this region. Indian subcontinent is also considered a malaria endemic zone. Twenty-five million pregnant women are currently at risk for malaria, and, according to the World Health Organization (WHO), malaria accounts for over 10,000 maternal and 200,000 neonatal deaths per year.[3] Malaria in pregnancy also contributes to significantly higher rates of miscarriage, intrauterine demise, premature delivery, low birth weight neonates.

EPIDEMIOLOGY

Malaria is a parasitic infection caused by the 4 species of *Plasmodium* that infect humans: *vivax, ovale, malariae*, and *falciparum*. Of these, *Plasmodium falciparum* is the most harmful causing severe complications. The infection is transmitted by the female anopheles mosquito; therefore, factors that influence mosquito breeding, such as temperature, humidity, and rainfall, affect malaria incidence.[2]

PATHOPHYSIOLOGY

Malaria is transmitted to human host when an infected mosquito takes a human blood meal and the *Plasmodium* sporozoites are transferred from the saliva of the mosquito into the capillary bed of the host. The parasite migrates to the liver within 30 minutes and multiplies within the hepatocytes to form merozoites which are then released in the circulation and invades erythrocytes. Subsequently, merozoites differentiate into ring trophozoites and then to schizonts and enters the circulation after rupturing the wall of erythrocytes. This cycle repeats in 72 hours in *Plasmodium malariae* and in 48 hours in other species resulting in periodic fever spikes.

The ability of *P. falciparum* to cause adherence of erythrocytes to vascular walls leads to sequestration of infected cells in small blood vessels, causing end organ damage via hemorrhage or infarct. Renal failure and cerebral ischemia are two dreaded complications of falciparum malaria. Phagocytosis of infected blood cells occurs in the spleen contributing to profound anemia and folic acid deficiency.

It has been established that repeated malarial infections lead to some immunity. Therefore, malaria-naive and immunocompromised patients are prone to more severe infection. This puts pregnant women, children, travellers to endemic regions, and persons with coexisting HIV infection at highest risk for morbidity and mortality secondary to malarial infection.

Fetomaternal Risk

Pregnant women are not only at increased risk of malarial infection, but also 3 times more likely to suffer from severe disease as a result of malarial infection compared with their nonpregnant counterparts, and have a mortality rate from severe disease that approaches 50%.[4] The majority of sequele in pregnancy results from two main factors: the immunocompromised state of pregnancy and placental sequestration of infected erythrocytes.

Pregnant women infected with malaria develop severe anemia due to destruction of infected erythrocytes in spleen and sequestration of the same in placenta. In Africa, it has been estimated that malaria is responsible for 25% of severe anemia during pregnancy (defined as hemoglobin less than 7 gm/dL)[5]. Women with severe anemia are at higher risk for morbidities such as congestive heart failure, fetal demise, and mortality associated with post-partum hemorrhage.

Hypoglycemia is also commonly seen during malaria in pregnancy possibly as a result of infected erythrocytes in the placenta stimulating pancreatic β-cell production of insulin, leading to hyperinsulinemia and hypoglycemia.

Miscarriage, intrauterine growth restriction, preterm labor, congenital infection and perinatal death are frequent in pregnancies infected with malaria. The greatest degree of placental infestation is seen in women who have the highest level of immunity, leading to milder maternal symptoms and a disproportionate increase in fetal complications.

DIAGNOSIS

Malaria can be uncomplicated or severe. Uncomplicated malaria is characterized by a *cold stage*, consisting of chill and shivering, and a *hot stage*, with fever, headache, muscle aches and sweating. Symptoms generally last for 6 to 10 hours and occur every 2 to 3 days, depending on the infecting species. Severe malaria, the second subtype, is generally caused by *P. falciparum* infection and is characterized by renal failure, hemolysis and severe anemia, jaundice, pulmonary edema, acute respiratory distress syndrome, thrombocytopenia and cardiovascular collapse.

Diagnosis of malaria is confirmed by identification of the parasite on a thick or thin blood smear obtained by finger prick and fixed with Giemsa stain. More recent advances in diagnosis have been made with the introduction of rapid diagnostic tests (RDTs) using dip stick or strip with monoclonal antibodies against parasitic antigen. Most of the RDTs report sensitivities above 90% for detection of malaria, with increasing sensitivity as the level of parasitemia increases. Alternative laboratory tests as quantitative buffy coat centrifugal hematology, immunoflorescence, ELISA, PCR techniques are also available for detection of malaria antigen. However, complexity and cost of these tests prevents their routine use.

TREATMENT[6]

Uncomplicated Malaria

Pregnant women diagnosed with uncomplicated malaria caused by *P. malariae, P. vivax, P. ovale*, or chloroquine-sensitive *P. falciparum* infection, treatment with chloroquine (treatment schedule as with nonpregnant adult patients) is recommended. Alternatively, hydroxychloroquine may be given.

For uncomplicated malaria caused by chloroquine-resistant *P. falciparum* infection, treatment with either mefloquine or a combination of quinine sulfate (600 mg 8 hourly) and clindamycin (450 mg 8 hourly) is recommended. Quinine treatment should continue for 7 days for infections acquired in South-East Asia and for 3 days for infections acquired elsewhere; clindamycin treatment should be continued for 7 days regardless of where the infection was acquired. For chloroquine-resistant *P. vivax* infection, prompt treatment with mefloquine is recommended.

Doxycycline and tetracycline are generally not indicated for use in pregnant women unless the benefits of adding them to quinine outweigh the risk. According to its US labels, atovaquone/proguanil and artemether-lumefantrine are classified as pregnancy category C medications and are generally not indicated for use in pregnant women because there are no adequate, well-controlled studies in pregnant women. However, for pregnant women diagnosed with uncomplicated malaria caused by chloroquine-resistant *P. falciparum* infection, atovaquone-proguanil or artemether-lumefantrine may be used if other treatment options are not available or are not being tolerated, and if the potential benefit is judged to outweigh the potential risks.

For *P. vivax* or *P. ovale* infections, primaquine phosphate for radical treatment of hypnozoites, should not be given during pregnancy. Pregnant patients with *P. vivax* or *P. ovale* infections should be maintained on chloroquine prophylaxis for the duration of their pregnancy. The chemoprophylactic dose of chloroquine phosphate is 300 mg base orally once per week. After delivery, pregnant patients with *P. vivax* or *P. ovale* infections who do not have G6PD deficiency should be treated with primaquine.

Severe Malaria

Patients who are considered to have manifestations of more severe disease should be treated aggressively with parenteral antimalarial therapy regardless of the species of malaria seen on the blood smear.

Artesunate IV 2.4 mg/kg at 0, 12, and 24 hours, then daily thereafter is the recommended treatment. When the patient is well enough to take oral medication, she can be switched to oral artesunate 2 mg/kg (or IM artesunate 2.4 mg/kg) once daily, plus clindamycin. If oral artesunate is not available, a 3 day course of atovaquone-proguanil or a 7-day course of quinine and clindamycin at 450 mg 3 times a day should be administered.

Alternatively, Quinine IV 20 mg/kg loading dose (no loading dose if patient already taking quinine or mefloquine) in 5% dextrose over 4 hours and then 10 mg/kg IV over 4 hours every 8 hours plus clindamycin IV 450 mg every 8 hours (maximum dose quinine 1.4 g). When the patient is well enough to take oral medication she can be switched to oral quinine 600 mg 3 times a day to complete 5–7 days and oral clindamycin 450 mg 3 times a day for 7 days (an alternative rapid quinine-loading regimen is 7 mg/kg quinine dihydrochloride IV over 30 minutes using an infusion pump followed by 10 mg/kg over 4 hours). Serum electrolyte, blood glucose, renal and liver function, hematological parameters should be closely monitored. Supportive treatment for maintaining adequate fluid and electrolyte balance for prevention of hypoglycemia and for control of temperature is necessary.

PREVENTION

Pregnant women should avoid travelling in chloroquine resistant *P. falciparum* endemic areas. If travel is unavoidable, use of insecticidal sprays and mosquito nets are recommended.

Chemoprophylaxis for travel in areas without choloroquine resistant strains should be with chloroquine (300 mg base once a week, 2 weeks prior to travel up to 4 weeks after leaving the endemic area). In endemic areas where chloroquine resistant *P. falciparum* exist, chemoprophylaxis should be given with mefloquine (250 mg/week) following the same schedule.

REFERENCES

1. Centers for Disease Control and Prevention Web site, authors. Malaria facts. [Accessed August 1, 2009]. http://www.cdc.gov/malaria/facts.htm. Updated April 11, 2007.
2. The Global Fund Web site, authors. Malaria [Accessed August 1, 2009].http://www.theglobalfund.org/documents/publications/diseasereport/disease_report_malaria_en.pdf.

3. World Health Organization Web site, authors. Global Malaria Programme: pregnant women and infants. [Accessed July 30, 2009]. http://apps.who.int/malaria/ pregnantwomenandinfants.html.
4. Monif GRG, Baker DA (Eds). Infectious Disease in Obstetrics and Gynecology. 6th ed. New York: Parthenon. 2004;pp. 280-6.
5. Desai M, ter Kuile FO, Nosten F, et al. Epidemiology and burden of malaria in pregnancy. Lancet Infect Dis. 2007;7:93-104.
6. World Health Organization, authors. Guidelines for the Treatment of Malaria. Geneva: World Health Organization; 2006.

Chapter 15

Toxoplasmosis in Pregnancy

Hiralal Konar, Picklu Chaudhuri

OVERVIEW

Toxoplasmosis is a parasitic infection caused by an intracellular parasite, *Toxoplasma gondii.*

In immunocompetent individuals, the infection is mild and subclinical. Vertical transmission of infection to the fetus occurs almost solely in women who acquire the primary infection during gestation and can result in significant disease in fetus—newborn and even fetal or neonatal death.

PATHOGENESIS

Toxoplasma exists in three distinct forms: tachyzoites or arc form, found in the blood during acute infective phase; tissue cyst form, found in different organs of human and other animals during latent or quiescent phase and oocyst form, found only in the digestive tract of domestic and feral cats.

The infection can be transmitted by three routes: firstly through ingestion of raw or undercooked meat containing the tissue cysts; secondly through ingestion of unwashed fruits, vegetables or water contaminated with feces of the cats containing oocysts and thirdly vertical transmission from infected mother to the fetus.

MATERNAL AND FETAL OUTCOME

Toxoplasmosis is a mild, harmless self-limiting infection in immuncompetent pregnant women. It is asymptomatic in 90% of the cases. Nonspecific symptoms such as malaise, low grade fever, muscle pain are experienced by a few. Discrete, nontender, nonsuppurative posterior cervical or axillary lymphadenopathy may be seen during acute infective stage. A recent study revealed that 52% of mothers who gave birth to congenitally infected offspring could not recall experiencing an infection-related illness during pregnancy or an identifiable epidemiological risk factor.[1]

Transmission to the fetus occurs in women who acquire their primary infection during gestation. In rare cases, congenital transmission has occurred in chronically infected women whose infection was reactivated because of their immunocompromised state, e.g. from AIDS or treatment with corticosteroids for their underlying disease. The degree of fetal affection depends on the trimester during which the maternal infection occurred and also on availability of treatment to the mother.

Thiebaut and colleagues[2] in a recent meta-analysis, established a correlation between time of infection and fetal affection. It was found that earlier the infection is acquired; lower is the risk of transmission. However, where transmission does occur, there is greater risk of major fetal defects in women who acquired the infection early compared with women who had infection in later part of pregnancy. The estimated risk of transmission as shown in this meta-analysis was 15%, 44% and 71% at 13, 26 and 36 weeks of gestation respectively.

The problems encountered in the newborn are visual defects due to chorioretinitis, hearing loss, mental and psychomotor retardation, seizures, hydrocephalus, cerebral calcification, hematological abnormalities and hepatosplenomegaly. Intrauterine fetal death is the sequel in severe infection.

DIAGNOSIS

Identification of acute infection in the pregnant women is a challenge as the disease is often without significant signs and symptoms. Universal screening is also not cost-effective and not practised even in high resource countries. If clinical suspicion of acute infection occurs during pregnancy, serological tests are done to confirm diagnosis.

Serology

The detection (and quantification) of *T. gondii* antibodies in serum is used to establish whether a pregnant woman has been infected or not. If serological test results suggest a recently acquired infection, an effort is made to determine whether the infection was acquired during gestation or shortly before conception. IgG and IgM antibodies are usually detected by different methods as ELISA, DAT (direct agglutination test) or IFA (immunofluorescent assay). IgM appears sooner than IgG after an acute infection and declines rapidly. IgG appears within 1–2 weeks after acquisition of infection, peaks at 1–2 months, then declines at a variable rate, and persists for life. Interpretation of serological test done during pregnancy is given in Table 1.

Polymerase Chain Reaction (PCR)

Amplification of *T. gondii DNA* in amniotic fluid at 18 weeks of gestation or later has been used successfully for prenatal diagnosis of congenital toxoplasmosis. Amniotic fluid examination by PCR should be considered for pregnant women who: (1) have serological test results diagnostic or highly suggestive of an infection acquired during gestation or shortly before conception; (2) have evidence of fetal affection by ultrasonographic

Table 1: Interpretation of serological test results (done during pregnancy)

IgG test results	IgM test results	Interpretation	Further tests required	Fetal risk
Negative	Negative	No recent or past infection	Serial testing to detect sero-conversion may be done	Nil unless fresh primary infection occurs
Positive	Negative	<18 weeks—most probably infection was acquired before pregnancy. ≥ 18 weeks—difficult to comment on the time of infection.	Nil	<18 weeks—nil ≥ 18 weeks—unpredictable
Negative	Positive	As IgM remains positive for a variable interval after acute infection, the time of infection is unpredictable	The tests should be repeated in 1–3 weeks. a. IgG becomes positive, it denotes seroconversion, i.e. a recent infection during pregnancy b. If IgG is still negative, it is considered insignificant	a. If repeat test shows IgG-positive: risk of vertical transmission b. if IgG continues to be negative, no risk to fetus
Positive	Positive	Same as above	Confirmation to be done in reference lab	Same as above

examination (e.g. ventriculomegaly or hepatic or brain calcifications); or (3) are significantly immunosuppressed and at risk of reactivation of latent infection (with the exception of women with AIDS). A definitive study of the routine use of PCR of amniotic fluid obtained at 18 weeks of gestation or later was reported in France to have an overall sensitivity of 64% for the diagnosis of congenital infection in the fetus, a negative predictive value of 88%, and a specificity and positive predictive value of 100%.[3]

Isolation of the Parasite

Acute infection can be diagnosed by demonstration of tachyzoites in amniotic fluid or in tissue obtained from placental biopsy by immunoperoxidase technique.

Ultrasound

Ultrasound is recommended for women with suspected or diagnosed acute infection acquired during or shortly before gestation. Ultrasound may reveal the presence of fetal abnormalities, including hydrocephalus, brain or hepatic calcification, splenomegaly and ascites.

TREATMENT FOR PATIENTS WITH SUSPECTED OR DIAGNOSED *T. GONDII* INFECTION ACQUIRED DURING GESTATION

Spiramycin

When serological test results are consistent with a recently acquired infection and it cannot be excluded that acquisition of the infection has occurred during the first 18 weeks of gestation or shortly before conception, an attempt to prevent vertical transmission of the parasite through treatment with spiramycin is recommended. Spiramycin is a macrolide antibiotic administered orally at a dosage of 1.0 g (or 3 million U) every 8 hours (total dosage of 3 g or 9 million U per day). The drug is administered until delivery even in those patients with negative results of amniotic fluid PCR, because of the theoretical possibility of fetal infection from a placenta that was infected earlier in gestation.

The use of spiramycin has been reported to decrease the frequency of vertical transmission in a number of studies.[4-6] However, Spiramycin does not readily cross the placenta and thus is not reliable for treatment of infection in the fetus. In recent years, the effectiveness of spiramycin to prevent congenital toxoplasmosis has become controversial. Members of the European Multicentre Study on Congenital Toxoplasmosis (EMSCOT) have raised the question of the value of such treatment.[2,7] These investigators have suggested that carefully designed studies are necessary to clarify whether spiramycin is efficacious in prevention of congenital toxoplasmosis.

Pyrimethamine, Sulfadiazine and Folinic Acid

The combination of pyrimethamine, sulfadiazine, and folinic acid is recommended as treatment for pregnant women who acquire the infection after 18 weeks of gestation and for those in whom fetal infection has been confirmed (i.e. by positive result of amniotic fluid PCR) or is highly suspected (e.g. because of fetal abnormalities consistent with congenital toxoplasmosis detected by ultrasound examination). This drug regimen is used in an attempt to treat the infection in the fetus and, in some instances, with the hope of preventing transmission, especially in those women for whom amniocentesis for PCR testing cannot be performed and whose infection was acquired after 18 weeks of gestation. Pyrimethamine is potentially teratogenic and should not be used in the first trimester of pregnancy. The drug produces reversible, usually gradual, dose-related depression of the bone marrow. All patients who receive pyrimethamine should have complete blood cell counts frequently monitored. Folinic acid (not folic acid) is used for reduction and prevention of the hematological toxicities of the drug.

PREVENTION

Primary Prevention

Heath education regarding the preventive measures need to be imparted to women who are pregnant, who are willing for pregnancy and general public as well. The specific measures are:

Meat to be cooked "well" or thoroughly to 67°C (153°F). Meat should not be "pink" in the center (Meat that is smoked, cured in brine, or dried may still be infectious).

1. Mucous membrane contact should be avoided when handling raw meat. Hands should be washed thoroughly after contact with raw meat.
2. Contact with materials potentially contaminated with cat feces, especially when handling cat litter or gardening should be avoided. Wearing gloves is recommended when these activities cannot be avoided.
3. Disinfection of emptied cat-litter box should be done with near-boiling water for 5 minutes before refilling.
4. Fruits and vegetables should be washed before consumption.

Secondary Prevention

Early identification of women who acquire *T. gondii* infection during gestation, and if fetal infection is detected by prenatal testing, therapeutic options, including termination of pregnancy and antibiotic treatment of the fetus in utero are the secondary preventive measures.

REFERENCES

1. Boyer KM, Holfels E, Roizen N, et al. Risk factors for *Toxoplasma gondii* infection in mothers of infants with congenital toxoplasmosis: implications for prenatal management and screening. Am J Obstet Gynecol. 2005;192:564-71.
2. Thiebaut R, Leproust S, Chene G, Gilbert R. Effectiveness of prenatal treatment for congenital toxoplasmosis: a meta-analysis of individual patients' data. Lancet. 2007;369:115-22.
3. Romand S, Wallon M, Franck J, Thulliez P, Peyron F, Dumon H. Prenatal diagnosis using polymerase chain reaction on amniotic fluid for congenital toxoplasmosis. Obstet Gynecol. 2001;97:296-300.
4. Forestier F. Les fetopathies infectieuses: prevention, diagnostic prenatal, attitude pratique. Presse Med. 1991;20:1448-54.
5. Hohlfeld P, Daffos F, Thulliez P, et al. Fetal toxoplasmosis: outcome of pregnancy and infant follow-up after in utero treatment. J Pediatr. 1989;115:765-9.
6. Couvreur J, Desmonts G, Thulliez P. Prophylaxis of congenital toxoplasmosis: effects of spiramycin on placental infection. J Antimicrob Chemother. 1988;22:193-200.
7. Gilbert R, Gras L, European Multicentre Study on Congenital Toxoplasmosis. Effect of timing and type of treatment on the risk of mother to child transmission of *Toxoplasma gondii*. BJOG. 2003;110:112-20.

Chapter 16

Recurrent Urinary Tract Infections in Pregnancy

Kusum Gopal Kapoor, Tripti Sinha

Women in general and pregnant women in particular, are vulnerable to urinary tract infections. More than 50% have had one episode of such infection at some time in their life. In one series over a six month period, 27 % college students had one recurrent episode and 3% had 2 episode of urinary infection.[1] In approximately 3–5% of women, there are multiple recurrences over many years.[2] Such recurrent infections over a period of time can have a detrimental effect on the long-term renal function. Additionally, the cost of UTI is high in terms of lost time at work and cost of medical care.

Factors contributing to the susceptibility of women to UTI include a short urethra, proximity of the vagina and perineum with their contaminant bacterial flora to the external urethral meatus, urethral massage and trauma during sexual activity—all facilitating the introduction of uropathogens into the lower urinary tract.

In pregnancy, further factors come into play. Pregnancy itself is an immunocompromised state. Anatomical factors like the pressure of the enlarging gravid uterus on the bladder and lower part of the ureter coupled with the physiological hormonal relaxant effect of progesterone on the smooth muscle of the urinary tract aggravate the urinary stasis and/or unmask or worsen the vesicoureteric reflux, thus predisposing to recurrent urinary tract infections. Glycosuria provide nutrients for growth of uropathogens and aminoaciduria affects their adherence to the uroepithelium.

Urinary infections can complicate up to 20% pregnancies and are a frequent cause of antepartum admissions.[3] During pregnancy, lower urinary tract infections have a 25–40% chance of progressing to pyelonephritis. About 1 in 5 women with pyelonephritis will develop evidence of multiple system derangement from endotoxemia and sepsis syndrome including acute respiratory insufficiency.[4] UTIs in pregnancy also cause pregnancy-specific complications like premature contractions and labor as well as pre-eclampsia. Hence, screening for asymptomatic bacteriuria and urinary tract infections during pregnancy is a cost-effective intervention because of its direct positive obstetric outcome and wider public economic benefits.

Host factors for recurrent UTI include local pH and cervicovaginal antibody changes in the vagina, greater adherence of uropathogens to uroepithelium and pelvic anatomic difference, e.g. shorter urethra-to- anus distance. Maternal family history of recurrent UTIs is often obtained, indicating a familial predisposition to some extent.

IMPORTANT DEFINITIONS IN RELATION TO URINARY TRACT INFECTION (TABLE 1)

- **Significant bacteriuria/Asymptomatic bacteriuria:** Defined as isolation of a single microorganism with at least 100,000 CFU/ML (colony–forming units/mL). Most clinicians consider this to be clinically significant and prescribe treatment. Some recommend using CFU/mL of 10,000/mL or greater to increase the sensitivity of the test. Treatment of significant bacteriuria in nonpregnant state is usually not recommended except in diabetics.[5] In pregnancy, however, screening at the time of first prenatal visit and treatment is recommended to prevent serious renal infection. During pregnancy, incidence varies from 2–8%. Less than 1% women will develop acute cystitis and one-fourth of these women will subsequently develop acute pyelonephritis.
- **Urinary tract infection:** Bacteria in urinary tract causing its inflammation.
- **Symptomatic bacteriuria:** Urinary tract infection causing local or systemic symptoms.
- **Uncomplicated UTI:** Occurs in a healthy host in the absence of structural or functional abnormalities of the urinary tract.
- **Complicated UTI:** UTI, often recurrent, due to associated host factors which tend to perpetuate the urinary tract infection and are difficult to eradicate (Table 1).
- **Recurrent UTI:** Three or more episodes of UTI after complete clinical resolution in a twelve months period.
  - **Relapse/persistent infection**—Chronic infection by the same organism

Table 1: Host factors that classify a urinary tract infection as complicated	
Anatomic abnormalities	→ Cystocele, diverticulum, fistula, polycystic kidneys, urethral valves
Iatrogenic	→ Indwelling/intermittent catheterization, nosocomial antibiotic-resistant infections, surgery (renal transplant, nephrostomy tube, ureteral stent)
Voiding dysfunction	→ Vesicoureteric reflux, neurological (e.g. multiple sclerosis), pelvic floor dysfunction, high post-void residue, incontinence
Urinary tract obstruction	→ Bladder outlet obstruction, urethral stricture, ureteropelvic junction obstruction
Others	→ Pregnancy, urolithiasis, diabetes mellitus, immuno-suppression states, chronic renal failure

- **Re-infection**—Infection develops after a symptomatic cure (the initial infecting bacteria persist in the fecal flora after elimination from the urinary tract and subsequently recolonize the introitus and bladder) or if it is caused by a different pathogen.
- ⊃ **Indications for specialist referral:**
  - Women with risk factors for complicated UTI
  - Surgical correction of a cause of UTI
  - When the diagnosis of recurrent uncomplicated UTI is uncertain.

Surrogate markers for UTI include past history of UTI and positive dipstick tests, microscopy showing bacteria, pus cells and sometimes red blood cells in urine and symptomatology specific urinary complaints (dysuria, urgency, frequency, overt hematuria, hazy or malodorous urine, recent nocturia, suprapubic pain, costovertebral angle tenderness, absence of vaginal discharge or irritation) and non-specific complaints (fever, often with chills, nausea, vomiting, reduced appetite).

UROPATHOGENS IN URINARY TRACT INFECTION

1. *Escherichia coli:* Specific sero-groups are most commonly involved (80–85%). They possess virulence factors specific for colonization and invasion of urinary epithelium. Some of these include adhesions such as P-fimbria and S-fimbria which enhance binding to vaginal and uroepithelial cells by forming a biofilm which resists body immune response. They also bind to erythrocyte membrane and inhibit serum bactericidal activity by expression of the DRA gene cluster associated with ampicillin resistance. Other serogroups express an increase in K antigen production which protects them from phagocytosis. Greater adherence of type I to uro-epithelial cells in diabetes may be due to impaired cytokine secretion and blunted leucocyte response.
2. *Staphylococcus saprophyticus:* (5–10%)
3. *Group B Streptococcus:* In diabetics
4. *Proteus mirabilis:* Associated with catheterization, spinal cord injuries and structural abnormalities of urinary tract.
5. *Klebsiella pneumonia:* In diabetics.
6. *Pseudomonas aeruginosa:* Associated with catheterization, 4, 5 and 6 are commonly associated with catheterization.
7. *Enterobacter.*
8. *Entercoccus.*
9. *Staphylococcus aureus:* Due to blood-borne infection.
10. *Miscellaneous including Mycoplasma and anaerobic bacteria.*

DIAGNOSIS OF UTI IN PREGNANCY

Lower urinary tract infection (cystitis, urethritis) is clinically manifested by dysuria, urgency, frequency, suprapubic cramping pain or burning sensation, low backache, nocturia and hematuria. The urine is often described as cloudy, blood-stained and/or foul smelling (level 1 evidence Grade A recommendation). Symptoms generally start after sexual intercourse and last on an average six days. Their severity varies from mild to severe. With the presence of one typical symptom, there is a 50% probability of a urinary infection being present; with a combination of symptoms (dysuria, frequency, and absence of vaginal discharge), the probability rises to 90%. Hence, history alone is often sufficient to confirm diagnosis of UTI. Symptoms resolve promptly with antibiotics. Nocturia and persistence of symptoms between UTI episodes are strong negative predictors of recurrent infection.

Ascending infection causing upper urinary tract infection (pyelo-nephritis) causes back pain and costovertebral angle tenderness. Severe infections are accompanied also by systemic symptoms of malaise, fever, nausea and vomiting. Isolated lower urinary tract infection is not associated with vaginal discharge or irritation. Women who have had an episode of UTI often report with a self-diagnosis of a repeat infection based on their previous symptomatology.

Complicated causes of UTI must be ruled out on history and physical examination followed by relevant investigations.

INVESTIGATIONS

When working up a suspected case of recurrent urinary tract infection, the aim is to confirm or exclude significant microbial infection in the urinary tract and other conditions which predispose to the recurrence.

- **Urinalysis**—presence of bacteria, leucocytes, red blood cells in significant numbers are associated with urinary tract infections, and treatment may be started empirically.
- **Urine dipstick testing**—positive tests for nitrites and leucocyte esterase may indicate urinary tract infection. However, history and physical examination supported only by urine dipstick is not sufficient to exclude UTI. A useful clinical decision aid is dysuria coupled with more than a trace of leucocytes and a positive nitrite dipstick result and is strongly associated with a urinary tract infection and justifies the initiation of empirical antibiotic treatment while awaiting results of culture and sensitivity.
- **Culture and sensitivity** must be performed when the patient is symptomatic and in two weeks from sensitivity-adjusted treatment to confirm UTI, guide further treatment and exclude persistence (Level 4, Grade C recommendation). A clean-catch mid-stream urine bacterial count of 1×10^5 sample should be considered positive culture while the patient is symptomatic (1×10^4 CFU/mL for catheter sample; 1×10^2 CFU/mL for suprapubic aspirated urine).
- Only women with suspected risk factors for complicated UTI apart from pregnancy should be evaluated by **cystoscopy** and **imaging (abdomino-pelvic ultrasound)**. There is a very low pre-test overall probability of positive findings in all women presenting with recurrent UTI. Hence, these

investigations are not routinely recommended by various bodies like the Society of Obstetricians and Gynecologists of Canada, American College of Radiology and European Association of Urology.

- **Uroflowmetry** and determining **post-void residual (PVR) urine in bladder** are optional tests but are usually not needed. In combination with clinical parameters, abnormalities in these tests may suggest complicated UTI. In comparison, no significant difference in PVR and urine flow rates is noted between women with recurrent uncomplicated UTI and controls.

DIFFERENTIAL DIAGNOSIS OF RECURRENT URINARY TRACT INFECTIONS[6]

- Genital herpes
- Interstitial cystitis
- Irritant cystitis
- Overactive bladder
- Sexually transmissible infections
- Vaginitis
- Urethritis.

PROPHYLACTIC MEASURES AGAINST RECURRENT UNCOMPLICATED UTI

- **Conservative measures** including limiting spermicide and vaginal diaphragm use and pre- and postcoital voiding lack evidence for their efficacy but are unlikely to be harmful (Level 4 evidence, Grade C recommendation). Other hygiene modifications include wiping from front to back after using the toilet and urinating every 3–4 hours to prevent urinary stasis.[7] Using showers instead of bubble baths, cotton under-wears instead of nylon to reduce bacterial growth near urethra and avoiding perfumed soaps can also minimize chances of recurrence though there are no good quality studies to support such advice.[8] Evidence regarding vaginal diaphragms, douching and tampon use is also flimsy. The combined oral contraceptive pill and condoms without spermicides do not increase the risk for UTIs.

- **Cranberry products** (juice and capsules) have conflicting evidence regarding their efficacy (Level 1 evidence, Grade D recommendation.[9] They prevent *E.coli* from adhering to the bladder epithelium. They interfere with certain medications and should be taken after medical advice only. Long-term tolerance is also an issue with gastrointestinal upset occurring in more than 30 % women. The dose recommended varies from 150–750 mL.

- **Continuous antibiotic prophylaxis** is effective at preventing UTI (Level 1 evidence, Grade A recommendation). The prescribed antibiotic should have a safe track record during pregnancy and be avoided if possible during first trimester.

- **Postcoital prophylaxis** within 2–3 hours of coitus is also effective at preventing UTI (Level 1 evidence, Grade A recommendation).
- **Self-start antibiotic therapy** with a 3 day treatment dose antibiotic at the onset of symptoms is another safe option (Level 1 evidence, Grade A recommendation).
- **Vitamin C intake** to acidify urine and make it hostile for bacterial growth.
- **Limiting the intake of substances that irritate and inflame the bladder**—epithelium like caffeine and chocolates is another simple lifestyle intervention to reduce recurrence rates.

MANAGEMENT OF RECURRENT URINARY TRACT INFECTIONS

The aim of management is to treat the current infection by effective anti- microbials and confirm its eradication by subsequent culture tests. Symptomatic relief is also required for most patients, e.g. relief from dysuria and febrile episodes. Additionally, any associated remediable factors perpetuating the infection should be dealt with during or after pregnancy as appropriate to give long-term relief from recurrence and minimize renal damage.

Antibiotics considered as first-line agents during pregnancy include nitrofurantoin, amoxicillin, amoxicillin-clavulanic acid, cephalexin and cefuroxime. Second-line drugs include fosfomycin, trimethoprim and the 4-fluoroquinolnes. Recommended dosage is shown in Table 2.

Drugs absolutely contraindicated in pregnancy include sulfonamides, chloramphenicol and tetracycline. Trimethoprim in first trimester can cause facial and cardiac defects and should be used with caution. Fluoroquinolones can cause neural tube defects, hypospadias, maldescended testis, inguinal hernia, atrial septal defect and bilateral hip dysplasia. Hence, risk versus benefits should be weighed carefully before using it in pregnancy and is best to be not used in first trimester. Nitrofurantoin is safe but its use may be restricted during last few weeks due to risk of hemolytic anemia in fetus or neonate due to glutathione instability.

Table 2: Recommended doses of antibiotics during pregnancy

Drug	Dosage
Nitrofurantoin monohydrate/macrocrystals	100 mg po bd for 5–7 days
Amoxycillin	500 mg po bd for 5–7 days
Amoxycillin-clavulanic acid	500/125 mg po bd for 3–7 days
Cephalexin	500 mg po bd for 3–7 days
Cefuroxime	250 mg po bd for 3–7 days
Ciprofloxacin	500 mg po bd for 3–7 days
Fosfomycin	3 g single dose with 3–4 oz water

After completion of the prescribed course, a test-of-cure urine culture should be undertaken to confirm infection eradication. This may be followed by continuous/postcoital antibiotic prophylaxis for six to twelve months, the choice of antibiotic being determined by the local susceptibility profile, adverse effects and cost considerations.

Behavioral modifications relating to toilet and sexual hygiene and contraceptive practice after pregnancy may also reduce recurrence rates of urinary tract infection in the long-term.

REFERENCES

1. Foxman B. Recurring urinary tract infection: Incidence and risk factors. Am J Public Health.1990;80(3):331-3.
2. Hooton TM. Recurrent urinary tract infection in women. Int J Antimicrob Agents. 2001;17:259-68.
3. Bacak SJ, Callaghan WM, Dietz PM, Crouse C. Pregnancy–associated hospitalizations in the United States, 1999-2000. Am J Obstet Gynecol. 2005;192:592-7.
4. Hill JB, Sheffield JS, McIntire DD, Wendel GD Jr. Acute pyelonephritis in pregnancy. Obstet Gynecol. 2005;105:18-23.
5. American College of Obstetricians and Gynecologists Guidelines; 2003.
6. Bogart, et al. Symptoms of interstitial cystitis, painful bladder syndrome and similar diseases in women [published correction appears in J Urol. 2007;177(6):2402]. J Urol. 2007;177(2):450-6.
7. Dielubanza EJ, Schaeffer AJ. Urinary tract infections. The Medical Clinics of North America. 2011 Jan;95(1): 27-41.doi10.1016/j,mcna.2010.08.023.
8. Nicolle LE. Uncomplicated urinary tract infection in adults including uncomplicated pyelonehritis. Urol Clin North am. 2008;35(1):1-12. v. doi: 10.1016/j.ucl.2007.09.004.
9. Cranberries for preventing urinary tract infections. Cochrane database of systematic review (Online) 10: CD001321.PMID 23076891.

Pregnancy After Kidney Transplantation

Pankaj Hans

INTRODUCTION

For a woman with a functioning kidney graft, to undergo a successful pregnancy is the best possible proof of rehabilitation from end stage renal disease (ESRD). Pregnancy in kidney transplant (KT) patients was considered hazardous in the past. This concept has been revisited over the past years.

But pregnancy in a renal allograft woman is not without risk, as there is high incidence of abortion, hypertension and pre-eclampsia, premature rupture of membranes, infections, prematurity and intrauterine growth retardation. Besides this, acute rejection is also more common during pregnancy. So all the pregnancies in renal allograft women should be considered high risk and should be managed at tertiary care center by maternal fetal medicine specialist in conjunction with nephrologist and neonatologist. Careful counseling and monitoring should be done to avoid unnecessary complications.

One of the many perceived benefits of kidney transplantation has been restoration of pituitary-ovarian function and fertility in women of reproductive age. Fertility potential rapidly improves within 6 months after successful KT. The first reported successful pregnancy in a kidney transplant recipient occurred in a kidney recipient from an identical twin sister in 1958. Over the last five decades, pregnancy in renal allograft recipients has become more common, with over 14,000 such pregnancies documented since 1958.

The number of patients receiving an organ transplant and the incidence of pregnancy in the kidney transplant patient population has increased over the past decade. Advances in surgical techniques and immunosuppressive therapy have improved the survival and quality of life in organ transplant patients. Thus, the number of women within the reproductive age group with organ transplants has also increased. This development demands a heightened awareness of the factors relevant to organ transplant and pregnancy.

Renal transplant patients and their physicians must consider renal allograft recipient-specific issues as early as the pretransplant evaluation. These include changing fertility, contraception, pregnancy risks and complications for the mother and fetus, and immunosuppressive regimens. Post-transplant, recipients have higher fertility rates and are at risk of unplanned pregnancies. Contraception and preconception counseling should play an integral role in pre- and post-transplant education. Multidisciplinary prenatal care can help in successful outcome.

If a transplanted kidney is functioning well, the patient's chances of having a healthy baby are about as good as for a woman without kidney disease. Moreover, pregnancy while having optimal graft function is unlikely to have adverse effects on kidney function. Pregnancies in kidney transplanted women are often unproblematic. Nonetheless, such patients should always be considered to be at high risk. Pregnancy after KT presents a potential risk to the allograft, to the mother, and to her offspring.

FERTILITY ISSUES

As renal function improves following kidney transplantation, endocrine functions generally improve which leads to normal menstruation and ovulatory cycles; resuming fertility in most women. However, irregular bleeding is still a major concern among women with transplanted kidneys. In a study of menstrual problems after kidney transplantation, Ghazizadeh et al reported normal menstruation in 49%; oligomenorrhea, hypomenorrhea, or amenorrhea in 31.2%; and hypermenorrhea in 19.8% of 114 patients.

About 1 in 50 women of childbearing age with functioning grafts become pregnant.

CONTRACEPTION ISSUES

Optimal contraception is important to initiate before transplantation in women of childbearing age. Contraception should be used before transplantation, because there have been several reports of women who were pregnant in the peritransplantation period. The peritransplantation period is not the optimal time for pregnancy because this is the time for highest use of potentially fetotoxic or teratogenic medications and a time when optimization of immunosuppression is essential.

The best contraception has historically been considered to be barrier method, but because of potential for contraception failure, the American Society of Transplantation Consensus Conference report recommended that transplant recipients be advised that barrier methods and intrauterine devices are not optimal forms of contraception. Intrauterine devices are not optimal because they require an intact immune system for efficacy. Progestin-only oral contraceptives as well as estrogen/progestin are probably acceptable for use in this patient population as long as hypertension is well controlled.

The best contraceptive agent to use after transplantation depends on considerations, made between the patient and her physician, of the desirability of pregnancy and consideration of the risks and benefits of each contraceptive method.

PREGNANCY ISSUES

The optimal timing of pregnancy depends on individual circumstances of the transplant recipient. Historically, the recommendation was to wait till 2 years after successful transplantation. This recommendation has been replaced by the American Society of Transplantation Consensus Opinion that as long as graft function is optimal, defined as a serum creatinine 1.5 mg/dL, with 500 mg/24 hours protein excretion, and no concurrent fetotoxic infections or use of teratogenic or fetotoxic medications, and immunosuppressive dosing is stable at maintenance levels, the patient can safely proceed with pregnancy. Given the increasing age of the transplant population, these recommendations might even be liberalized to waiting 6 months after transplantation in specific situations. There have been no specific recommendations for male transplant recipients with regard to post transplantation intervals and fathering a child.

Pregnancies that occur 5 or more years after transplantation may result in persistent impairment of postpartum renal function. This decrease in renal function seems to be related to poor tolerance to the stress of pregnancy by a kidney weakened by chronic rejection.

A major concern for kidney transplant recipients is whether pregnancy will worsen renal function and lead to graft loss. Overall, in the majority of recipients studied, pregnancy does not appear to cause irreversible problems with graft function if the function of transplanted organ is stable prior to pregnancy.

In early reports, the overall risk of graft loss was reported to be 10–20 percent.

Recently, the UK renal transplant registry reported the outcome of 188 pregnancies among kidney transplant recipients from 1994 to 2001. There were live births in 79% of pregnancies. Two-year post-pregnancy graft survival was 94% for patients in that cohort, compared to 93% among matched controls. A univariate survival analysis, however, suggested an association between drug-treated hypertension during pregnancy and poorer post-pregnancy graft survival. In patients with pre-pregnancy serum creatinine more than 1.7 mg/dL, a trend toward increased post-pregnancy serum creatinine was identified.

As in women with renal insufficiency who have not received kidney transplantation, the serum creatinine level at the time of conception is an important determinant of successful pregnancy in women with kidney transplant. The outcome of pregnancy depends on pre-pregnancy renal function. If a woman has a pre-pregnancy serum creatinine level of less than 1.4 mg/dL, the chances of having a successful pregnancy are 96 percent. However, if pre-pregnancy creatinine is more than 1.4 mg/dL, the outlook for a successful pregnancy drops to 70–75 percent and one-third of these pregnancies end in therapeutic or spontaneous abortions.

Potential causes of worsening renal function in a pregnant transplant patient include pre-eclampsia, acute or chronic rejection, recurrent kidney disease, dehydration, obstruction of the transplant ureter by the pregnant uterus, infection and medication toxicity.

The long term effects of pregnancy on renal graft is less clear but one of the few studies done on this suggests that pregnancy does not adversely affect the long term survival of the renal graft as well as the patient.

OUTCOME

According to one meta-analysis, the overall post-transplant live birth rate was 73.5%, and the overall post-transplant miscarriage rate was 14.0% compared to 66.7% and 17.1% respectively for the general US population. However, complications of pre-eclampsia (27.0%), gestational diabetes (8.0%), cesarean section (56.9%) and preterm delivery (45.6%) were higher than the general US population (3.8%, 3.9%, 31.9% and 12.5%, respectively). Pregnancy outcomes were more favorable in studies with lower mean maternal ages and obstetric complications were higher in studies with shorter mean interval between transplant and pregnancy.

Prematurity is a frequent condition in post-transplant conceptions. The severity of this risk depends on maternal renal function, the interval from transplant to conception and blood pressure control. Higher pre-pregnancy creatinine, maternal anemia, and uncontrolled hypertension are associated with higher incidence of prematurity and its complications like intrauterine growth retardation (IUGR) and low birth weight (LBW).

The UK renal transplant registry report provided obstetric data for 121 live births after kidney transplantation. 50% of these were preterm termination of pregnancy. Elective caesarean section or induction of labor was required for 64% and 24% of pregnancies, respectively. The main reasons were hypertension or pre-eclampsia 36%, deteriorating renal function 24%, intrauterine growth retardation 20%, and fetal distress 11%. Of infants, 52% had a low birth weight (LBW) and 22% had a very low birth weight (VLBW).

Factors Associated with Favorable Pregnancy Outcomes

- Good general health for about 2 years after transplantation
- No graft rejection in the last year
- Adequate and stable graft function
- No acute infections that might affect the fetus
- Maintenance of immunosuppression at stable doses
- Patient compliance with treatment and follow-up
- Normal blood pressure or blood pressure well controlled with one medication
- Normal allograft ultrasonography results.

Comorbid Factors that may Worsen Pregnancy Outcomes

- Etiology of the original disease that necessitated transplantation (i.e. chances of recurrence)

- Chronic allograft dysfunction
- Renal insufficiency
- Cardiopulmonary diseases
- Hypertension (HTN)
- Diabetes mellitus (DM)
- Obesity
- Maternal infection with HBV, HCV, or cytomegalovirus (CMV).

IMMUNOSUPPRESSIVE MEDICATIONS

Immunosuppressive medications are required to be continued during pregnancy in transplant recipients to prevent graft rejection. Immuno-suppressive therapy based on cyclosporine or tacrolimus, with or without steroids and azathioprine may be continued in renal transplant women during pregnancy. Other drugs such as mycophenolate mofetil and sirolimus, are not recommended based on current information available. Commonly used immunosuppressive medications are shown in Table 1.

Recommendations regarding breastfeeding while on immunosuppressive medications are evolving. The American Association of Pediatrics support

Table 1: The US Food and Drug Administration (FDA) classification for commonly used immunosuppressive medications

Drugs	FDA safety classification	Comments
Corticosteroids (prednisolone, methylprednisolone)	B – No evidence of risk in humans	Prednisolone does not appear to have teratogenic activity in humans at therapeutic doses. In utero exposure of human fetuses to a high prednisolone dose (>40 mg/day) increased the rate of spontaneous abortion, intrauterine fetal death, perinatal mortality, IUGR and LBW. Administration of glucocorticoid throughout the pregnancy may cause adrenal suppression but this is rare with doses < 15 mg/day. Thymic hypoplasia without a significant immuno-deficiency, depressed hematopoiesis, lymphopenia, hyponatremia and hyperkalemia have also been related to in utero exposure to prednisolone.
Cyclosporine	C – Risks cannot be ruled out	Cyclosporine treatment is associated with an increased incidence of abortions, stillbirths, prematurity, LBW and IUGR. Severe B cell depletion was described in newborns from renal transplant recipients receiving cyclosporine, azathioprine and prednisolone,

Contd...

Contd...

Drugs	FDA safety classification	Comments
		and this depletion persisted at three months of life. Despite known nephrotoxicity, infants antenatally exposed to cyclosporine had normal renal functions. A few isolated cases of minor abnormalities have been described, including osseous hypoplasia (leg and foot).
Tacrolimus	C – Risks cannot be ruled out	Preterm birth is common. Transient hyperkalemia and transient renal impairment are common. Cases of congenital malformation have been reported without any consistent pattern of affected organs.
Sirolimus	C – Risks cannot be ruled out	Few data are available on in utero exposure to sirolimus. It is contraindicated in pregnancy.
Azathioprine	D – Positive evidence of risk	The major reported side-effects are spontaneous abortions, prematurity, IUGR and LBW. Infants of mothers administered azathioprine during pregnancy often presented with neonatal leukopenia, thrombocytopenia, thymic hypoplasia, and decreased serum IgG, IgM, and/or IgA levels. These immunological abnormalities were transient and usually resolved at 1 year of age.
Mycophenolate Mofetil	D – Positive evidence of risk	Mycophenolate mofetil is contraindicated in pregnancy. It is associated with high incidence of structural malformations, including hypoplastic nails and shortened fifth fingers, microtia and cleft lip and palate.

LBW: low birth weight; IUGR: intrauterine growth retardation

breastfeeding by mothers taking prednisone and warns against breastfeeding by those taking cyclosporine. Studies are needed for other drugs. Until these studies are available, expert consensus is that breastfeeding need not be seen as absolutely contraindicated.

MANAGEMENT OF KIDNEY TRANSPLANT RECIPIENT

Medical Management

- The patient should monitor her blood pressure daily
- Hypertension (HTN), which is a common problem in this patient group, should be aggressively managed
- Angiotensin converting enzyme (ACE) inhibitors and angiotensin receptor blockers (ARB) are contraindicated

➲ Methyldopa is the drug of choice. Clonidine and calcium channel alpha-blockers may be used as second-line therapy

➲ Graft function should be monitored closely; biopsy should be considered if rejection is suspected

➲ In the case of acute rejection, steroids are the preferred drugs. Steroids are considered safe, while the safety of antilymphocyte antibodies and rituximab is not known.

Obstetrical Management

➲ The pregnancy of a transplant recipient should be managed by an obstetrician experienced in high-risk pregnancies, in collaboration with a transplant physician and perinatologist or neonatologist

➲ Frequent evaluation is recommended (preferably every 2 weeks)

➲ The immunocompromised state in transplant recipients put them at increased risk for infections. There is an increased risk of maternal-fetal transmission of infections and its potential risk to the mother as well as the fetus needs to be considered

➲ Delaying delivery until the onset of labor in patients who have had a transplant is generally thought to be the most prudent step, provided the mother and fetus show no signs of distress

➲ Vaginal delivery is preferred and is usually delayed until the onset of labor, unless maternal or fetal indications for induction exist

➲ At the time of delivery, instrumentation should be minimized

➲ Cesarean delivery is indicated only for obstetrical reasons

➲ In the case of cesarean delivery, the exact location of the graft should be known to avoid injury to the allograft

➲ The transplanted kidney (which is usually in the pelvis) does not obstruct the birth canal and rarely causes labor dystocia

➲ Care must be taken to avoid fluid overload and infection

➲ Prophylactic antibiotics should be administered for all surgical procedures

➲ No anesthetic agent for general or regional anesthetics is contraindicated

➲ Pelvic osteodystrophy was described in patients with prolonged exposure to corticosteroids. This may necessitate cesarean delivery

➲ The dose of steroids should be increased at the onset of labor to overcome the stress of labor and prevent postpartum transplant rejection.

RISKS OF PREGNANCY TO FEMALE KIDNEY DONORS

The issue of kidney donation and subsequent pregnancy has been mostly ignored. Several small self-reporting surveys of women who became pregnant after donation indicated little cause for concern. A recent abstract presented at The American Society of Nephrology meeting brought out the possibility that donation may increase the risk for pre-eclampsia in post-donation pregnancies. Further data is needed before any firm conclusion is drawn.

RISKS TO THE INFANT BORN TO A TRANSPLANT RECIPIENT FEMALE

- Prematurity occurs in up to 50% of cases. It is associated with an increased risk for neonatal death, cerebral palsy, deafness, learning disability, and low IQ
- Intrauterine growth retardation (IUGR) occurs in up to 20% of cases
- Infants born may have low birth weight
- Immunosuppression is noticed in these infants, including low immunoglobulin levels and lymphocyte counts. Most of these deficits seem to normalize by the 6th month of life with no noted impact on the infant's health
- Although the rate of congenital malformations is similar to that in the general population, the number of pregnancies reported is still small; therefore, no definite decision can be made about a possible correlation between these malformations and immunosuppressive medication
- Risk is increased for congenital infections including toxoplasmosis, HBV, HCV and CMV
- Risk is increased for autoimmune diseases.

INDIAN DATA

In India, pregnancy in a renal allograft recipient is still a less common event and considered risky. However, the situation is changing gradually and anecdotal case reports showing successful outcomes have been published from India. These case reports show that if pregnancy is planned in a patient with good general health, and the patient understands the importance and need for regular follow up, and stature compatible with good obstetric outcome and the time interval between transplantation and conception has exceeded more than 1–2 years, and patient has normal renal function (serum creatinine < 1.5 mg/dL), hypertension which is absent or satisfactorily controlled, no or minimal proteinuria, no evidence of active graft rejection or pelvicalyceal distension then the outcome of pregnancy is likely to be satisfactory. But if these criteria are ignored, the outcome of these pregnancies could be catastrophic, leading to morbidity, graft dysfunction and even mortality.

In India, regretfully many of these pregnancies are not planned, the allograft recipients being unaware that they could conceive and therefore take prenatal care quite late in gestation. Pregnancy after renal transplantation needs multidisciplinary care. In one report from a center in India, 83.3% women had good perinatal outcome. Good outcome can be expected in India when periconceptional renal parameters are normal and pregnancy is not complicated by hypertensive disorders.

SUMMARY

Although pregnancy is likely to end in a live birth in the majority of organ transplant recipients, there are potential risks to the graft, to the mother and to the fetus. Pregnancy in this population should be planned with combined care from surgeons, nephrologists, obstetricians, pediatricians and dietitians to offer the best chance of a favorable outcome in the mother and the fetus. Timing of pregnancy should be based upon whether graft function is optimal and not necessarily upon the time since the transplant. Most pregnancies in women with kidney transplants are successful but rates of maternal and neonatal complications remain high.

IMPORTANT MESSAGE

- Counseling for all the renal allograft recipients of childbearing age is important
- Pregnancy and delivery of a normal child is possible in a renal allograft recipient, provided careful planning and monitoring of pregnancy is accomplished
- If pregnancy is planned and monitored appropriately, outcome is likely to be good, and these women can be reassured that pregnancy is unlikely to substantially alter their graft function, but unplanned and inappropriately monitored pregnancies can cause morbidity, graft dysfunction and even mortality
- In India, in the renal transplant population—social factors also have a marked influence on the patient's decisions for pregnancy
- Antenatal care must incorporate serial assessment of renal function, control of blood pressure, early diagnosis and management of rejection, infection, anemia and meticulous fetal surveillance
- Vaginal delivery is feasible, since the renal allograft is not an obstacle to delivery; caesarian section is required for obstetric reasons only
- The long-term outcome of children of renal allograft mother is excellent.

SUGGESTED READING

1. Ahmad M. Outcome of Pregnancies in Renal Allograft Recipients. J Assoc Physicians India. 2003;51:208-10.
2. Hirachan P, Pant S, Chhetri R, Joshi A, Kharel T. Renal transplantation and pregnancy. Arab J Nephrol Transplant. 2012;5(1):41-6.
3. McKay DB, Josephson MA. Pregnancy after kidney transplantation. Clin J Am Soc Nephrol. 2008;3 Suppl 2:S117-25.
4. McKay DB, Josephson MA. Pregnancy in recipients of solid organs—effects on mother and child. N Engl J Med. 2006;354(12):1281-93.
5. Mukherjee S. Transplantation and Pregnancy. link - http://emedicine.medscape.com/article/429932-overview (accessed on 5-7-2013).

Chapter

18

Rh Isoimmunization

Dipika Deka, K Aparna Sharma

INTRODUCTION

Rhesus (Rh) negative woman who gives birth to an Rh positive baby is at a risk of developing antibodies against the Rh positive RBCs usually in a subsequent pregnancy, and rarely in the index pregnancy, depending on the amount of fetomaternal hemorrhage and formation of antibodies in the maternal Reticuloendothelial system (RES). Or if she gets exposed to red blood cells (RBCs) carrying the Rh antigen because of a mismatched transfusion. It is the Rh positive fetus who is at risk of anemia due to the hemolysis, resulting from the transplacental passage of antibodies against Rh +ve fetal cells in the maternal blood due to fetomaternal hemorrhage that occurs during pregnancy and in all cases at delivery. These antibodies coat the Rh positive cell and cause hemolysis, resulting in fetal anemia and hyperbilirubinemia. The severity of affection can vary from mild fetal anemia to severe anemia and fetal hydrops in utero, and from mild jaundice to kernicterus due to severe hyperbilirubinemia in the neonatal period.

Because of the widespread availability of antenatal and postnatal Rh (D) immuneoglobulin, there has been a significant reduction in the frequency of maternal Rh isoimmunization. The risk of RhD alloimmunization during or immediately after a first pregnancy is about 1–1.5%.[1,2] Administration of antenatal anti-D at 28–32 weeks gestation to women in their first or non-immunized further pregnancies can reduce this risk to about 0.2% without, to date, any adverse effects. Though this policy is unlikely to confer benefit or improve outcome in the present pregnancy, fewer women will have RhD antibodies in their next pregnancy.

However, isoimmunization still occurs[3,4] particularly in India and low income countries where prophylaxis is not available, delayed or inadequate. Retrospective review of cumulative reporting to the UK confidential hemovigilance scheme, Serious Hazards of Transfusion (SHOT), between 1996 and 2011 (15 years) showed a total of 1211 errors related to the administration of anti-D immunoglobulin, particularly regarding omission or late administration (157/249 or 63% reported in 2011). Anti-D immunoglobulin errors comprised 13.7% (249/1815) of all SHOT reports in 2011. Failure to recognize women who already had RhD sensitization occurred in 19 cases, and was followed by suboptimal monitoring of the pregnancy. Nine of the infants suffered hemolytic disease of the fetus and newborn (HDFN): One resulted in neonatal death and three required red cell transfusion.

Early detection of pregnant women with Rh isoimmunization, appropriate monitoring and timely fetal and neonatal interventions can insure a favorable outcome in majority of pregnancies. Ideally, alloimmunized pregnant women should be referred to a maternal-fetal medicine specialist with experience in managing this condition and with the expertize to perform intrauterine fetal blood transfusions.[5,6]

MANAGEMENT

Initial Approach

An Rh(D)-negative fetus is not at risk of complications from maternal anti-D antibodies; therefore, the first step in antenatal management of maternal Rh negative pregnancy is to test paternal blood group, which will help predict the fetal Rhesus type.

Testing for paternal blood group: The biologic father of the baby is tested for his Rh (D) type at booking, and if Rh (D)-positive, zygosity maybe determined early in the course of evaluation, though in practice this is not routinely done. Homozygotes always pass the Rh (D) antigen to their offspring; heterozygotes have a 50 percent chance of having Rh (D)-negative offspring. Quantitative polymerase chain reaction (PCR) DNA testing reliably identifies the presence of one or two paternal *RHD* genes.

Cell free fetal DNA testing to determine fetal Rh(D) type: Cell free fetal DNA (cffDNA) may be detected in the maternal circulation as early as 38 days of gestation; the amount of DNA increases with advancing gestational age and disappears soon after delivery. Fetal Rh (D) status can be determined by evaluation of cffDNA sequences in maternal plasma using a reverse transcriptase PCR.[7]

Testing amniocytes to determine fetal Rh (D) type: If the paternal phenotype is heterozygous for Rh (D) or unknown and cffDNA testing is not available, Then fetal blood genotype can be determined by PCR on uncultured amniocytes. This is not done routinely, but if amniocentesis is done for genetic condition, this can be done.[8,9]

First Immunized Pregnancy

Monitoring maternal anti-D titers by ICT— The indirect Coomb's titer is used to detect not only the presence, but also the degree, of alloimmunization. Antibody titers are interpreted as screening tests. A positive anti-D titer means that the fetus is at risk for hemolytic disease. It does not however signify that the fetus is affected or will get affected definitely. Variation in titer results between laboratories and intra-laboratory is common.

Critical Titer

Indirect Coomb's Test (ICT) Critical titer refers to the titer associated with a risk for severe fetal anemia. The critical titer will vary among institutions and methodologies; however, in most centers, an anti-D titer between 8 and 32 is considered critical; at AIIMS, it is ICT titer of 1:16. Below the critical titer, there is a risk of mild to moderate, but not severe, fetal or neonatal hemolytic anemia.

In the first affected pregnancy, serial antibody titers are determined every four weeks after 20 weeks of gestation as long as the titer remains below the critical titer. If the critical titer is reached or exceeded, then further assessment to determine whether severe fetal anemia is present is required as for immunized pregnancy. Checking maternal titers is of no significance now and should be discontinued.

Subsequent Pregnancies with Rh(D) Positive Fetus

In general, pregnancies after the delivery of Rh +ve baby will involve a greater severity of fetal/neonatal hemolytic disease due to secondary immunological maternal antibody response from the entry of Rh +ve fetal cells into the maternal circulation at delivery. Fetal RES is mature by 16–18 weeks after which Rh +ve fetal cells may be hemolyzed. For this reason, the severity of fetal anemia is assessed at beginning as early as 16 weeks of gestation.

ASSESSMENT OF FETAL ANEMIA

Doppler's assessment of the fetal middle cerebral artery (MCA) peak systolic velocity is currently the best non-invasive method for prediction of fetal anemia.[10,11] Other ultrasonographic parameters that have been used to predict the presence of severe fetal anemia are placental thickness, umbilical vein diameter, hepatic size, splenic size, polyhydramnios, etc but none have proven to be sufficiently reliable for clinical practice. Ultrasound detection of hydrops is a late sign of severe fetal anemia.

Middle Cerebral Artery-peak Systolic Velocity (Fig. 1)

Doppler's assessment of the fetal MCA peak systolic velocity (PSV) in alloimmunized pregnancies is based on the principle that the anemic fetus preserves oxygen delivery to the brain by increasing cerebral flow of low viscosity blood.

The sensitivity of increased MCA-PSV (above 1.5 multiples of the median [MoMs]) for the prediction of moderate or severe anemia in a landmark study was 100 percent (95% CI 86–100), either in the presence or absence of hydrops, with a false positive rate of 12 percent.[1] Ideally, MCA-PSV is measured when

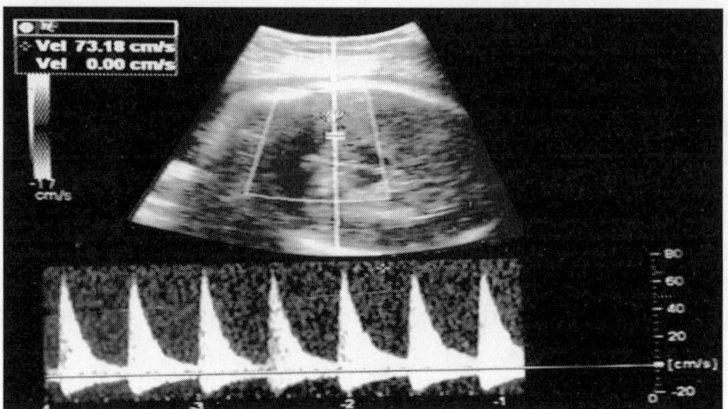

Fig. 1: Raised MCA-PSV in Rh isoimmunized fetus

the fetus is in a quiet behavioral state. MCA-PSV increases across gestation and results should be adjusted for gestational age. Measurements can be initiated as early as 16 weeks of gestation if there is a past history of early severe fetal anemia, otherwise Doppler evaluation is begun later since intrauterine, intravascular transfusions are very difficult before 20 weeks of gestation. The optimal interval between examinations has not been determined, but should be one to two weeks based on clinical experience and what is known about progression of fetal anemia in this setting.

Other Methods

- **Spectral analysis of amniotic fluid:** In the past, amniocentesis to determine amniotic fluid bilirubin levels was the usual method for indirectly estimating the severity of fetal anemia. However, with the availability of noninvasive Doppler monitoring, its use has now become very limited.
- **Fetal blood sampling:** Ultrasound-directed fetal blood sampling (i.e. percutaneous umbilical blood sampling, cordocentesis, funipuncture) allows direct access to the fetal circulation to obtain important laboratory values such as hematocrit, direct Coomb's, fetal blood type, reticulocyte count and platelet count. Because this procedure is associated with a 1 to 2 percent rate of fetal loss, fetal blood sampling is usually done immediately before the intrauterine transfusion, keeping the blood and setup for transfusion ready.

INDICATIONS FOR FETAL BLOOD TRANSFUSION OR DELIVERY

Severe fetal anemia can be defined as a hematocrit below 30 percent or two standard deviations below the mean hematocrit for the gestational age. MCA-PSV of > 1.5 MoM is a good predictor of severe fetal anemia requiring blood transfusion or delivery.[10,11]

Severe fetal anemia is an indication for intervention because fetal cardiac failure will eventually develop. Intrauterine transfusions for severe fetal anemia are generally performed between 18 and 34 weeks of gestation. Before 18 weeks, fetal transfusions are rarely successful due to limited visualization and the small size of the relevant anatomic structures. Prior to 20 weeks of gestation, intraperitoneal fetal transfusion is technically easier than intravascular transfusion. When technically possible, the intravascular transfusion is preferred because the therapeutic effects are more rapid and reliable. After 34 weeks, the procedure is generally considered riskier than late preterm delivery for neonatal treatment of severe anemia.

Intrauterine Fetal Blood Transfusion (IUT) (Figs 2 and 3)

Preparation/Requirements specific to IUT include:

- Type O Rh(D) negative RBCs are transfused
- Donor units are screened for antibody to cytomegalovirus (CMV); the units must be negative
- The donation should be relatively fresh to enhance the level of 2, 3-diphosphoglycerate (DPG). The red cells used for IUT should not have been stored for more than five days

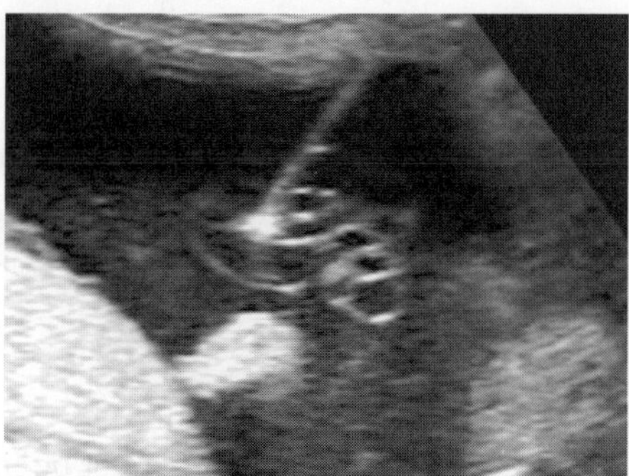

Fig. 2: Needle in umbilical vein for IUT

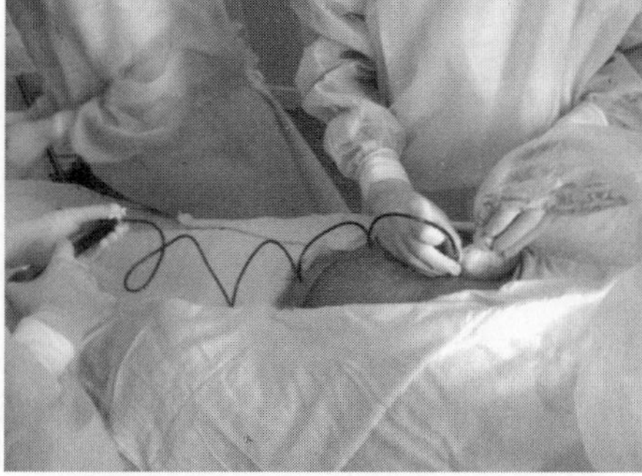

Fig. 3: Packed cells being transfused through needle
(For color version, see Plate 1)

- The red cell units for IUT should undergo irradiation with 25 Gy of gamma radiation to the central portion of the donor bag to prevent a graft-versus-host reaction
- Leukodepletion should be done as it reduces CMV risk
- Units are washed and tightly packed to a final hematocrit of 75 to 85 percent to reduce the volume administered to the fetus at the time of IUT.

Access Site

- Direct vascular access—Intravascular transfusion (IVT) is the preferred route especially in the presence of hydrops. It can be done either at the placental end or the fetal end of the cord or the intrahepatic portion of the umbilical vein. It is generally preferred to intraperitoneal transfusion (IPT) because IVT is significantly more effective in hydropic fetuses and the effects of transfusion are more rapid. Puncture of the intrahepatic portion of the umbilical vein has several advantages. There is a low incidence of fetal bradycardia, probably due to absence of inadvertent umbilical artery puncture at this anatomical level, and additionally blood loss from the cord puncture site is compensated, at least in part, by its subsequent absorption from the peritoneal cavity. A disadvantage is that IVT using the intrahepatic umbilical vein may result in a greater degree of fetal pain. The fetal movement may dislodge the needle.
- Peritoneal cavity—Intraperitoneal transfusion (IPT) provides indirect access to the fetal circulation. It utilizes the principle that fluid and cells in the peritoneal cavity are absorbed through the diaphragmatic lymphatics. In the hydropic fetus, however, a functional blockage of the lymphatic system probably exists and prevents good absorption of RBCs after IPT.

Special Circumstances

Several circumstances deserve special mention:
- Gestational age less than 22 weeks—If IUTs must be initiated early in the second trimester (<22 weeks), an IPT is often the best approach
- Fetal ascites—If fetal ascites is present, blood placed by IPT will not be absorbed. In these cases, IVT by targeting the umbilical cord, intrahepatic portion of the umbilical vein, or in extreme cases, the fetal heart, is warranted.

Intravascular Blood Transfusion

The volume of blood to be transfused can be calculated by the Mandelbrot's formula given by:

Volume transfused (mL) = Volume of fetoplacental unit (mL) × (final – initial hematocrit) divided by the hematocrit of the transfused blood.

The fetoplacental volume (mL) is calculated from the ultrasound estimate of the fetal weight according to the formula (1.046 + fetal weight in grams × 0.14).

Technique of IVT

- In case of fetuses who have crossed the period of viability, an operation theatre back up should be there to delivery in case of some complication
- Patients are usually instructed to avoid oral intake for six to eight hours before the procedure and an IV access should be secured
- The uterus is displaced to the left to reduce the risk of maternal hypotension and the abdomen is prepared and draped as for a surgical procedure. A single dose of prophylactic antibiotic can be administered half an hour before the IUT
- Under continuous ultrasound guidance using a curvilinear 2-D transducer covered with a sterile sleeve, the cord insertion site is identified and then a 20-gauge six-inch needle is directed into the umbilical vein
- An initial 2 mL sample of blood is withdrawn for Hb, hematocrit (hct), blood group
- After withdrawing a blood sample, a short acting paralytic agent can be given to minimize fetal movement. Alternatively, more commonly, fetal paralysis is achieved by giving an intramuscular injection into the fetal buttock or shoulder. Options include vecuronium (0.1 mg per kg of ultrasound estimated fetal weight) or atracurium besylate (0.4 mg per kg of estimated fetal weight), drugs which are associated with minimal fetal cardiovascular effects. Both agents cause fetal paralysis for up to two hours
- Transfusion is given using a three way connector and preloaded syringes of 10 mL each. During the infusion, the transfused blood can be seen streaming away from the needle in the umbilical vein as it mixes with fetal blood
- The fetal heart rate should be monitored periodically using color flow or pulsed Doppler ultrasound. Bradycardia usually responds to slowing or stopping the transfusion, needle removal, maternal oxygen administration and repositioning in the left lateral decubitus position. If bradycardia persists for more than 30 seconds, the procedure needle should be removed and the fetal heart rate continuously monitored by ultrasound. Maternal atropine injection should be given. If severe bradycardia persists for more than three minutes, emergency caesarean delivery may be required if the fetus is more than 28 weeks gestation
- Post-transfusion monitoring—after the infusion has been completed, another fetal blood sample is obtained at the end of the procedure for post-transfusion hemoglobin and hct
- Fetal heart rate monitoring is continued until resumption of fetal movement and a reactive tracing is documented. An ultrasound examination is scheduled for the following day, as most cases of fetal loss occur within the first 24 hours post-procedure.

Intraperitoneal Transfusion

The calculation of volume can be done by subtracting 20 from the gestational age in weeks and multiplying by a factor of 10. Thus, a 30 weeks fetus would receive 100 mL of blood. Blood in the peritoneal reservoir can be expected to be absorbed over a 7- to 10-day period.

Timing of second IUT and subsequent transfusions: After the first IUT, a decline in fetal hematocrit of approximately 1 percent per day can be expected if the fetus is not hydropic (1.88 percent if the fetus is hydropic). Therefore, a second IUT is planned 10 to 14 days after the first IUT, depending upon the final hematocrit achieved at the conclusion of that transfusion. Predicting the fetal hematocrit after a transfusion is an inexact process given fluid shifts from the extravascular to the intravascular compartment, bleeding from the cord puncture site when the needle is removed, and possibly from decreased survival of adult RBCs in the fetal circulation.

After the first two or three transfusions, the interval between subsequent procedures can usually be lengthened to three to four weeks because of the suppression of fetal erythropoiesis, and replacement by Rh –ve blood which is not at risk of early hemolysis.

Last transfusion—most centers perform fetal transfusions for up to 35 weeks of gestation. The last transfusion can be planned at around 34 weeks if possible so that the delivery can be done at around 37 week. Vaginal delivery can be performed for non-anemic fetus as these are usually parous woman.

Complications

The risks of IVT are best illustrated by a large series reported from a single hospital.[12] This series of 740 IVTs in 254 patients described the following procedure related complication rates:
- Perinatal death: 1.6 percent per procedure
- Emergency cesarean delivery: 2.0 percent per procedure
- Infection: 0.3 percent per procedure
- Premature rupture of membranes: 0.1 percent per procedure
- Inadvertent arterial puncture: 3 percent
- Bradycardia or tachycardia: 5 percent of procedures (but 57 percent of procedures resulting in perinatal death or emergency delivery)
- Bleeding from puncture site: 0 to 17 minutes.

The total procedure related complication rate, corrected for procedures with more than one complication, was 3.1 percent.

FETAL MONITORING

Doppler ultrasound measurement of the peak systolic velocity of the fetal middle cerebral artery is useful not only for monitoring for fetal anemia before first transfusion, but has also been investigated for the timing of the second intrauterine transfusion. Published data and anecdotal clinical experience do not support the use of middle cerebral artery Doppler assessment to time serial IUTs beyond the first two transfusions or after 35 weeks of gestation.

Fetal wellbeing of these potentially anemic and hypoxic fetuses is by fetal kick count, biophysical profile and umbilical artery Doppler as in other high-risk pregnancies.

TIMING OF DELIVERY

Elective delivery by induction of labor or cesarean section is undertaken after at least 34 weeks of gestation, preferably at 38 weeks of gestation depending on the presence of hydrops at initial diagnosis and fetal well being. The delivery should take place in a center with excellent NICU facilities and expertize of neonatal exchange transfusion.

OUTCOME

Survival—Overall survival after IUT is about 80–90 percent, but varies with the presence of hydrops, and the experience of the treating physician.[13] Survival of hydropic fetuses is lower than that of fetuses who are not hydropic at first IUT (70 versus 90 percent). Survival is also lower when severe anemia occurs at less than 20 weeks of gestation.

Neurologic Outcome

The long term neurological outcome in treated fetuses has been a matter of concern. The long-term follow-up after intrauterine transfusions (LOTUS) study is the largest study to assess the incidence and risk factors for neurodevelopmental impairment in children with hemolytic disease of the fetus/newborn treated with IUT.[14] This incidence of severe neurodevelopmental delay (3.1 percent) was similar to that of the normal Dutch population (2.3 percent). However, the incidence of cerebral palsy (2.1 percent) was higher than expected in a normal population (0.7 percent with delivery between 32 and 36 weeks and 0.2 percent with delivery at 37 weeks of gestation or greater).

CONCLUSION

The use of anti-D has revolutionized prognosis in Rh negative pregnant women. Immunized pregnancies still occur, with grave fetal outcome. Early referral to fetal medicine specialist, ultrasound monitoring for early detection of fetal anemia, timely intrauterine blood transfusion and delivery at a tertiary center with neonatal intensive care facilities can result in up to 90% favorable outcome in these very high-risk pregnancies.[13,15]

REFERENCES

1. Crowther CA, Middleton P, McBain RD. Anti-D administration in pregnancy for preventing Rhesus alloimmunization. Cochrane Database Syst Rev. 2013 Feb 28.

2. Crowther CA, Keirse MJ. Anti-D administration in pregnancy for preventing rhesus alloimmunization. Cochrane Da tabase Syst Rev. 2000;(2).

3. Bolton-Maggs PH, Davies T, Poles D, Cohen H. Errors in anti-D immunoglobulin administration: Retrospective analysis of 15 years of reports to the UK confidential hemovigilance scheme. BJOG. 2013 Jun;120(7):873-8.

4. Deka D. Causes of Rh-isoimmunization in India (FOGSI Rhogam Project, 2000-2001). Fogsifocus. 2006;42-6.

5. Deka D, Buckshee K, Garg P, Verma A. Successful management of very early hydrops fetalis due to Rh-isoimmunization by 7 serial intrauterine transfusions. Journal of Obst & Gyne of India. 1999;49(3):81-2.

6. Deka D, Buckshee K, Kinra G. Intravenous immunoglobulin as primary therapy or adjuvant therapy to intrauterine fetal blood transfusion: A new approach in the management of severe Rh-immunization. J Obstet Gynecol Res. 1996 Dec;22(6):561-7.

7. Arora S, Kabra M, Deka D, Kriplani A. Molecular Analysis of Fetal RhD Status Using Cell Free DNA in Maternal Circulation. Int J Hum Genet, Supplement No. 2006;2:50-1.

8. Deka D, Arora S, Kabra M, Roy KK, Malhotra N. Amniocentesis for Rh Grouping by PCR : A Major Breakthrough in Anti-D Prophylaxis and Management of Rh Negative Pregnancies. Journal of Obst & Gynae of India. March 2004, 54(2);151-4.

9. Deka D, Takkar D. Rh negative fetus in a patient with severe Rh-isoimmunization and previous 5 hydropic fetuses- need for antenatal determination of fetal Rh group. Journal of Obstet & Gynae of India. 2001;51(1):121.

10. Mari G, Deter RL, Carpenter RL, et al. Noninvasive diagnosis by Doppler ultrasonography of fetal anemia due to maternal red-cell alloimmunization. Collaborative Group for Doppler Assessment of the Blood Velocity in Anemic Fetuses. N Engl J Med. 2000; 342:9.

11. Sharma N, Deka D, Dadhwal V, Mittal S. Identification of Fetal Anemia Due to Rh-isoimmunization by Middle cerebral artery peak systolic velocity (MCA-PSV) Doppler Measurements. Perinatology 2009, Vol 11 (1):9-14.

12. Van Kamp IL, Klumper FJ, Oepkes D, et al. Complications of intrauterine intravascular transfusion for fetal anemia due to maternal red-cell alloimmunization. Am J Obstet Gynecol. 2005;192:171.

13. Dadhwal V, Deka D, Gurunath S, Mittal S, Paul VK, Deorari A. Treatment of Fetal Anemia in Rh Isoimmunized pregnancies with Intrauterine Fetal Blood Transfusion. J Obstet Gynaecol India. March/April 2010;60(2):135-40.

14. Lindenburg IT, Smits-Wintjens VE, van Klink JM, et al. Long-term neurodevelopmental outcome after intrauterine transfusion for hemolytic disease of the fetus/newborn: The LOTUS study. Am J Obstet Gynecol. 2012; 206:141.

15. Papantoniou N, Sifakis S, Antsaklis A. Therapeutic management of fetal anemia: Review of standard practice and alternative treatment options. J Perinat Med. 2013: 41(1):71-82.

Preterm Labor

Shanti HK Singh, Smita Kumari, Sushma Singh

This is defined as "regular uterine contractions, which cause progressive dilatation and effacement of cervix before 37th completed weeks of gestation".

The lower limit for the onset of preterm labor for our country is 28 weeks. It is the most common cause of preterm delivery.

RISK FACTORS

- Previous history of preterm labor
  - Very young or advanced maternal age
    - Low BMI
    - Smoking or cocaine abuse
  - Low socioeconomic status
- Previous history of induced abortion or MTP
- Maternal stress.

Pregnancy Complications

- Antepartum hemorrhage
- Pre-eclampsia and eclampsia
- Multifetal gestation
- Polyhydramnios
- Uncontrolled diabetes mellitus
- Intrauterine growth restriction
- Preterm rupture of membrane
- Intrauterine death.

Infections

- Bacterial vaginosis
- Chlamydial infection
- Urinary tract infection
- Group B streptococcal infection.

Anatomical

- Congenital malformation of uterus, e.g. bicornuate uterus, subseptate uterus
- Submucous fibroid
- Cervical incompetence.

Idiopathic

A majority of cases of preterm labor are without apparent or detectable cause and are often referred to as idiopathic preterm labor.

PATHOGENESIS OF PRETERM LABOR

- Premature activation of fetal hypothalamic-pituitary adrenal axis
- Decidual hemorrhage
- Infection and inflammation leading to increase in cytokines IL-1,6,8 and TNF-alfa and which stimulates release of prostaglandin
- Pathological uterine distension (increase in gap junction).

COMPLICATIONS OF PREMATURE BABY

- Respiratory distress syndrome (RDS)
- Intraventricular hemorrhage
- Necrotizing enterocolitis
- Retinopathy of prematurity (due to prolonged inhalation of 100% oxygen)
- Neonatal jaundice
- Failure to thrive
- Cerebral palsy.

PREDICTORS OF PRETERM LABOR

- Assessment of risk factors, e.g. previous history of preterm labor, multiple pregnancy, polyhydramnios, etc.
- Vaginal examination to assess cervical change—it is a traditional method used to detect cervical changes but quantifying change is often difficult
- USG visualization of cervical length and dilatation—USG evaluation provides more objective approach for cervical assessment. 80–100% women who deliver a preterm baby have cervical length <30 mm. When the cervical length is <15 mm, 50% cases deliver within one week
- Detection of fetal fibronectin in cervicovaginal secretion. Fibronectin is glue like glycoprotein, which binds choriodecidual membrane
- It is normally present in cervical secretion between 24–34 weeks, its presence in cervical secretion before 24 and after 34 weeks signifies onset of labor
- Bedside test can also be done

- It has negative predictive value, level <50 ng/mL rules out preterm labor in the next two weeks
- Vaginal examination gives false-positive result for 24 hours.
- Presence of FFN fetal fibronectin (FFN) in cevicovaginal secretion at a level higher than 50 ng/mL and cervical length less than 25 mm are strong predictors of preterm labor.

DIAGNOSIS OF PRETERM LABOR

Three important criteria to document preterm labor are:
  a. Regular uterine contractions at least 1 in 10 minutes or 4 in 10 minutes with progressive cervical change
  b. Cervical dilatation >2 cm
  c. Cervical effacement >80% along with symptoms of pelvic pressure, vaginal discharge and backache.

Based on the findings preterm labor is divided into three groups.
  1. Threatened preterm labor
     - Cervical dilatation < 1 cm
     - Cervical effacement <80%
     - Cervical length < 25 mm
  2. Early preterm labor
     - Cervical dilatation >1 cm but <3 cm
     - Cervical effacement >80%
     - Cervical length <25 mm
  3. Advanced preterm labor
     - Cervical dilatation > 3 cm
     - Cervical effacement >80%
     - Cervical length <25 mm

MANAGEMENT OF PRETERM LABOR

Management depends upon six main factors:
  1. Status of membranes
  2. Dilation of cervix
  3. Gestational age
  4. Cause of preterm labor
  5. Availability of NICU
  6. Corticosteroids

All causes of preterm labor should be managed in tertiary care center equipped with NICU facility.

Investigations that may be needed are:
  1. Complete blood count and urine analysis for evaluating infection
  2. Amniocentesis to assess fetal pulmonary maturity
  3. USG—to assess AFI, determine gestational age, TVS for cervical length and funneling of membranes
  4. Cervicovaginal swab for FFN.

These are three modalities of treatment:
- Prophylactic
- Management of acute preterm labor
- Neonatal care.

PROPHYLACTIC MANAGEMENT

- Reduce/eliminate risk factors if possible
- In multifetal gestation rest and sedatives are very important
- In cervical incompetence, prophylactic cervical cerclage can be done.
  - Rescue or emergency cerclage can also be done during pregnancy in early preterm labor provided the contraindications are excluded, e.g. evidence of infection, dead or congenitally malformed fetus or preterm premature rupture of membranes
- Supplemental progesterone
  - Inj 17-hydroxyprogesterone (250 mg) intramuscularly at weekly interval starting from 16th to 20th week, up to 36 weeks can be given in women with previous history of preterm labor before 34 weeks.
  - It has been approved by FDA.
- Treat infections like urinary tract infections.
  - In bacterial vaginosis, vaginal clindamycin 2% or oral metronidazole 500 mg BD for 7 days early in 2nd trimester significantly reduces the rate of spontaneous preterm labor.
- Strict glycemic control and prevention of infection in diabetic mother.

MANAGEMENT OF ACUTE PRETERM LABOR

- Bed rest and hydration—commonly recommended without proven efficacy
- Corticosteroids
- Antibiotics
- Tocolytics

Steroids

Single course antenatal steroid between 24 and 34 weeks to accelerate pulmonary maturity and reduce risk of respiratory distress syndrome (RDS), intraventricular hemorrhage (IVH) and necrotizing enterocolitis (NEC).

In 1998, ACOG recommended steroids in PPROM in the absence of infection to reduce the risk of RDS, IVH and NEC.

Dose and Drugs

- Inj betamethasone 12 mg IM 12th hourly for 24 hours, or
- Inj dexamethasone 6 mg IM every 12th hourly for 4 doses
- Maximum effect is from 24 hours after last dose up to 7 days.

Repeated doses are not recommended, as it increases risk of sepsis in PPROM, restricts fetal body and brain growth and cause adrenal suppression.

Antibiotics

ACOG advices screening of all women for group B *Streptococcus* (GBS) infection.

All patients with preterm labor are considered at high-risk for neonatal GBS sepsis and should receive prophylactic antibiotics.

The treatment goal is to prevent neonatal sepsis and not to prevent preterm birth.

Role of Tocolytics

It is usually used for short-term course to complete the course of corticosteroid and also for in utero transfer to a tertiary care center.

Maintenance tocolysis beyond 48 hours is not recommended as it is associated with significant risk.

Candidates for Tocolysis

- No contraindication to the drug
- Fetal status is reassuring
- Cervical dilatation is < 4 cm
- Gestational age is between 24 to 34 weeks.

Contraindications for Tocolysis

- Severe PIH
- Uncontrolled DM
- Placental abruption
- Cardiopulmonary disease
- Maternal hyperthyroidism
- Severe anemia
- Chorioamnionitis
- Congenitally malformed fetus.

Drugs Used for Tocolysis

1. *Nifedipine:* A cheap calcium channel blocker, can be given orally, and has a low incidence of side effects (hypotension, dizziness, flushing). It is often considered the first line of therapy.
2. *Beta agonists (ritodrine, terbutaline):* Side effects are tachycardia, hypotension, tremor, palpitations, chest discomfort, hypokalemia and hyperglycemia.
3. *Magnesium sulfate:*
   - Side effects are nausea, flushing, fatigue, diaphoresis, respiratory depression, cardiac arrest
   - It has been shown that magnesium sulfate in preterm babies reduces the risk of neurological damage.

4. *Indomethacin causes:* Maternal gastrointestinal upset, premature closure of the ductus arteriosus, and oligohydramnios.
5. *Atosiban, an oxytocin antagonist:* It increases fetal and neonatal morbidity and mortality so it is not commonly used.

More than one tocolytic agent should not be combined as it significantly increases the side effects.

MANAGEMENT OF ACUTE PRETERM LABOR

Labor should be managed gently as preterm baby cannot sustain stress and strain of normal labor because of immature development of the autoregulatory system.

1st Stage

- Continuous electronic fetal monitoring to detect fetal hypoxia early is recommended
- Epidural analgesia is preferred as it has a relaxant effect on pelvic floor muscles, and avoids compression on the fetal head
- Moist oxygen inhalation should be given when needed
- Cesarean section should be done for obstetric indication only
- Premature breech before 34 weeks should be delivered by cesarean section to avoid compression and decompression injury on fetal head as the lower segment is not completely formed. Lower segment vertical or 'J" shaped incision may be used.

2nd Stage

- Gentle and slow delivery should be done in between contractions.
- Episiotomy and forceps may be used to avoid compression and to provide a protective cage for the fetal head.
- Forceps may be applied as it provides a protective cage for immature fetal head.
- Early cord clamping should be done to avoid fluid overload to avoid cardiac overload on immature cardiovascular system.
  Cord should be kept long as exchange transfusion may be needed
- Pediatrician must be present during delivery and baby may be shifted to NICU for better management.

SUGGESTED READING

1. Cunniglam FG (Ed), et al. Preterm birth. In Williams obstetrics. 23rd ed. New York:McGrow-Hill. 2010;pp 804-31.
2. Effect of corticosteroids for fetal maturation on perinatal outcomes. NIH Consensus Statement. 1994;12(2):1-18.

3. Hubert PJ. Atosiban. Cline Obsbet Gynaecol. 1995;38:722-4.
4. Mc Combs J. Update on tocolytic therapy. Ann Pharmacother. 1995;29:515-22.
5. Preterm labour. Technical bulletin no 206. Washington DC;ACOG 1995. (contraindications to tocolysis. Complications).
6. Simhans HN, Carilis. Prevention of preterm delivery. British J of Obs and Gynecol. 2007;(supp 1):1-3.

Polyhydramnios and Oligohydramnios

Amrita Sharan

The amniotic fluid surrounding the growing fetus provides a protective milieu, cushioning the fetus against mechanical and biological injury, supplying nutrients and facilitating its growth and movement.

Either an abnormal increase—hydramnios or polyhydramnios, or a decrease—oligohydramnios, is associated with increased maternal morbidity and increased perinatal morbidity and mortality.

SOURCE OF AMNIOTIC FLUID

The major source of amniotic fluid is thought to be the amniotic epithelium, but there are other sources also. During the first half of pregnancy, the composition of amniotic fluid resembles the fetal extra cellular fluid (fetal plasma) as there is free diffusion of fluid to and fro from the fetus. In the second half of pregnancy, rapid diffusion across fetal skin is impaired by keratinization of the skin. Thereafter, fetal urine and lung secretions are the two main sources of amniotic fluid. At term, the fetal urine contributes 400–500 mL per hour.

There is rapid turnover of fluid, around 500 mL enters and leaves the amniotic sac every hour. Removal of fluid depends largely on fetal swallowing and intramembranous transport via the skin, placental and cord surface.

VOLUME OF AMNIOTIC FLUID

Liquor amnii volume varies with gestational age:

10 weeks	—	25 to 30 mL
12 weeks	—	50 mL
20 weeks	—	250 to 400 mL
36 weeks	—	1,000 mL
38–40 weeks	—	800 mL
42 weeks	—	400 mL
43 weeks	—	200 mL

HYDRAMNIOS (OR POLYHYDRAMNIOS)

Definition

It is defined anatomically as a state when liquor amnii exceeds 2,000 mL (Fig. 1).

Clinically, it is defined as excessive accumulation of liquor amnii causing discomfort to the patient and/or when an imaging aid is required to substantiate the clinical diagnosis of lie and presentation of the fetus.

Sonographically, it is diagnosed when the amniotic fluid index (AFI) is more than 24 cm (> 95th percentile for gestational age) and when the largest vertical pocket is more than 8 cm. Largest vertical pocket of 8-11 cm is considered mild, 12–15 cm moderate and > 16 cm as severe polyhydramnios.

Incidence

It varies from 1–2%, being more common in multigravidae than in primigravidae. Minor degrees of hydramnios (2–3L) are common whereas hydramnios sufficient to cause symptoms (over 3–4 L) occurs less commonly, probably 1 in 1,000 pregnancies.

Whatever, the source of excessive liquor, it does not as a rule; differ in composition from normal cases.

Etiology

In many cases (60%) it is idiopathic and no cause can be found.

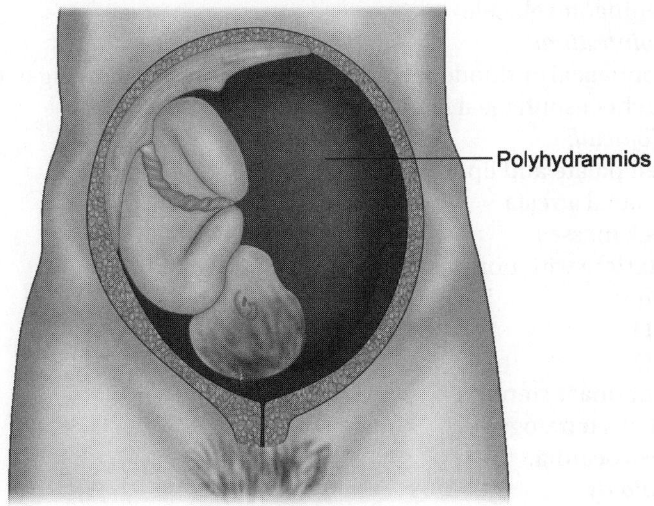

Fig. 1: Polyhydramnios

Maternal Causes

- Diabetes mellitus—50% of diabetic pregnancies have hydramnios. It is due to fetal polyuria, which is secondary to maternal and fetal hyperglycemia and therefore, polyhydramnios is seen when the maternal diabetes is poorly controlled.
- Multiple pregnancies—hydramnios occurring in mid-pregnancy should always arouse a suspicion of monozygotic twins.
- Cardiac or renal disease leading to edema of the placenta and increased transudation.
- Women undergoing hemodialysis during pregnancy may develop hydramnios due to decreased oncotic pressure resulting from frequent removal of solutes from the vascular compartment, which favor a shift of fluid into the amniotic cavity.

Fetal Causes

1. Congenital fetal malformation (both structural and chromosomal) is associated with hydramnios in 20% cases.
   Central Nervous System:
   - Anencephaly—hydramnios is associated in 59% cases and it is due to:
     a. Transudation from the exposed meninges
     b. Absence of fetal swallowing reflex
     c. Possible suppression of fetal antidiuretic hormone leading to excessive urination.
   - Open spina bifida
   - Hydrocephalus
   - Meningomyelocele
   Gastrointestinal:
   - Esophageal or duodenal atresia—preventing swallowing of liquor
   - Tracheoesophageal fistula
   Craniofacial:
   - Cleft palate and lip
   - Choanal atresia
   - Neck masses
   All interfere with normal swallowing.
   Cardiac:
   - VSD
   - ASD
   - Pulmonary stenosis
   - Fallot's tetralogy
   - Dextrocardia.
   Aneuploidy
2. Hydrops fetalis in Rh isoimmunization.

Placental Causes

Chorioangioma of the placenta causing increased transudation.

Types of Polyhydramnios

Acute Polyhydramnios

Extremely rare, onset is acute, occurs earlier in pregnancy and is generally associated with uniovular twins. Preterm labor, before 28 weeks is frequent. Fetal prognosis is guarded because of prematurity and high incidence of congenital abnormalities.

In severe twin-to-twin transfusion syndrome (TTTS), laser ablation may cure the cause of TTTS whereas repetitive amnioreduction until AFI is normal, may improve the perinatal outcome.

Chronic Polyhydramnios

10 times more common than acute variety, occurs later in pregnancy usually between 32 and 40 weeks. Accumulation of liquor is gradual and the maternal symptoms are less marked than in the acute type. Fetal prognosis is good in the idiopathic group but the prognosis is guarded when there is association of erythroblastosis or diabetes or congenital anomalies.

In recent times the incidence of polyhydramnios of severe magnitude is decreasing because of:
- Early detection and control of diabetes
- Rh isoimmunization is preventable
- Genetic counseling in early months and detection of congenital abnormalities with USG and their termination.

Clinical Presentation

Depends on the degree of hydramnios and the rapidity of its onset.

Acute Polyhydramnios: This variety may present with features of acute abdominal catastrophe, the uterus being hard and tender, causing great distress to the patient. This condition may be confused with abruptio placentae.

Chronic Polyhydramnios: In this variety the patient may complain of an unmanageable girth, shortness of breath, considerable digestive discomfort, edema of lower extremities and increasingly troublesome varicose veins. Occasionally hyperemesis in late pregnancy and features of preeclampsia may be present.

Ultrasonography—(Figs 2A and B):
- There is a large, echo-free space between the fetus and the uterine wall
- Largest vertical pocket > 8 cm
- Amniotic fluid index > 24 cm
- Fetal congenital malformation can be diagnosed
- Multiple pregnancy can be detected
- Lie and presentation of the fetus can be noted.

Other Investigations

- CBC
- Urine analysis

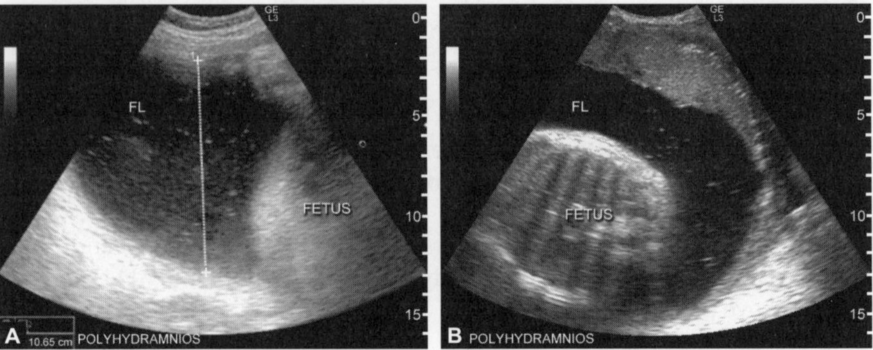

Figs 2A and B: Ultrasound findings in polyhydramnios

- Rh typing ABO grouping
- Blood sugar level 2 hours after 75 gram glucose given orally
- If fetal hydrops is noted on ultrasound, maternal antibody screen for D, C, Kell and Duffy antigens should be done to exclude alloimmunization
- If no antibodies are detected, evaluation of causes of non-immune hydrops should be done—serological test for syphilis, TORCH titers
- Heterozygosity for alpha thalassemia may need to be excluded by electrophoresis
- Invasive testing—amniocentesis may be required for:
  - Fetal karyotype
  - Estimation of alpha-fetoprotein to detect open neural tube defect
  - Isolation of viruses by PCR and
  - Diagnosis of metabolic disorders.

  If rapid karyotyping is needed, cordocentesis provides result in 48–72 hours as compared to amniocentesis which takes 2–3 weeks.

Differential diagnosis—polyhydramnios has to be distinguished from the following conditions:
- Multiple pregnancy, they are often present together
- Pregnancy with huge ovarian cyst
- Hydatidiform mole—USG can show characteristic features of mole
- Maternal and fetal ascites
- Acute hydramnios may simulate abruptio placentae with concealed hemorrhage.

Complications of Polyhydramnios

Maternal Complications

- Increased incidence of pre-eclampsia and diabetes
- Malpresentation
- Preterm labor
- PROM and cord prolapse

- Accidental hemorrhage
- Uterine inertia and PPH
- Increased operative delivery
- Increased puerperal morbidity.

Fetal Complications

There is increased perinatal mortality—50% due to:
- Prematurity
- Congenital abnormality, cord prolapse
- Hydrops fetalis
- Accidental hemorrhage

Management of Polyhydramnios

The treatment is tailored according to the magnitude of polyhydramnios and the underlying cause:
- In mild hydramnios, conservative treatment with bed rest and close observation throughout pregnancy will suffice in most cases
- In many cases, the excess quantity of fluid diminishes as pregnancy advances and the condition may resolve spontaneously
- In severe polyhydramnios, the patients are dealt as 'high-risk' and managed in well-equipped hospitals.

Management is aimed to:
- To relieve the symptoms
- To detect the causes
- To avoid the complications.

Supportive Therapy

- Bed rest with a back rest if necessary
- Treatment of associated conditions like pre-eclampsia, diabetes, etc.
- Prostaglandin synthetase inhibitors:
  a. **Indomethacin**—25 mg 6 hourly given to the mother has been found to decrease the amniotic fluid volume by decreasing the fetal urine production mainly. Maternal side effects are mainly ductus arteriosus constriction leading to right ventricular hypertrophy and pulmonary hypertension, with long-term use.

     The constructive effect of indomethacin has been shown to increase with advancing gestational age, with rate of fetal compromise, approaching 50%. As the majority of fluid reduction occurs in the first week of treatment with indomethacin, the drug may be discontinued once the amniotic fluid volume has been reduced by more than two thirds of the pretreatment level. This strategy reduces the fetal complication.
  b. **Sulindac**—another prostaglandin inhibitor having milder effect on ductal constriction is being evaluated for use.

Investigations

Investigations are done to exclude twin pregnancy, congenital fetal malformations and also to detect Rh-isoimmunization, diabetes, nonimmune hydrops, etc.

Further Management

It depends on:
- Presence of fetal malformation
- Gestational age
- Response to treatment
- Associated complicating factors.

When polyhydramnios is associated with congenital fetal abnormality, termination of pregnancy is to be done irrespective of period of gestation.

When congenital fetal abnormality is absent, maternal well-being is unaffected and responses to conservative treatment are good, pregnancy is to be continued awaiting spontaneous delivery at term.

In uncomplicated cases (no demonstrable fetal congenital abnormality), unresponsive to supportive treatment and associated with maternal distress, management depends on the period of gestation.

- Pregnancy < 37 weeks—repeated amnioreduction till fetal maturity. Slow decompression is done at the rate of 500 mL per hour up to 1–1.5 liter. This amount of fluid removal is sufficient to relieve the mechanical pressure.
- Pregnancy > 37 weeks—induction of labor is done. Amnioreduction is to be done first, lie and presentation of the fetus corrected, stabilizing oxytocin drip is started after controlled low rupture of membranes. This minimizes sudden placental separation and cord prolapse.

Labor is Closely Monitored

- Avoid oxytocin before ARM for risk of amniotic fluid embolism
- Do active management of 3rd stage of labor to prevent PPH and retained placenta
- Examine the baby thoroughly for any congenital anomaly.

OLIGOHYDRAMNIOS (SYN: OLIGOAMNIOS)

Definition

It is defined anatomically as a condition where liquor amnii is decreased in amount to the extent of less than 200 mL at term (Fig. 3).

Sonographically, it is defined when the maximum vertical pocket of liquor is less than 2 cm or when amniotic fluid index (AFI) is < 5 cm (< 10th percentile).

Incidence

Varies between 0.5% to > 5% depending on the definition of oligohydramnios used and the population studied.

The incidence increases in postdated pregnancies, noted in as many as 11%.

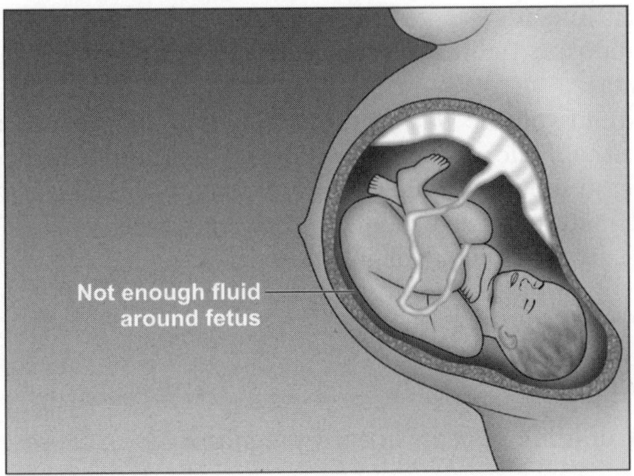

Fig. 3: Oligohydramnios

Etiology

Exact cause is not known, but there are certain conditions, which are associated with oligohydramnios.

Maternal Conditions

- Hypertensive disorders of pregnancies
- Uteroplacental insufficiency
- Postdated pregnancy
- Preterm premature rupture of membranes
- Dehydration—reports have confirmed a significant increase in amniotic fluid volume in women with oligohydramnios after oral or intravenous hydration
- Autoimmune disorders
- Maternal medication like prostaglandin synthetase inhibitor, ACE inhibitor. **Idiopathic**—isolated oligohydramnios may occur in late pregnancy in patients with no other risk factors associated with oligohydramnios.

Fetal Conditions

- Fetal chromosomal or structural anomalies. The incidence of structured malformations and aneuploidy with oligohydramnios ranges between 7–37% and 4.4–30.7%.
- Intrauterine growth restrictions
- Renal anomalies with oligohydramnios includes:
    - Bilateral renal agenesis
    - Multicystic dysplastic kidneys
    - Bladder outlet obstruction
- Infantile polycystic kidneys
- Increased incidence of musculoskeletal, digestive and cardiac anomalies have been reported

- Intrauterine infection
- Amnion nodosum (failure of secretion by the cells of the amnion covering the placenta).

Amniotic fluid volume was reported to increase after successful version from breech to cephalic presentation—also it was found to be decreased after vibro acoustic stimulation, which increases fetal swallowing activity.

Increased maternal serum alphafetoprotein levels have been found in women with second trimester oligohydramnios.

Effects of Oligohydramnios

Early Pregnancy

When oligohydramnios occurs in early pregnancy it can cause:
- Abortion
- Fetal deformities:
    - Amniotic adhesion or bands may cause deformities like amputation of fetal limbs or constriction and obstruction of the umbilical cord
    - Pressure deformities such as club feet.
- Pulmonary hypoplasia
- The skin becomes dry, leathery and wrinkled.

Late Pregnancy

Severe oligohydramnios can create several problems:
- It is a sign of fetal jeopardy as in cases of IUGR
- Fetal hypoxia may result from close adaptation between the fetus and the uterine wall leading to pressure on umbilical cord and obstruction to the flow of blood to and from the fetus
- Meconium aspiration syndrome—meconium passed in the amniotic sac is not diluted in case of severe oligohydramnios and aspiration of thick meconium causes aspiration pneumonia after birth.

Labor

- Fetal distress
- High perinatal mortality
- Increased maternal morbidity due to high incidence of operative intervention.

Diagnosis

Clinically
- Uterine size is much smaller than period of amenorrhea
- Less fetal movement
- Uterine is full of fetus due to scanty liquor
- Malpresentation (breech) is common
- Evidences of intrauterine growth restriction of the fetus.

Sonographically

- Diagnosis of oligohydramnios is confirmed by ultrasonography
- Maximum vertical pocket of liquor < 2 cm
- AFI < 5 cm
- Once oligohydramnios is diagnosed, detailed examination of fetal anatomy particularly renal tract is undertaken. Also, fetal growth parameters are assessed to exclude fetal growth restriction. Amnioinfusion with normal saline can help to improve diagnosis of structural malformation
- Doppler velocimetry of the umbilical artery should be performed and S/D ratio recorded to identify the fetus at risk.

Management

There is no specific treatment for oligohydramnios. Management depends on two factors:

a. Associated pregnancy complications
b. Gestational age.
   - Presence of fetal congenital anomaly needs delivery irrespective of gestational aged
   - When remote from term, the endeavor is to prolong pregnancy with close fetal monitoring
   - Nearer term, pregnancy termination is planned in women whose fetus is at risk of adverse perinatal outcome either because of pregnancy complications like IUGR and hypertension or if the umbilical artery doppler is abnormal
   - Continuous intrapartum fetal heart rate monitoring should be done to detect early signs of hypoxia and perform timely intervention
   - Isolated oligohydramnios in the third trimester with a normal fetus should be managed conservatively
   - Maternal hydration, oral or intravenous has been shown to increase amniotic fluid volume
   - Now evidence is accumulating on the benefits of antepartum and intrapartum amnioinfusion in women with oligohydramnios.

CONCLUSION

Until we can find means to prevent and treat oligohydramnios effectively in utero, the mainstay in the management is to provide intensive fetal surveillance and timely intervention when fetal compromise is evident.

SUGGESTED READING

1. DC Dutta's Textbook of Obstetrics, 7th Ed.
2. Essentials of Obstetrics, 2nd Edition.
3. Holland and Brews Manual of Obstetrics.
4. Ian Donald's Prac Obst Problems, 6th Ed.

Prolonged Pregnancy

Archana Kumari

DEFINITION

Typical pregnancy duration can vary between 37 and 42 weeks. The adjectives post-term, prolonged, postdates and postmature is often loosely used interchangeably to describe pregnancy which has crossed upper limit of normal. The term postdates is inadequate as there is no definition of the dates to which the term refers. Prolonged pregnancy refers to those pregnancies which have advanced beyond the expected date of delivery (EDD). The term postmature is reserved for the relatively uncommon specific fetal syndrome of intrauterine growth retardation associated with prolonged gestation in which infant has recognizable feature of a pathologically prolonged pregnancy. International definition of prolonged pregnancy endorsed by ACOG (2004) is one that exceeds 42 completed weeks (294 days or more) from onset of last menstrual period. Therefore, post-term or prolonged pregnancy is preferred expression for an extended pregnancy.

INCIDENCE

A great deal of controversy surrounds the incidence with estimates ranging from 4–19% (Divon and Feldman, 2008). Incidence of post-term pregnancies is 7.5% when based on menstrual dating, 2.6% when dating is based on early USG evaluation and 1.1% when ultrasound and dates coincide (Boyd et al).

ETIOLOGY

- Inaccurate dating
- Idiopathic
- High socioeconomic status with sedentary lifestyle
- Primiparity
- Prior post-term pregnancy (recurrence rate is about 50%)
- Genetic factors—studies on monozygotic and dizygotic twins and their subsequent development of prolonged pregnancy have found that maternal and not the paternal genes influence the rate of prolonged pregnancy and account for in as many as 30% of these pregnancies

- Gender of the fetus—males are more likely to be post-term.
- Rare fetoplacental factors include anencephaly, adrenal hypoplasia, X-linked sulfatase deficiency, fetal osteogenesis imperfecta.

Lack of development of fetal hypothalamus in anencephaly negates the production of corticotropin releasing hormone (CRH) and stimulation of pituitary-adrenal-placental axis necessary for initiation of parturition. Placental sulfatase plays a critical role in the synthesis of placental estrogens that are required for development of gap junctions and increased expression of oxytocin and PG receptors in the myometrial cells.

TYPES

Two types can be recognized based on functional efficacy of the fetoplacental unit:

- The first type (accounts for 90%) is the one in which placental function is unaffected. The fetus continues to grow and does not have any stigmata of post maturity. Fetal macrosomia and cephalopelvic disproportion (CPD) occur more frequently.
- The second type (accounts for 10%), the function of placenta is adversely affected. The dysmature placenta reveals the presence of infarcts, fibrin deposits and calcification with reduced reserve. Fetus suffers from hypoxia. In such women uterine sensitivity to oxytocin is often reduced and induction of labor often fails.

PATHOPHYSIOLOGY

Amniotic Fluid Changes

Quantitative: Amniotic fluid volume decreases from 1 liter at 36 weeks to less than 200 mL at 42 weeks. The mechanism seems to be diminished fetal urine production, which in turn may be related to reduced fetal renal blood flow.

Qualitative: After 38 to 40 weeks amniotic fluid becomes milky and cloudy because of abundant flakes of vernix caseosa. Phospholipid composition changes because of large number of lamellar bodies released from fetal lungs. L:S ratio becomes 4:1 or greater. Color of the fluid has green or yellow discoloration when fetus passes meconium.

Placental Changes

Post-term placenta shows a decrease in diameter and length of chorionic villi, fibrinoid necrosis and accelerated atherosis of chorionic and decidual vessels. Infarcts (foci of calcium deposition) are present in 10 to 20% of term placenta and 60 to 80% of post-term placenta, and are more common at the placental borders. Smith and Baker (1999) reported that placental apoptosis (programmed cell death) was significantly increased at 41–42 completed weeks compared to that at 36–39 weeks. The clinical significance is however unclear. Morphological changes that occur with placental senescence can be observed by ultrasound. However, correlation between USG signs of placental senescence and the functional capacity of the placenta is poor.

Fetal Changes

The velocity of fetal weight gain peaks at approximately 37 weeks. Although, growth velocity slows at that time, most fetuses continue to gain weight. The incidence of fetal macrosomia, those weighing more than 4000 g is 10% at 38–40 weeks and it is 43% at 43 weeks (Arias F). Approximately 5–10% fetus undelivered after their EDD show wasting of subcutaneous fat, characteristic of intrauterine malnutrition.

COMPLICATIONS

Prolonged pregnancy is associated with significant adverse consequences to the fetus and the mother.

Fetal Complications

During Pregnancy

- Oligohydramnios
- Fetal hypoxia due to placental inefficiency

During Labor

- Increased incidence of asphyxia and acidosis (intrapartum fetal distress)
- Cord compression due to oligohydramnios
- Difficult and prolonged labor due to macrosomia and non-molding of head
- Shoulder dystocia
- Stillbirth

After Birth

- MAS (meconium aspiration syndrome)
- Hypoglycemia and polycythemia
- Post-maturity syndrome
- Neonatal death

Maternal Complications

Adverse consequences of mother are related to the large size of infant, and includes injury to birth canal due to difficult labor, increased rate of cesarean birth with associated risks of bleeding, infection and injury to surrounding organs.

Intrapartum Fetal Distress

Approximately 25% of prolonged pregnancies are delivered by cesarean due to non-reassuring fetal heart rate patterns detected by electronic monitoring. The common patterns observed are:

- One or more prolonged decelerations
- Severe variable decelerations with slow recovery and episodes of fetal bradycardia with loss of beat to beat variability
- Saltatory baseline
- Less commonly repetitive late deceleration.

The more common cause of non-reassuring heart pattern is umbilical cord compression secondary to the oligohydramnios (Lenovo et al, 1984). In minority of cases, they are the result of placental insufficiency (Silver et al, 1988).

Perinatal Mortality

It is calculated as number of stillbirths per 1000 live births or per 1000 total births. But according to Smith (2001) correct assessment of population at risk for perinatal mortality in a given week should consist of all ongoing pregnancies in the denominater rather than just the total birth in a given week. This cumulative probability of perinatal death is called perinatal risk index. Delivery at 38 weeks has the lowest risk index for perinatal death. After this, risk increases steadily with each week of gestation. There is general consensus that PMNR increases several fold when pregnancy is prolonged beyond 42 weeks.

Fetal Trauma

Difficult vaginal delivery with varying degrees of fetal trauma occur commonly in prolonged pregnancy especially those associated with fetal macrosomia. Shoulder dystocia is the most feared complication which can result in brachial plexus injury, fracture of humerus or clavicle, or severe asphyxia with neurological damage. Cephalic hematomas and skull fractures may also occur during vaginal delivery of large babies.

Post-maturity Syndrome

It is (also called fetal dysmaturity) one of the features associated with prolonged pregnancy which occurs in 5–10% of the cases. Post-mature fetuses have decreased subcutaneous fat and wrinkled, patchy, peeling skin due to loss of vernix. They have long thin body, long hair and long fingernails suggesting wasting and advanced maturity. The infant is open-eyed, unusually alert and appears old and worried. Most such post mature infants are not technically growth restricted, because their birth weight seldom falls below 10th percentile for the gestational age. On the other hand, severe growth restriction which logically must have preceded completion of

42 weeks may be present. This complication should be discovered prior to labor as these fetuses tolerate labor poorly and are acidotic at birth.

Meconium Aspiration Syndrome

It occurs more frequently when thick meconium, fetal tachycardia, and absence of fetal heart rate (FHR) accelerations are present. Patients with thin meconium at the beginning of labour may have thick meconium and MAS at the time of birth.

DIAGNOSIS

Diagnosis of prolonged pregnancy is based on—history, examination and investigations.

History

The single most important event for diagnosis is the date of LMP and assesment of the reliability of gestational age. The reliability of EDD is excellent if one or more of the following criterias are met:

- Three or more normal menstrual cycle before LMP and no use of OCP
- Pregnancy achieved with infertility technique with known date of conception
- EDD calculated from menstrual history coincides with EDD from ultrasound examination performed between 12 to 20 weeks of gestation
- EDD established from ultrasound crown-rump length between 7–11 weeks of gestation
- EDD corresponds to 36 weeks since the patient has a positive serum or urine pregnancy test
- EDD established from 2 or more ultrasound 3–4 weeks apart between 12–28 weeks.
- Fetal heart tones were documented 20 weeks before the EDD by means of non electronic fetoscope, or 30 weeks before EDD if fetal heart was detected with Doppler.

When menstrual history is uncertain and early USG or pregnancy test has not been done; the date of quickening, early months PV finding, serial measurements of fundal height in the antenatal record, history of false labor pain around EDD may be helpful in ascertaining the gestational age.

A number of symptoms warrant an immediate evaluation in female nearing term or suspected term. These include—any perceived decrease in fetal movements, loss of fluid, any pain or other discomfort that appears abnormal.

Examination

- Maternal weight—stationary or falling
- Girth of abdomen decreases due to decreasing liquor

- Obstetric palpation—height of uterus decreases, liquor appears less (uterus full of fetus), fetal head hard in consistency, fixed or engaged
- Pelvic examination—ripeness of cervix is indicative of term pregnancy, but unripe cervix does not exclude prolonged pregnancy.

Investigations

- Ultrasound evaluation
- Antenatal fetal surveillance tests—NST, BPP, MBPP, CST.

USG Evaluation

Ultrasound done at the end of pregnancy is unreliable for estimation of gestational age. It should be done to know about **amniotic fluid volume, fetal size and weight, fetal malformations** and **placental grading.**

- **Amniotic fluid volume:** USG is reliable technique for estimation of amniotic fluid volume. An AFI of less than 5 cm indicates oligohydramnios. Evidences show that perinatal mortality increases dramatically with progressive severity of oligohydramnios. Lenovo et al have demonstrated that umbilical cord compression due to oligohyramnios is the most common cause of intrapartum fetal distress in these patients.
- **Fetal size:** A significant part of neonatal morbidity associated with prolonged pregnancy is the result of fetal macrosomia. USG can confirm the clinical impression of fetal macrosomia and help the obstetrician in making decision about management of these patients.
  - The abdominal circumference is the most important measurement in estimating fetal weight. Fetus is macrosomic if AC measurement is two or more SD above the mean
  - Majority of macrosomic fetus have subcutaneous fat thickness, measured at the anterior abdominal wall, that exceeds 10 mm. Babies with less than 6 mm of subcutaneous fat are rarely macrosomic
  - When oligohydramnios is present and mother is obese, visualization of fetal structure is difficult, and measurements are inaccurate.
- **Fetal abnormalities:** USG should be done to look for fetal defects, in those rare patients with prolonged pregnancy who did not have USG early in gestation.
- **Placental grading:** Poor neonatal outcome is more frequent in patients with advanced degree of placental maturity, than in patients of same gestational age with less mature placenta.

Antenatal Fetal Surveillance Tests

Two important questions related to antenatal fetal monitoring are—when to initiate testing and what should be the interval between testing.

ACOG recommends initiating these tests at 42 weeks (294 days) or more followed by twice weekly monitoring. To be safe, most obstetricians prefer to begin fetal monitoring at 41 weeks. In most cases, monitoring is recommended when pregnancy extends beyond due date (40 weeks) and to continue as long as women is undelivered.

Regarding interval, the classical concept has been that one week interval is adequate. However, there is evidence (Clement et al, 1987) that in prolonged pregnancy, amniotic fluid volume can drop precipitously even within few days or 24 hours period. The frequency of fetal surveillance must be related to the risk of fetal mortality and morbidity; risk that increases with gestational age. For this reason, testing should be done at 40 weeks and 41 weeks and twice weekly after 41 weeks.

- **Non stress test (NST):** It is performed 2–3 times per week, and is most commonly employed for the evaluation of prolonged pregnancy by obstetricians. However, NST was designed for detection of placental insufficiency and is inadequate to diagnose oligohydramnios or to predict fetal trauma which are both relatively frequent complications of prolonged pregnancy. Therefore, use of NST alone is not ideal.

- **Biophysical profile (BPP) and Modified Biophysical profile (MBPP):** Both these tests are better than NST for evaluation of prolonged pregnancy. But there are problems associated with these tests.

  Firstly, when oligohydramnios is diagnosed as the largest pocket lesser than or equal to 2 cm, patients with grossly decreased fluid may be classified as normal. When AFI less than or equal to 5 cm is taken as diagnostic criteria, pregnancy with low normal fluid may be classified as having oligohydramnios. Secondly, BPP test result is numeric score which assigns equal number of points to all its components—fetal movement, fetal breathing movements, fetal tone, reactive NST and normal AFV. In prolonged pregnancy, decreased amniotic fluid which is a variable of critical importance will cause a decrease of only 2 in total score, and test may be falsely interpreted as normal. To avoid this problem, test is always regarded abnormal when AFV is decreased (Manning et al, 1990). Third problem is that fetal movement, fetal tone, fetal reactivity are variables that are affected by relatively advanced fetal hypoxia, and ideal test should diagnose early rather than late stages of fetal compromise.

- **Contraction stress test (CST):** Checks the fetal response to reduced oxygen during uterine contractions. In theory, CST combined with evaluation of AFV is the best test for fetal surveillance in prolonged pregnancy. The reason is that, in chain of events leading to fetal acidosis and hypoxia, late decelerations are one of the first signs to appear. One advantage of CST is that contraction induced during the test will help to ripen the cervix and initiate labor. However, CST requires time and has high proportions of false positive result.

MANAGEMENT AND TREATMENT

Information provided by history, physical examination and fetal surveillance tests will identify some group of patients who need to be delivered.

- Women with medical or obstetric complications of pregnancy (diabetes and hypertension)
- Women with oligohydramnios
- Estimated fetal weight between 4000 gm to 4500 gm
- Suspected fetal compromise
- Fetal congenital abnormalities
- Women with ripe cervix
- Women with senescent placenta

Expectant treatment—is justified in a small group of women who are:

- <41 weeks
- Unripe cervix
- Normal AFV
- Normal size baby
- Normal CST, NST, BPP.

The main objective of expectant treatment in these cases is to allow spontaneous onset of labor and cervical ripening to occur during a period of 1 week or rarely up to a maximum of 2 weeks.

There is universal agreement that a well dated pregnancy should be terminated at 42 weeks due to adverse prognosis of the fetus as well as risk to the mother. On the other hand, approach to managing pregnancies between 41 and 42 weeks of gestation remains an open question (Wennerholm et al, 2009). The main argument in research literature against a policy of routine induction between 41 to 42 weeks, that it increases the rate of cesarean delivery without decreasing maternal and/or neonatal morbidity. But majority of data (Rand et al, 2000, Gulmezogle et al, 2006), suggest that routine induction of labor at 41 weeks in well dated low risk pregnancy does not increase cesarean rates and it rather decrease the perinatal mortality and morbidity.

Therefore, expectant treatment is appropriate between 40–41 weeks of gestation which includes twice weekly assessment of fetal status by NST and BPP, amniotic fluid volume and assessment of cervical ripening. Oral rehydration therapy with hypotonic fluids and water may have a role in the management of oligohydramnios (Malhotra and Deka, 2002). Induction of labor is best choice in those which decreased AFV or when cervix becomes ripe. Cesarean is best choice when there are signs of fetal distress or weight greater than 4500 g.

Methods to Ripen Cervix

- PGE2 gel for intracervical application
- Vaginal or oral of PGE1 tablet (misoprostol)
- Mechanical dilation by Laminaria tent or Foley's catheter
- Glycerol trinitrate vaginal tablets.

In case of scarred uterus, care should be taken to avoid using too high dose or too short dosing intervels as both can result in uterine tachysystole and subsequent fetal distress.

INTRAPARTUM MANAGEMENT

Labor is a dangerous time for post-term fetus, therefore, it should be intensively monitored using partograph and continuous cardiotocogram. Once labor is induced, obstetricians should be ready to deal with complications during intrapartum period which includes meconium, fetal macrosomia and fetal distress.

The farther the pregnancy progresses beyond 40 weeks, the more likely the presence of thick meconium. This is due to increased uteroplacental insufficiency which leads to hypoxia in labor and activation of vagal system. Decision to do amniotomy is problematic as further decrease in fluid enhances the possibility of cord compression. Conversely amniotomy identifies thick meconium. In the presence of thick meconium, when women are remote from delivery, cesarean section should be done. Traditionally, saline amniofusion and aggressive nasopharyngeal and oropharyngeal suction as soon as head is delivered has been used to reduce the incidence of meconium aspiration syndrome (MAS). Recent studies, however, suggest that such procedures do not effectively prevent MAS. ACOG does not recommend routine intrapartum suctioning in vigorous baby. However, if depressed baby has meconium, the intubation should be done with tracheal suctioning by experienced persons.

In view of fetal macrosomia an important part of delivery plan is to be prepared for undertaking shoulder dystocia drill.

Fetal distress—Nonreassuring FHR pattern like variable deceleration, absence or decreased variability, prolonged bradycardia are frequently observed in prolonged pregnancy. Amniofusion with 300–500 mL of warmed normal saline though does not prevent meconium aspiration, remains a reasonable treatment for repetitive variable deceleration, regardless of meconium status. If amniofusion fails to correct abnormal FHR, delivery should be by cesarean section.

SUGGESTED READING

1. ACOG. Practice Bulletin: Clinical management guidelines for obstetricians-gynecologists. No 55, September 2004 (replaces practice pattern No 6, October 1997). Management of postterm pregnancy. Obstet Gynecol. 2004;104:639-46.
2. Arias F. Predictability of complications associated with prolongation of pregancy. Obstet Gynecol. 1987;70:101.
3. Boyd ME, Usher RH, McLean FH, et al. Obstetric consequences of postmaturity. Am J Obstet Gynenol. 1988;158:334.
4. Clement D, Schifrin BS, Kates RB. Acute oligohydramnios in postdated pregnancy. Am J Obstet Gynenol. 1987;157:884.
5. Divon MY, Feldman- Leidner N. Postdates and antenatal testing. Semin Perinatal. 2008;32(4):295.
6. Gulmezoglu AM, Crowther CA, Middleton P. Indution of labour for improving birth outcomes for women at or beyond term. Cochrane Database Syst Rev 2006; issue 4:CD004945. DOI10. 1002/1461858.

7. Lenovo KJ, Quirk JG, CunninghamFG, et al. Prolonged pregnancy: observations concerning the causes of fetal distress. Am J Obstet Gynenol. 1984;150:465.
8. Malhotra B, Deka D, Maternal oral hydration with hypotonic solution (water) increases amniotic fluid volume in pregnancy. J Obstet Gynecol India. 2002;52(1):49.
9. Manning FA, Morrison I, Harman CR, et al. The abnormal fetal biophysical profile score. V. predictive accuracy according to score composition. Am J Obstet Gynecol. 1990;162:918-24.
10. Rand L, Robinson JN, Economy KE, et al. Post term induction of labour revisited. Obstet Gynecol. 2000;96:779-83.
11. Silver RK, Dooley SI, MacGregor SN, et al. Fetal acidosis in prolonged pregnancy can not be attributed to cord compression alone. Am J Obstet Gynecol. 1988; 159:66.
12. Smith GCS. Lifetime analysis of the risk of perinatal death at term and at postterm in singleton pregnancy. Am J Obstet Gynecol. 2001;184:489-96.
13. Smith SC, Baker PN. Placental apoptosis is increased in postterm pregnancy. Br J Obstet Gynecol. 1999;106:861.
14. Wennerholm UB, Hagberg H, Brorsson B, Bergh C. Induction of labour versus expectant management for postdate pregnancy: is there sufficient evidence for a change in clinical practice? Acta Obstet Gynecol Scand. 2009;88(1):6-17.

Chapter 22

Fetal Distress in Labor

Abha Rani Sinha, Anita Verma

INTRODUCTION

The term fetal distress is commonly used, much maligned, and little understood. It denotes disruption of normal fetal oxygenation ranging from mild hypoxia to profound asphyxia. The term hypoxia refers to reduction in tissue oxygenation and asphyxia implies combination of hypoxia and metabolic acidosis.

INCIDENCE

Exact incidence is not known mainly because there is no consensus on definition. Incidence of birth asphyxia though is said to be in the range of 40% of instrumental deliveries and 30% of cesarean sections.[1,2]

PATHOGENESIS

During labor → uterus contracts → transient decrease in blood supply and oxygen to the fetus → uterus relaxes → oxygenation restored to fetus. A normal fetus with good metabolic reserve can withstand this assault to a certain extent. A compromised fetus with low metabolic reserve or a normal fetus with repetitive hypoxic assaults will develop hypoxia which is initially completely reversible.

Initially, fetus responds by:
- Decreasing heart rate
- Decreasing body movements
- Redistributing blood supply to vital organs
- Switch to anerobic metabolism from aerobic glycolysis.

  This results in accumulation of lactic acid and pyruvic acid leading to metabolic acidosis which leads to:
- Accumulation of H⁻ ions which initially stimulate sinoauricular nodes leading to fetal tachycardia. Later they depress the node causing bradycardia.
- The parasympathetic nerves are also stimulated leading to increased peristalsis and relaxation of anal sphincter causing 'meconium staining' of liquor.
- Prolonged hypoxia may lead to neurological injury and even still birth.

ETIOLOGY

Factors associated with increased risk of fetal distress in labor:
- Antenatal maternal conditions
  - Hypertension/PIH
  - Diabetes
  - Antepartum hemorrhage
  - Severe maternal medical diseases
- Antenatal fetal condition
  - Growth restricted fetus
  - Prematurity
  - Post-maturity
  - Oligohydramnios
  - Isoimmunization
  - Multiple pregnancies
  - Malpresentation
  - Abnormal umbilical cord Doppler velocimetry
- Intrapartum maternal conditions
  - Vaginal bleeding in labor
  - Intrauterine infection
- Labor
  - Rupture uterus
  - Premature rupture of membrane
  - Induced/Augmented labor
  - Hypertonic uterus
  - Cord prolapse
- Fetal condition
  - Meconium staining of liquor
  - Suspicious FHR on auscultation
  - Shoulder dystocia
  - Nuchal cord

DIAGNOSIS

Proper history and examination will alert an obstetrician to fetuses at risk to develop distress during labor. These high-risk fetuses will require rigorous monitoring.

A number of methods and tools are being used to identify fetal distress as early as possible, i.e. when fetal hypoxia is still in reversible phase.

Intermittent Auscultation

NICE, RCOG recommends:[3]
- Every 15–30 minutes in active phase and 5 minutes in second stage of labor
- FHR should be monitored during contraction and thirty seconds after contraction.

FHR thus obtained is considered non-reassuring if:

- The average heart rate between contractions is less than 100 beats per minute (bpm)
- The heart rate is less than 100 bpm 30 seconds after contraction
- There is unexplained average heart rate of more than 160 bpm between contractions
- When tachycardia persists through three or more contractions (10 to 15 minutes) despite corrective measures.

Electronic Fetal Monitoring

Electronic fetal monitoring (EFM) was introduced in early 1970 and adopted by obstetricians with alacrity as it provided significant improvement in fetal assessment. But EFM was later found to have high sensitivity and low specificity. 95% babies having normal patterns on EFM will have a good Apgar score but only 50% babies with abnormal patterns will have a low Apgar score,[4] leading to an error in judgment and an increase in cesarean rates. However, it is still the most widely used method for intra partum fetal monitoring in western countries.

Cardiotocography

Cardiotocography (CTG) tracings forms the backbone of fetal monitoring in labor. Continuous EFM is recommended in:

- All high-risk pregnancies
- In low-risk pregnancy if FHR on intermittent auscultation is abnormal
- It is also recommended for meconium stained liquor. The chances of developing acidosis are greater with thick meconium than thin meconium.

Admission CTG is not preferred for low risk pregnancy.

It is interpreted as follows:

- **Baseline FHR:** The normal range of baseline FHR is 110–160 bpm. An uncomplicated moderate bradycardia that is, 110–119 bpm and moderate tachycardia, i.e. 161–179 bpm, is probably not associated with adverse fetal outcome. But FHR above 180 or below 100 is definitely abnormal.
- **Baseline variability (beat to beat):** Normal baseline variability is between 5 to 25 beat per minute. This denotes healthy influence of autonomic nervous system on cardiovascular function. Variability of less than 5 beat per minute is indicative of:
    - Fetal hypoxemia
    - Sleep status of fetus
    - Epidural analgesia
    - Drugs given in labor
    - Extreme prematurity
    - CNS abnormality.

Baseline variability of more than 25 bpm is called saltatory pattern and is considered benign if present with long and short term variability.

- **Acceleration:** Increase in heart rate of 15 beats or more from baseline lasting more than 15 seconds and associated with fetal movement is indicative of integrity of somatic nervous system. If more than 2 such accelerations are present in 15 minutes it is reassuring. However, significance of its absence is unclear. Its absence may be due to:
  - Sleep status of fetus
  - Medication
  - Infection.

- **Deceleration:** FHR falling below the baseline level by 15 beats or more and lasting more than 15 seconds is termed deceleration.
  - Early deceleration (Fig. 1)—This is when deceleration coincides with a contraction, the peak of contraction coinciding with nadir of deceleration (mirror image). This is rarely more than 40 beats. It is seen in late first or second stage of labor. It may be due to head compression.
  - Late deceleration (Fig. 2)—Slowing of FHR coinciding with the peak or at the end of contraction is called late deceleration. The recovery

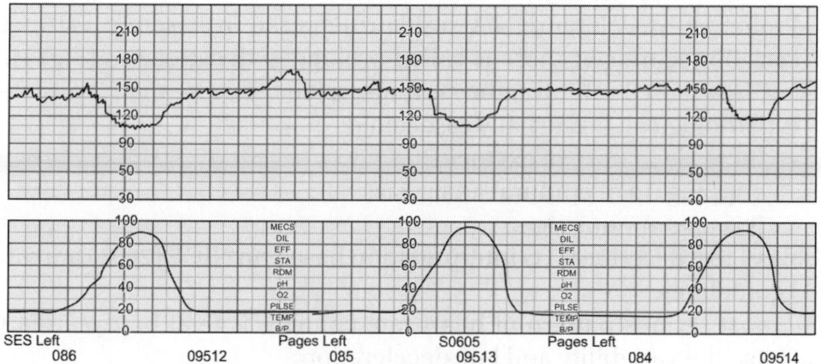

Fig. 1: Early deceleration

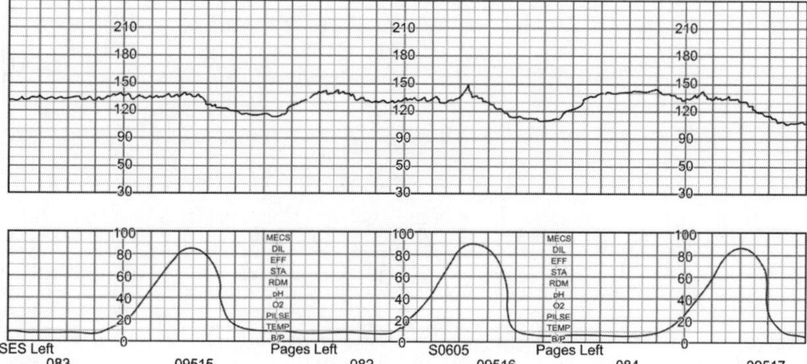

Fig. 2: Late deceleration

is gradual and magnitude is rarely more than 40 beats. This indicates uteroplacental insufficiency.

- Variable deceleration (Fig. 3)—These are periodic slowing down and recovery of FHR and have got no relation to contraction. It is said to be due to cord compression. Another character is 'shouldering', i.e. initial acceleration followed by deceleration which is again followed by a little acceleration. It is a typical characteristic of cord compression.
- Atypical variable deceleration:

  Its features are:
  - Loss of primary or secondary rise in baseline rate
  - Slow return to baseline rate after contraction
  - Prolonged secondary rise in base line rate
  - Loss of variability during deceleration
  - Biphasic deceleration
  - Continuation of baseline rate at lower level
  - Deceleration that has a depth of more than 60 beats and duration more than 60 seconds. This is considered severe.

    This results from a combination of cord compression and decreased uteroplacental flow.
- Prolonged deceleration—A sudden decrease in baseline FHR which lasts 90 seconds or more is called prolonged deceleration (Fig. 4). If it last less than 3 minutes, they are suspicious; if more than 3 minutes. It is pathological. It is usually associated:
  - Increase in dose of oxytocin
  - Topping up of epidural analgesia.

    It is an ominous sign.

Tables 1 to 3 describe CTG interpretation based on NICE (2001) and RCOG (2001) guidelines.[5,6]

The most serious pattern of heart rate changes is fetal bradycardia with loss of baseline variability and late deceleration.

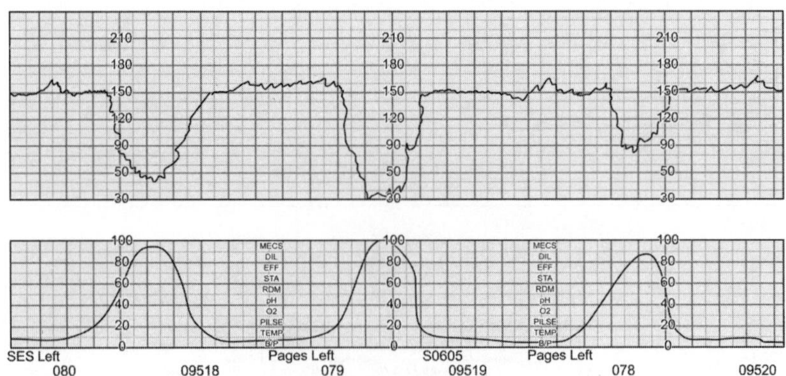

Fig. 3: Variable deceleration

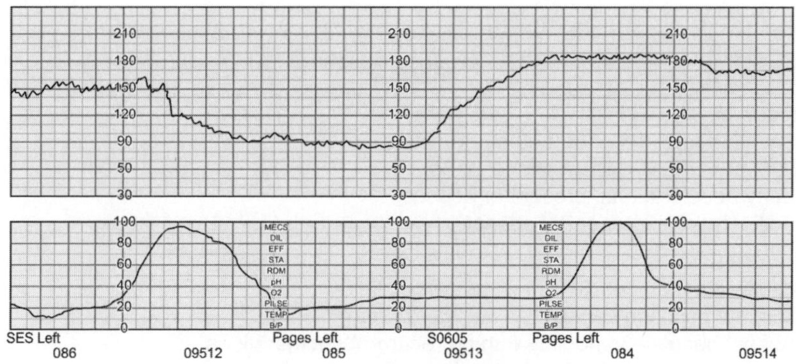

Fig. 4: Prolonged deceleration

Table 1: Classification of the individual features of the FHR trace
(NICE 2001; RCOG 2001)

Feature	Baseline (bpm)	Variability (bpm)	Decelerations	Accelerations
Reassuring	❖ 110–160	≥5	None	Present
Non-reassuring	❖ 100–109 ❖ 161–180	<5 for ≥40 but <90 minutes	❖ Early deceleration ❖ Variable deceleration ❖ Single prolonged deceleration up to 3 minutes	May or may not be present
Abnormal	❖ <100 ❖ >180 ❖ Sinusoidal pattern ≥10 minutes	<5 for ≥90 minutes	❖ Atypical variable deceleration ❖ Late deceleration ❖ Single prolonged deceleration >3 minutes	The absence of accelerations with an otherwise normal CTG is of uncertain significance

Table 2: Classification of CTG based on the features of FHR trace
(NICE 2001; RCOG 2001)

Category	Definition
Normal	A CTG whose features fall into the reassuring category
Suspicious	A CTG whose features fall into one of the non-reassuring categories while the remainder are reassuring
Pathological	A CTG whose features fall into two or more non-reassuring categories or one or more abnormal categories

Table 3: Three-tiered fetal heart rate interpretation system (ACOG practice bulletin 2010)[7]
Category I   ❖ Baseline rate: 110–160 beats per minute   ❖ Late or variable decelerations: absent   ❖ Early decelerations: present or absent   ❖ Accelerations: present of absent
Category II   Baseline rate   ❖ Minimal baseline variability   ❖ Absent baseline variability with no recurrent decelerations   ❖ Marked baseline variability   Accelerations   ❖ Absence of induced accelerations after fetal stimulation, periodic or episodic decelerations   ❖ Recurrent variable decelerations accompanied by minimal or moderate baseline variability   ❖ Prolonged deceleration more than 2 minutes but less than 10 minutes   ❖ Recurrent late decelerations with moderate baseline variability   ❖ Variable decelerations with other characteristic such as slow return to baseline, overshoots, or "shoulders"

Category III
 ❖ Absent baseline FHR variability and any of the following
   – Recurrent late decelerations
   – Recurrent variable decelerations
   – Bradycardia or
 ❖ Sinusoidal pattern

About 15% of CTG recordings in labor are non-reassuring (RCOG 2001). Therefore, additional methods have emerged to assess fetal wellbeing. They complement CTG and help in reducing unnecessary interventions.

Fetal Scalp Stimulation

If there is increase in FHR in response to painful stimuli (digital scalp stimulation, fetal scalp puncture), it is considered normal and fetus is unlikely to have acidosis.[8] However, absence of this response does not mean fetal compromise. Fetal monitoring should be continued inspite of positive result. If suspicious FHR persists, this test may even be repeated. Fetal scalp pH should be performed, if available in such circumstances.

Vibroacoustic Stimulation

Artificial larynx is used for vibroacoustic stimulation (VAS) of fetus. It is non-invasive. Rise in FHR for at least 15 seconds following VAS is considered a positive test. It indicates that fetus with non reassuring pattern on CTG monitoring is not hypoxic. However, 50% of fetuses born after negative testing were found to have normal blood gas at birth.[9]

Fetal Scalp Blood Sampling

Fetal scalp blood pH is considered 'gold standard' to detect fetal acidosis following non-reassuring FHR pattern. RCOG (2001)[5] recommends:

- pH >7.25—reassuring
- pH 7.20 to 7.25—suspicious or preacidotic. Repeat fetal scalp blood sampling (FBS) within 30 minutes
- pH less than 7.20—acidosis. Immediate delivery is indicated.

Limitation—This method requires:

- Dilatation of cervix
- Access to presenting part
- Ruptured membrane
- Requires large volume of fetal blood
- Is expensive.

It is contraindicated in:

- Maternal infections including HIV, hepatitis and herpes simplex
- In fetal bleeding disorders.

Fetal Scalp Blood Lactate Measurement

Measurement of fetal scalp blood lactate is more accurate for diagnosing fetal acidemia. A level more than 4.8 mmol/liter is considered pathological.[10] It requires lesser amount of blood and fewer scalp incisions and is quicker. The results looks promising. At present large trials are being conducted.

Fetal Pulse Oximetry

This offers to continuously measure oxygen saturation of fetus in the event of non-reassuring FHR pattern. It is noninvasive but requires cervix to be dilated at least 2 cm and membrane to be ruptured. Fetal oxygen saturation of more than 30% has not been associated with abnormal gas values of fetus, but a saturation of less than 30% requires immediate intervention.[11,12] It is being further evaluated and is the focus of several studies.

Fetal ECG Waveform Analysis (STAN)

ST wave analysis of fetal ECG provides information regarding ability of heart muscle to withstand stress of labor. An ST segment rise indicates response of fetus to hypoxia and a switch to anerobic myocardial metabolism. A negative ST segment indicates a fetus that is incapable of responding or has not had time to respond.[13,14]

Studies indicate that combine CTG monitoring with STAN lead to increased identification of fetal hypoxia. This too is still being evaluated.

Near Infrared Spectrometry (NIRS)

NIRS is a noninvasive optical technique measuring absorption of reflected light to detect and measure cerebral oxygenation. Preliminary studies have indicated significant correlation between fetal cerebral oxygen saturation and umbilical artery and vein pH at birth.[15,16] Its use is experimental at present.

MANAGEMENT

CTG remains the main tool for diagnosing fetal compromise. Pathological tracings necessitate prompt delivery within 30 minutes either by cesarean section or by operative vaginal delivery.

It is the non-reassuring or suspicious pattern which poses problem. Further tests to determine fetal academia is required. In the meanwhile assessment of the following is required:

a. Cause of hypoxia if possible
b. Fetal reserve
c. Progress of labor

Intrapartum resuscitation measures are to be instituted to buy time and to correct cause of hypoxemia if possible.

Intrapartum Resuscitation

Maternal Oxygenation

It is said to increase available oxygen from mother to fetus and helps in reducing fetal distress. This is of benefit only as a short term therapy.[17] Oxygen is administered by mask (8–10 L/min).

Change of Position

Lateral recumbent position helps to increase uteroplacental perfusion.

Discontinuation of Oxytocin

If there are suspicious or pathological FHR tracings, oxytocin should be stopped immediately. This improves fetal oxygenation if hypoxia was due to a uterine contraction.

Tocolysis

If there is uterine hyperstimulation, with abnormal CTG in the absence of oxytocin infusion, tocolysis helps in improving fetal oxygenation. Injection terbutaline 0.25 mg SC, glyceryl trinitrate as sublingual spray has been used with positive results. It is contraindicated if patient has tachycardia.

Intravenous Fluid

Bolus of 500 mL of crystalloid like Ringers' Lactate given over 20 minutes helps in increasing placental blood flow especially in hypovolemic and hypotensive women. It also has tocolytic effect on uterus for 15 to 20 minutes.[18] It should be used with caution in conditions where there is increased risk of pulmonary edema like pre-eclampsia, preterm labor treated with magnesium sulphate, corticosteroid and beta sympathomimetics. Prolonged use of oxytocin in large doses can also lead to fluid overload due to its antidiuretic action.

Glucose containing fluids are best avoided as they increase fetal lactate level.

Cord Prolapse

Pelvic examination should be done to exclude cord prolapse in the event of non-reassuring tracings. Steps should be taken to relieve pressure from cord immediately.

Amnioinfusion

Role of amnio infusion to dilute meconium in liquor is dubious and ACOG does not recommend it. However, it has a role in reducing cord compression in cases of oligohydramnios with variable decelerations.[19] A bolus of 200–300 mL of warm saline solution can be given through intrauterine pressure catheter in over 30 minutes. It should not be performed if there are late decelerations, fetal scalp pH less than 7.2, abruption placenta, placenta previa and known uterine anomalies.

Anesthesia in Fetal Distress

There is not much study on quickest and best anesthesia in patients with fetal distress. Evidence supports the use of regional anesthesia.[20]

Neonatal Care

Presence of a neonatologist is must when delivery of a hypoxic baby is anticipated. Intrapartum suction of oropharynx and nasopharynx is not recommended by ACOG at present as it does not prevent meconium aspiration syndrome. If baby is depressed, endotracheal intubation is to be done and tracheal suctioned done from beneath the glottis.[21,22]

CONCLUSION

- Fetal distress is a cause of obstetrician distress.
- Pathological CTG tracings necessitate delivery within 30 minutes.
- It is the non-reassuring patterns which pose problem in management.
- Further tests like fetal scalp stimulation, FBS, lactate measurement, etc. is required to further confirm fetal hypoxia.
- Intra partum resuscitation plays an important role in both suspicious and non-reassuring pattern groups to buy time before delivery.
- While there is no ideal test for assessing fetal acidemia, new trials are giving hope of finding one in near future.

REFERENCES

1. Okunwobi-Smith Y, Cooke-I, MacKenzie Iz. Decision to delivery intervals for assisted vaginal vertex delivery. Br J Obstet Gynaecol. 2000;107:467-71.
2. Wilkinson C, McIlwaine G, Boulton-Jones C, Cole S. Is a rising caesarean section rate inevitable ? Br J Obstet Gynaecol. 1998;105:45-52.
3. Liston R, et al. Intrapartun Fetal surveillance. J. Obstet and Gynae. 2007;152:524-39.
4. Schiermeier et al. Sensitivity and Specificity of intrapatem computerized FIGO Criteria for CTG and Fetal scalp pH during labour. Br J Obstet Gynaecol. 2008;115:1557-63.
5. Royal college of Obstetricians and gynaecologists. 2001. The use of electronic fetal monitoring: the use and interpretation of cardiotocography in intrapartum fetal surveillance. Evidence- best clinical guideline number 8; Royal College of Obstetricians and Gynaecologists, London.
6. NICE 2001. National institute for clinical excellence. The use of electronic fetal monitoring: The use and interpretation of cardiotocography in intrapartum fetal surveillance. NICE Inherited Clinical Guideline C, London: National institute of clinical excellence.
7. ACOG Practice Bulletin, Number 116, November 2010.
8. Clark SL, Gimovsky ML, Miller FC. The scalp stimulation test : a clinical alternative to fetal scalp blood sampling. Am J Obstet Gynaecol. 1984;148:274-7.
9. Spencer JAD, Deans A, Nicolaidis P, et al. Fetal heart rate response to vibroacoustic stimulation during low and high heart rate variability episodes in late pregnancy. Am J Obstet Gynaecol. 1991;165:86-90.
10. Kruger K, Halberg B, Blennow M. Predictive value of fetal scalp blood lactate concentration and pH as markers of neurological disability. Am J Obstet Gynaecol. 1999;5:1072-8.
11. Arikan GM, Scholz HS, Haeusler MCH, et al. Low Fetal oxygen saturation at birth and acidosis. Obstet Gynaecol. 2000;95:565-71.
12. Garite Tj, Dildi GA, Namara H Mc, et al. A multicenter controlled trial of fetal pulse oximetry in the intrapatum management of nonreassuring fetal heart rate patterns. Am J Obstet Gynaecol. 2000;183:1049-58.
13. Neilson JP. Fetal electrocardiogram for fetal monitoring during labour (Cochrane review). The Cochrane Library 1. Chichester, UK: John Wiley and Sons, Ltd; 2004.
14. Luttkus AK, Noren H, Stupin JH, et al. Fetal scalp pH and ST analysis of the fetal ECG as an adjunct to CTG. A multicenter, observational study. J Perinat Med. 2004;32:486-92.
15. Peebles DM, Edwards AD, Wyatt JS, et al. Changes in human fetal cerebral haemoglobin concentration and oxygenation during labour measured by near-infrared spectroscopy. Am J Obstet Gynaecol. 1992;166:1369-73.
16. Peebles DM. Cerebral Hemodynamics and Oxygenation in the fetus: The role of intrapartum near- infrared spectroscopy. Clinics in perinatology. 1997;24:547-65.
17. Maharaj D. Intrapartum fetal resuscitation: A Review. The Internet Journal of Gynaecology and Obstetrics. 2008;9(2).
18. Simpsom KR, James DC. Efficacy of intrauterine resuscitation techniques in improving fetal oxygen status during labour. Obstet Gynecol. 2005;105:1362-8.
19. Mino M, Puertas A, et al. Amnioinfusion in term labour with low amniotic fluid due to rupture of membranes: A new indication. Eur J Obstet Gynecol Reprod Biol. 1999;82:29-34.

20. Bonnet MP, Bruyere M, Moufouki M, De la Dorie A, Benhamou D. Anaesthesia, a cause of fetal distress? Annales Francaises d's Anesthesie et ded Reanimation. 2007;26(7-8):694-8.
21. The International Laison Committee on resuscitation (ILCOR). 2006;117(5): e978-e988.
22. Kattwinkei J, Periman JM, Aziz K, et al. Part 15: Neonatal resuscitation 2010 American heart association guideline. 2010;122(18 Suppl. 3):S909-S919.

Shoulder Dystocia

Abha Rani Sinha, Vinita Sahay

INTRODUCTION

Shoulder dystocia is an obstetric emergency associated with high perinatal mortality and morbidity shoulder dystocia is defined as a vaginal cephalic delivery that requires additional obstetric maneuvers to deliver the fetus after head has delivered and gentle traction has failed.[1] It is a condition when either the anterior or the posterior (rarely) fetal shoulder impacts on the maternal symphysis or on the sacral promontory respectively.

It is a specific case of dystocia whereby after delivery of the head, the anterior shoulder of infant cannot pass below the pubic symphysis. It is diagnosed when shoulder fails to deliver shortly after the fetal head. In shoulder dystocia it is the chin that passes against the walls of the perineum. Fetal demise can occur if the infant is not delivered, due to compression of the umbilical cord within the birth canal.

PELVIC ANATOMY RELATED TO SHOULDER DYSTOCIA

The maternal pelvis is composed of series of bones forming a circle protecting the pelvic organs. The front most bone is the symphysis pubis. It is this structure that a baby's anterior shoulder gets caught on during a delivery complicated by shoulder dystocia. The bone at the back of the maternal pelvis is sacrum. Because of its shape, it generally serves as a slide over which baby's posterior shoulder can descend freely during labor and delivery. The side walls of maternal pelvic, although very important in determining the ease of the process of labor in general, usually do not contribute to shoulder dystocia.

In normal vaginal deliveries in cephalic presentation vertex emerges first. During labor, the soft mobile bones of the fetal head can 'mould' their shape and to a slight degree overlap. This facilitates the fetal head fitting into and passing through the maternal pelvis. The baby's shoulders, likewise, being flexible usually follow the delivery of the baby's head quickly and easily. But for this to happen, the axis of the fetal shoulders must descend into the maternal pelvis at an angle oblique to the pelvis's anteroposterior dimension. This position affords the shoulders most room for their passage. If instead, the shoulders line up in a front to back orientation as they are brought to emerge from the mother's pelvis, there will often be insufficient room for them to squeeze through. The back of the mother's pubic bone then forms a shelf on which the baby's anterior shoulder can get caught. If this happens, the shoulders cannot deliver and shoulder dystocia results.

Shoulder dystocia can also occur if the posterior shoulder of a baby gets caught on its mother's sacrum. This is far less likely to impede the descent of the baby's posterior shoulder.

Incidence

There is wide variation in the reported incidence of shoulder dystocia.[2] The incidence of shoulder dystocia is generally reported to be between 0.5% and 1.5% with scattered reports listing both higher and lower values. Those studies involving the largest number of vaginal deliveries report incidences between 0.58% and 0.7%.[3]

The true incidence of shoulder dystocia, however, is very much dependent upon how it is defined, how it is reported and the characteristics of the population being measured.

Recurrent Shoulder Dystocia

The risk of recurrent shoulder dystocia is substantial, 10–15%. Moreover, women who have had a shoulder dystocia delivery that resulted in injury to the fetus have an even greater risk of having a recurrent shoulder dystocia and subsequent fetal injury.

Risk Factors

The risk factors for shoulder dystocia can generally be divided into three categories.
 A. Preconceptional.
     1. Previous shoulder dystocia.
     2. Maternal obesity.
     3. Maternal age.
     4. Abnormal pelvis.
     5. Multiparity.
 B. Antepartum.
     1. Macrosomia.
     2. Diabetes.
     3. Excessive maternal weight gain.
     4. Fetal sex.
     5. Post-dates.
 C. Intrapartum.
     1. Instrumental delivery (forceps or vacuum).
     2. Labor abnormalities.
     3. Oxytocin and anesthesia.
     4. Episiotomy.

Previous shoulder dystocia significantly increases the risk of repeat shoulder dystocia. It is seen more commonly with increased maternal age, obesity and multiparity but in reality these are only markers for the increased risk of more primary risk factors. There is no evidence linking the abnormal pelvis to shoulder dystocia.

There is a definite relationship between fetal size and shoulder dystocia.[4] The incidence of shoulder dystocia increases as birth weight increases over 4000 g. But approximately 50% of cases of shoulder dystocia occur in infants whose birth weight is less than 4000 g.

Rate relationship between birth weight and shoulder dystocia is as follows:

Birth weight (g)	Nondiabetic	Diabetic
<4000	0.1–1.1	0.6–3.7
4000–4449	1.1–10	4.9–23.1
>4500	4.1–22.6	20–50

Sensitivity and specificity of USG to detect fetal weight greater than 4500 g were 22–69% and 98–99%. Therefore, estimated fetal weight (EFW) using ultrasound biometry did not appear to be more accurate than clinical estimate based upon palpation using Leopold's maneuvers.

The chest to head and shoulder to head ratios are increased in infants of diabetic mothers thereby increasing the risk of shoulder dystocia independent of fetal weight. Maternal diabetes increases the likelihood of shoulder dystocia 2–6 fold over the nondiabetic population.[5]

Other Factors

- Maternal weight gain, fetal sex and post-dates are secondary risk factors.
- They do indicate an increased risk for shoulder dystocia but they are only relevant to the degree that they increase risk of fetal macrosomia.
- Since multiparity increases the number of precipitous labors, it may be a primary risk factor for shoulder dystocia.
- 50% of pregnancies complicated by shoulder dystocia have no risk factor. Thus the predictive value of any one or combination of risk factors for shoulder dystocia is low.

Recognition

The first step in treating shoulder dystocia is recognizing when it occurs. There are two main signs that a shoulder dystocia is present:

1. The baby's body does not emerge with standard moderate traction and maternal pushing after delivery of the fetal head.
2. One often described feature is the 'turtle sign' (Fig. 1), which involves the appearance and retraction of fetal head (analogous to a turtle withdrawing into its shell) and erythematous (red) puffy face indicative of

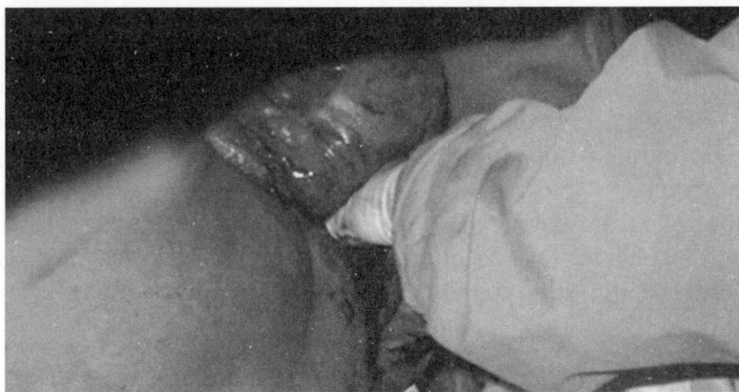

Fig. 1: Turtle sign
(For color version, see Plate 1)

facial flushing. This occurs when the baby's shoulder is obstructed by the maternal pelvis.

Procedures

A number of labor positions and/or obstetrical maneuvers are sequentially performed in an attempt to facilitate delivery at this point, including;

➲ McRoberts maneuver:[6] The McRoberts maneuver (Fig. 2) is employed in case of shoulder dystocia during childbirth and involves hyperflexing the mother's legs tightly to her abdomen. This widens the pelvis and flattens the spine in the lower back (lumbar spine). If this maneuver does not succeed, an assistant applies pressure on the lower abdomen (suprapubic pressure) and the delivered head is also gently pulled. The technique is effective in about 42% cases.

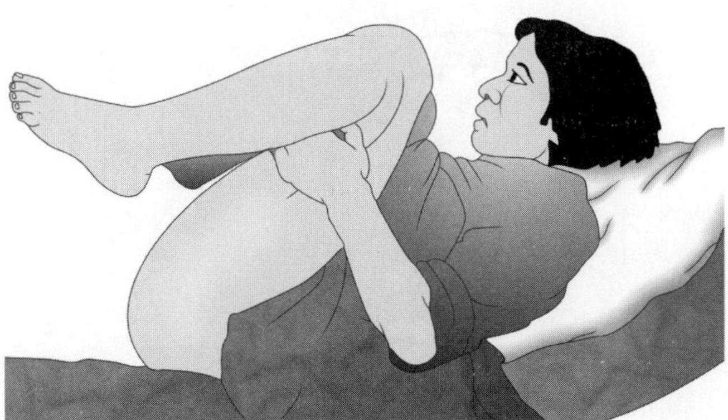

Fig. 2: McRoberts maneuver
(*Source:* McRoberts; http://altair.chonnam.ac.kr/~tbsong/medical/sh-dyst)

- Rubin ll[7] (Fig. 3) or posterior pressure on the anterior shoulder, which would bring the fetus in an oblique position with head somewhat towards the vagina.
- Wood's screw maneuver[8] (Figs 4 and 5), which leads to turning the anterior shoulder to the posterior and vice versa (somewhat the opposite of Rubin ll maneuver).
- Jacquemier's maneuver (also called Barnum's maneuver) shown in Figure 6 for delivery of the posterior shoulder first, in which the forearm and hand are identified in the birth canal and gently pulled.

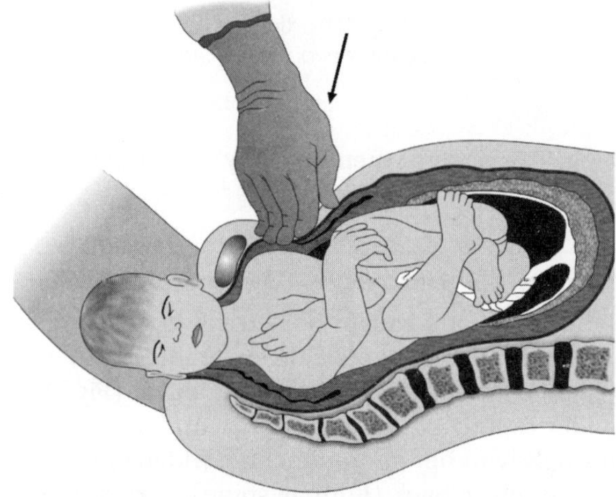

Fig. 3: Suprapubic pressure (or Rubin II)
[*Source:* Rubin I patientsafetyauthority.org/ADVISORIES/AdvisoryLibrary/
2009/dec16_6(suppl1)/Pages/18.aspx]

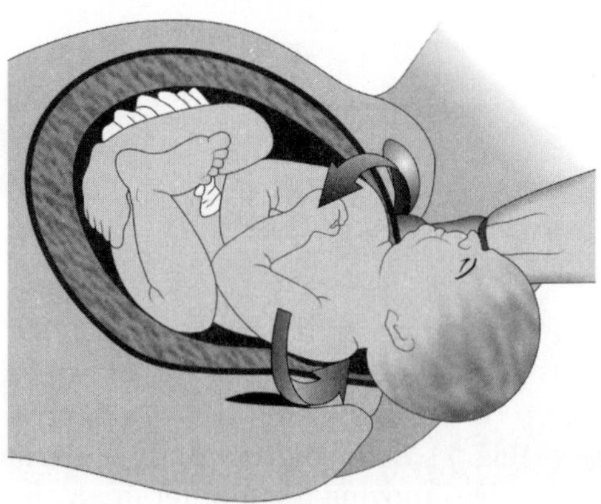

Fig. 4: Wood's screw maneuver (Rotate anterior shoulder)

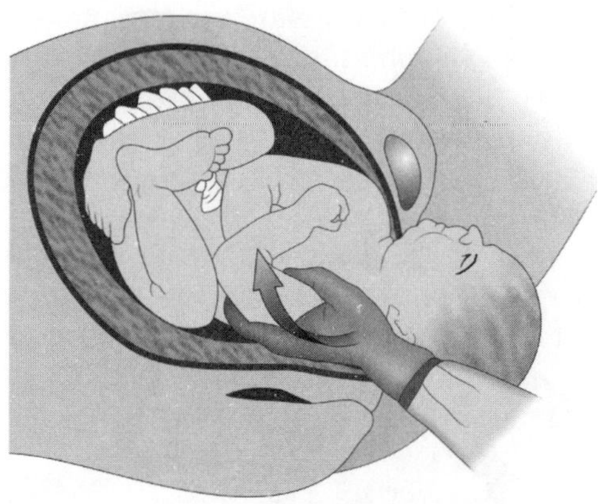

Fig. 5: Wood's screw maneuver (Rotate posterior shoulder)
(*Source:* Rotational; http://shoulderdystociainfo.com/resolvedwithoutfetal)

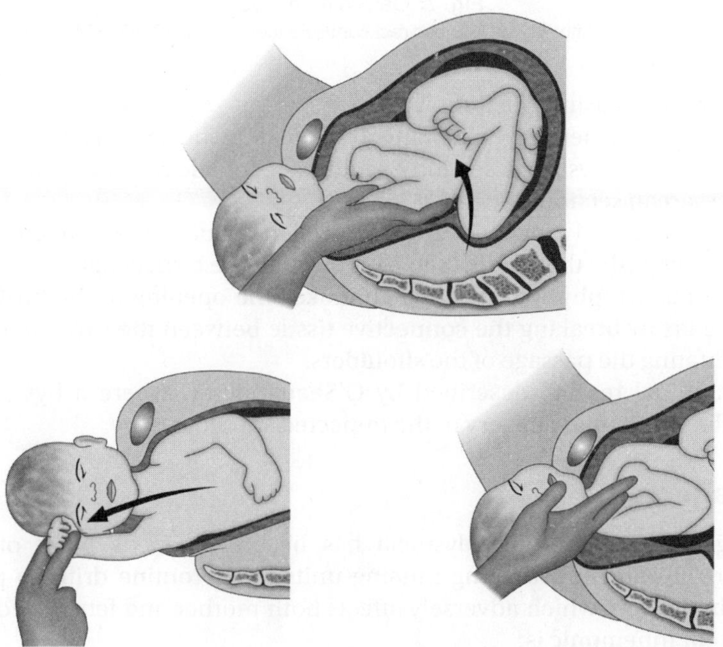

Fig. 6: Jacquemier's maneuver
(*Source:* Manual delivery of posterior arm; http://www.glowm.com/resources/glowm/
cd/pages/v2/v2c079)

⮕ Gaskin maneuver[9] (Fig. 7), named after a Certified Professional Midwife, Ina May Gaskin, involves moving the mother to an all four position with the back arched, widening the pelvic outlet.

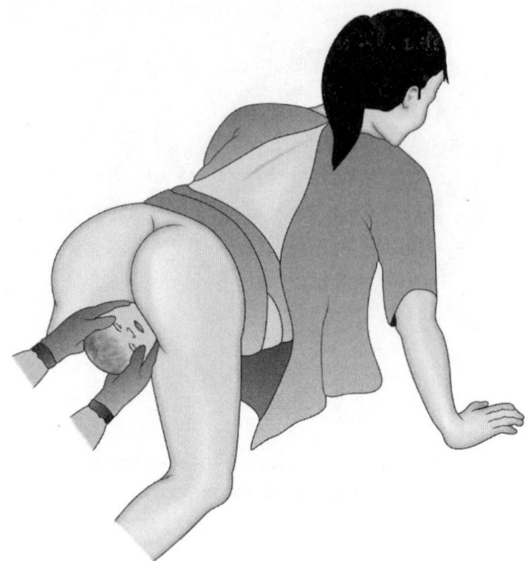

Fig. 7: Gaskin maneuver
(*Source:* Gaskin; http://www.sciencedirect.com/science/article/pii/S0889854505700899)

More drastic measures include:
- Zavanelli's maneuver[10] which involves pushing the fetal head back in and performing a cesarean section or internal cephalic replacement followed by cesarean section.
- Intentional fetal clavicular fracture, which reduces the diameter of the shoulder girdle that requires to pass through the birth canal.
- Maternal symphysiotomy,[11] which makes the opening of the birth canal more lax by breaking the connective tissue between the two pubic bones facilitating the passage of the shoulders.
- Abdominal rescue, described by O'Shaughnessy, where a hysterotomy facilitates vaginal delivery of the impacted shoulder.

Management

Management of shoulder dystocia has become a focus point of many obstetrical units encouraging nursing units to do routine drills to prevent delay in delivery which adversely affects both mother and fetus. A common treatment mnemonic is:

HELPER Mnemonic: It is a clinical tool that offers a structural framework for coping with shoulder dystocia. These maneuvers are designed to do one of three things:
1. Increase the functional size of the bony pelvis through flattening of lumbar lordosis and cephalad rotation of the symphysis—McRoberts maneuver.
2. Decrease the bisacromial diameter, the breadth of the shoulders of the fetus through application of suprapubic pressure.

3. Change the relationship of the bisacromial diameter with the bony pelvis through internal rotation maneuvers.

- H-Call for help
- E-Evaluate for episiotomy
- L-Legs (McRoberts maneuver)
- P-Pressure (suprapubic)
- E-Enter maneuver (internal rotation)

Rubin II

At vaginal examination apply pressure if shoulders move into the oblique diameter-attempt delivery

Rubin II +Wood's screw maneuver.

- If unsuccessful add Woods screw maneuver
- Reverse Wood's screw maneuver
- R-Remove the posterior arm
- R-Roll the patient

Another treatment mnemonic is ALARMER

- A-Ask for help: This involves requesting the help of an obstetrician, anesthetist and pediatrician for subsequent resuscitation of the infant
- L-Leg hyperflexion (McRobert's maneuver)
- A-Anterior shoulder disimpaction (pressure)
- R-Rubin maneuver
- M-Manual delivery of posterior arm
- E-Episiotomy
- R-Roll over on all fours

The advantage of proceeding in this order is that it goes from least to most invasive, thereby reducing harm to the mother in the event that the infant delivers with one of the earliest maneuvers. In the event that these maneuvers are unsuccessful, a skilled obstetrician may attempt some of the additional procedures listed above. Intentional clavicular fracture is a final attempt at non-operative vaginal delivery prior to Zavanelli's maneuver or symphysiotomy, both of which are considered extraordinary treatment measures.

Complications

A. Maternal[12]
   1. Postpartum hemorrhage
   2. Vaginal and vulval lacerations, cervical injury and rectovaginal fistula
   3. Symphyseal separation
   4. III or IV degree tears
   5. Uterine rupture
B. Fetal[13]
   1. Brachial plexus injury (complicating 2.3 to 16% of such deliveries)[14]
   2. Clavicular fracture
   3. Fetal death
   4. Fetal hypoxia
   5. Fracture of humerus

Prevention

Labor induction in women with gestational diabetes who require insulin may reduce the risk of macrosomia and subsequent shoulder dystocia.

Documentation

Careful documentation of instances of shoulder dystocia and their resolution is extremely important for two reasons:
1. Obstetricians want to learn as much as possible from instances of shoulder dystocia in order to develop the best technique for dealing with them.
2. Shoulder dystocia is so often the initiating cause of medicolegal action.[15]

Acker (1991) described what careful documentation of a shoulder dystocia delivery should include:
1. Exact time of events
2. Description of maneuvers used
3. Estimation of the traction forces exerted.

The note must be legible and must be written shortly after the events so that it is a contemporaneous medical progress note. Acker also recommends that the note have a specific form.

The best defence in a medical liability action is thoughtful, articulate, timely documentation of each decision in the course of treatment.

CONCLUSION

It cannot be determined with any degree of accuracy, which babies will be macrosomic and which babies will experience shoulder dystocia at delivery.

KEY POINTS

- Shoulder dystocia is one of the most frightening obstetric emergencies in the labor room, most of these cases occur with no warning
- Macrosomia and maternal diabetes appear to be the two risk factors most often associated with shoulder dystocia
- The most common injuries associated with shoulder dystocia are brachial plexus injury, fracture of humerus and fracture of clavicle
- An obstetrician must be prepared to recognize a shoulder dystocia immediately and proceed through an orderly sequence of steps to effect delivery in a timely manner
- The goal of management is to prevent fetal asphyxia while avoiding fetal injury.

REFERENCES

1. Resnick R. Management of shoulder dystocia girdle: Clin Obstet Gynecol. 1980;23:559-64.
2. Gherman RB. Shoulder dystocia: an evidence based evaluation of the obstetric nightmare: Clin Obstet Gynecol. 2002;45:345-62.
3. McFarland M, Hod M, Piper JM, Xenakis EM, Langer O. Are labour abnormalities more common in shoulder dystocia? Am J Obstet Gynecol. 1995;173:1211-4.
4. Acker DB, Sachs BP, Fridman EA. Risk factors for shoulder dystocia. Clin Obstet Gynecol. 1985;66:762-8.
5. Nesbitt TS, Gilbert WM, Herrchen B. Shoulder dystocia and associated risk factors with macrosomic infants born in California. Am J Obstet Gynecol. 1998;179:476-80.
6. Gonik B, Stinger CA, Held B. An alternate maneuver for management of shoulder dystocia. Am J Obstet Gynecol. 1983;145:882-4.
7. Rubin A. Management of shoulder dystocia. JAMA. 1964;189:835-7.
8. Woods CE, Westbury NYA. A principle of physics as applicable to shoulder delivey. Am J Obstet Gynecol. 1943;45:796-804.
9. Bruner JP, Drummond SB, Meenan AL, Gaskin IM. All fours maneuver for reducing shoulder dystocia during labour. J Repod Med. 1998;43:439-43.
10. Sandberg EC. The Zavanelli maneuver: a potentially revolutionary method for the resolution of shoulder dystocia. Am J Obstet Gynecol. 1983;152:479-84.
11. Van Roosmalen J. Shoulder dystocia and symphysiotomy. Eur J Obstet Gynecol Reproductive Biol. 1995;59:115-6.
12. Sheiner E, Leavy A, Hershkovitz R, Hallak M, Hammel RD, Katz M, et al. Determining factors associated with shoulder dystocia: a population based study. Eur J Obstet Gynecol Reprod Biol. 2006;126:11-5.
13. Gherman RB, Ouzounian JG, Goodwin TM. Obstetric maneuvers for shoulder dystocia and associated fetal morbidity. Am J Obstet Gynecol. 1998;178:1126-30.
14. Gherman RB, Goodwin TM, Souten I, Neumann K, Ouzounian JG, Paul RH. The McRoberts' maneuver for the alleviation of shoulder dystocia: how successful is it ? Am J Obstet Gynecol. 1997;176:656-61.
15. The '4 KG and over' enquiries: In: Confidential Enquiries into Still births and Deaths in Infancy. Sixth Annual Report. London Maternal and Child Health Research Consortium.

Chapter
24

Delayed Postpartum Hemorrhage

Archana Jha

INTRODUCTION

Postpartum hemorrhage (PPH) is an obstetric emergency that can follow vaginal or cesarean delivery. It is a major cause of maternal morbidity and mortality throughout the world, contributing to nearly 30% of pregnancy-related deaths annually, and one of the top three causes of maternal mortality in both high and low per capita income countries. Although, the absolute risk of death is much lower in high income countries (1 in 100,000 versus 1 in 1,000 births in low income countries), PPH is the leading cause of admission to the intensive care unit and most preventable cause of maternal mortality.

DEFINITION

The term 'postpartum' means 'after birth and related to it'. PPH is best defined as excessive bleeding that makes the patient symptomatic (e.g. pallor, lightheadedness, weakness, palpitations, diaphoresis, confusion, air hunger, syncope) and/or results in signs of hypovolemia (e.g. hypotension, tachycardia, oliguria, low oxygen saturation). Vaginal bleeding is usually noted, but in some cases it may be concealed as in cesarean section and broad ligament hematoma after a sulcus laceration.

Delayed or seceondary postpartum hemorrhage is defined as abnormal or excessive bleeding from the vagina between 24 hours and 12 weeks after giving birth. About one percent of postpartum women have a late postpartum hemorrhage with these signs:
- Bleeding that soaks more than one sanitary pad in an hour
- Bright red bleeding that occurs four days or more after delivery
- Blood clots bigger than a golf ball.

INCIDENCE

- The incidence of PPH varies widely, depending upon the criteria used to define the disorder.
- A reasonable estimate is 1 to 5 percent of deliveries
- Uterine atony was the most common cause of PPH.

CAUSES

Late postpartum hemorrhage may be caused by a uterus that does not contract normally, possibly as a result of fragments of the placenta or the amniotic sac that remain in the uterus after birth, an infection, or both. A late postpartum hemorrhage may also be caused by an inherited disorder that alters blood's ability to clot, such as von Willebrand disease. Sometimes, though, the cause is unknown.

The following lists the most common causes of early and late postpartum hemorrhage.

Early

- Uterine atony
- Lower genital tract lacerations (perineal, vaginal, cervical periclitoral, labial, periurethral, rectum)
- Upper genital tract lacerations (broad ligament)
- Lower urinary tract lacerations (bladder, urethra)
- Retained products of conceptions (placenta, membranes)
- Invasive placentation (placenta accreta, placenta increta, placenta percreta)
- Uterine rupture
- Uterine inversion
- Coagulopathy (hereditary, acquired).

Delayed

- Endometrial wall infection—Endometritis. When the site of placental implantation is not healed yet, infection in the uterus can cause the blood capillaries in the placental bed to start bleeding again.
- Poorly contracted uterus—The uterus may not contract well because of infection, retained placental fragments, or an unknown reason. As a result, bleeding can start again.
- Retained placenta—Remnants of placental tissue or fetal membranes retained in the uterus are common causes of delayed PPH.
- Sloughing of the placental bed—There is a possibility that the healed placental bed peels away (sloughs) and opens the blood capillaries again.
- Molar pregnancy—Although, it is uncommon for a woman to develop a molar pregnancy after delivery, its occurrence can have life-threatening complications; the rapidly growing mass of grape-like tissues in the uterus can cause profuse hemorrhage.

DIAGNOSIS

- Delayed or secondary PPH is a clinical diagnosis of exclusion, which may present as slight to heavy bleeding (and rarely hypovolemic shock), usually 7 to 14 days after birth.

- Small amount of bleeding may persist for several weeks and therefore some bleeding defined as a delayed or secondary PPH may be normal.
- Bleeding may also represent the initial menstrual period after childbirth, (result of an anovulatory cycle) and may be heavy, painful and prolonged.
- The time frame for secondary PPH also encompasses the period when contraception is commenced and vaginal bleeding is a common side effect of hormonal contraception.
- History of complications in previous pregnancies may reflect aberrant maternal-trophoblastic interaction, e.g. pre-eclampsia, IUGR, spontaneous miscarriage and especially retained placenta (retained products are more common in such women)
- Endometritis is suspected if the history includes uterine tenderness, fever or foul smelling lochia.
- Secondary PPH in the first week may be related to coagulopathy, especially von Willebrand disease.

ASSESSMENT

- Assessment should include thorough detailed history including parity, labor, and mode of delivery, third stage and puerperal complications.
- Temperature, pulse and blood pressure should be checked.
- Uterine size should be assessed.
- Clinical features may include bleeding per vaginam (may be offensive), abdominal cramping, uterine tenderness, pyrexia and an enlarged uterus.
- In women with pyrexia, other sources of infection, e.g. mastitis, urinary tract infection or septic pelvic thrombophlebitis need to be excluded.
- Clinical signs of blood loss (perfusion and hydration) should be assessed and compared with estimated blood loss.
- Speculum examination is done to check status of cervical os and obtain endocervical swab.
- Intravenous access should be established using 16 gauge cannulae and resuscitation commenced. Oxygen should be given via face mask.

INVESTIGATIONS

- Blood grouping, if not done earlier and cross-match 2-4 units red blood cells, if bleeding is marked
- Complete blood picture
- C-reactive protein should be estimated
- Serum β-hCG may be helpful to distinguish between trophoblastic disease and retained placental tissue or other causes when ultrasound is not informative
- Coagulation profile as indicated
- Midstream urine specimen
- Blood cultures if temperature $\geq$ 38°C
- Speculum examination and high vaginal swab for culture.

ULTRASOUND

- Ultrasound should be considered if there are concerns of retained placental tissue
- Ultrasound is useful to identify clot or other debris in uterine cavity and sub involution of the uterus
- Real time or color Doppler ultrasound may not differentiate placental tissue from blood clots, but it may show an empty uterus
- On color Doppler ultrasound, the rare uterine arteriovenous malformation appears as a hypervascular lesion with turbulent flow within the myometrium.

MANAGEMENT

- There are no randomized controlled trials for evidence based management of women with secondary postpartum hemorrhage.
- The pragmatic approach is stabilization, investigation to establish a cause for the bleeding and appropriate treatment.
- The mainstay of initial treatment is administration of a uterotonic agent. Antibiotics should be added and the need for surgical intervention considered if bleeding is heavy and ongoing. This necessitates urgent evacuation of the uterus.
- In most cases, endometritis can be effectively treated with antibiotics without surgical intervention (dilation and curettage).
- If curettage is recommended, the aim is to give antibiotics for 24 hours before the procedure (unless bleeding requires earlier intervention).

Management of PPH begins before excessive blood loss has occurred by carefully observing the rate of bleeding immediately after delivery. In contrast, active management of the third stage involves early cord clamping, prophylactic administration of uterotonic agents before placental delivery, and controlled cord traction.

A schematic approach to PPH is presented in Table 1. Immediately after placental delivery, bimanual massage of the uterus promotes uterine contraction and hemostasis. If uterine bleeding does not promptly diminish, the obstetrician should proceed in serial fashion to consider possible causes of bleeding and institute therapeutic interventions. If a maneuver is unsuccessful in stopping hemorrhage, an alternative should be attempted. When less invasive measures are not initially successful, it is usually fruitless to repeat them while the patient continues to bleed.

TREATMENT

All patients with suspected retained products require antibiotic cover because there is always an element of infection in these circumstances.

Give intravenous antibiotics if the woman is febrile and oral antibiotics if a febrile but endometritis is suspected. Continue until a diagnosis is made or symptoms subside.

Table 1: Management scheme for postpartum hemorrhage		
Diagnostic maneuver	*To determine etiology*	*Therapeutic maneuver*
Palpate uterus	Uterine atony	❖ Uterine massage ❖ Establish intravenous access (if not established) ❖ Oxytocin ❖ Methylergonovine ❖ Prostaglandin (carboprost or alternative) ❖ Catheterize bladder ❖ Obtain blood for transfusion (if not already available) ❖ Prevent/treat shock
Examine perineum, vagina, cervix	Lacerations	❖ Repair lacerations
Manually explore uterus	❖ Retained products ❖ Uterine inversion ❖ Uterine rupture	❖ Manual removal ❖ Dilatation and curettage ❖ Replace uterus ❖ Surgical replacement ❖ Laparotomy for repair or hysterectomy
Coagulation studies If above measures are unsuccessful, presume uterine atony, uterine rupture, or intra-abdominal laceration	Coagulopathy	❖ Specific factor ❖ Replacement ❖ Repeat prostaglandin ❖ MAST suit (if available) ❖ Uterine artery embolization or laparotomy ❖ Hypogastric artery ligation ❖ Hysterectomy

Intravenous

- ⮀ Ampicillin (or amoxycillin) 2 g IV initial dose then 1 g IV every 4 hours
- ⮀ Gentamicin 5 mg/kg IV daily (80 mg IV bid)
- ⮀ Metronidazole 500 mg (100 mL IV) every 8 hourly.

Allergy to Penicillin

- ⮀ Lincomycin 600 mg IV in 100 mL over 1 hour every 8 hours
- ⮀ Gentamicin 5 mg/kg (80 mg IV bid) daily.

Oral

- ⮀ Augmentin Duo Forte (amoxycillin 875 mg/clavulanic acid 125 mg) every twelve hours for five days.

Uterotonics

Administer bolus dose of one of the following:
- ⮀ Intravenous or intramuscular Syntocinon® 10 IU (Oxytocin)

- Intramuscular Syntocinon® 5 IU in combination with ergometrine maleate 0.5 mg (Syntometrine®)
- Ergometrine 500 µg in 1 mL. Intramuscular dose: Give 250 µg; intravenous dose: give 25–50 µg bolus and can repeat after 2–3 minutes
- Prepare and commence an oxytocin infusion (40 IU Syntocinon® in 1,000 mL sodium chloride 0.9%.) Consider misoprostol available as tablets 200 µg, 800 µg per rectum or Gemeprost 1 mg per rectum or intramyometrial prostaglandin F2α
- Misoprostol may be useful to help the uterus expel products of conception that are not adherent to the uterine wall such as blood clots.

Condition Stable

Admit for conservative management with bed rest and intravenous antibiotics as above.

Adherent material—If the woman's condition is stable, after discussion with a senior registrar/consultant, conservative management (bed rest and IV antibiotics) may be an option.

If bleeding has not settled after 24 hours of antibiotic treatment, consider surgical intervention [Examination under anesthesia (EUA) and curettage].

Stabilization of Marked Bleeding

- Evidence of shock suggests severe sepsis requiring urgent intervention
- Call for obstetric and anesthetic assistance
- Consider uterine massage to expel any clots
- Administer oxygen via face mask. Lay the woman flat. Gets IV access in both forearms using 16 G cannulae. Resuscitate with appropriate IV fluid, e.g. sodium chloride 0.9 %, Hartmann's solution (crystalloids) or Gelofusine® (gelatin-based colloid). When using crystalloid, the ratio of resuscitative IV fluid required to blood lost is 3:1
- To resuscitate more quickly, administer IV fluids using a pressure infusion device. Consider use of blood warmer and hot air blanket to avoid hypothermia
- Avoid hypotension by adequate fluid replacement in relation to ongoing measured blood loss, close observations including pulse, blood pressure, respirations, SpO_2, capillary refill and urine output.

UTEROTONIC AGENTS

Oxytocics

Prophylactic use of oxytocics postpartum reduces the risk of postpartum hemorrhage by approximately 40%. Ten to twenty units oxytocin in 1000 mL crystalloid is administered at 100 to 200 mL per hour through a previously established intravenous site. Direct intravenous bolus injection of as little as 5 units of oxytocin has been associated with hypotension; therefore, a continuous drip is preferable.

Ergot

Methylergonovine or ergonovine maleate 0.2 mg may be administered intramuscularly. There is no clear evidence suggesting superior efficacy of ergot derivatives over oxytocin, although ergot preparations appear to be associated with a higher incidence of hypertension and should not be used in hypertensive patients. Ergot derivatives should not be administered intravenously because of the potential for severe vasospasm and hypertensive crisis.

Prostaglandins

Prostaglandins F and E promote strong uterine contractions that are effective in the treatment of uterine atony unresponsive to either oxytocin or methylergonovine stimulation. Reported series in which prostaglandin was used selectively for uterine atony showed a success rate of approximately 85%. Prostaglandins may be less effective in the presence of chorioamnionitis or after a cesarean section.

Multiple forms of prostaglandin are available. The principal parenteral prostaglandin formulation is 15-methyl prostaglandin F2α, also known as carboprost, is given in an intramuscular dose of 0.25 mg carboprost every 15 minutes for up to five injections over 1.5 hours. Carboprost may also be injected directly into the myometrium and may have a faster onset of action by this route. If carboprost is not immediately available, other forms of prostaglandin are effective in controlling uterine atony. Prostaglandin E2 20 mg vaginal suppositories) may be administered vaginally or rectally. Recently, rectal administration of 1000 mcg (five 200 μg tablets) of misoprostol was described for treatment of severe postpartum hemorrhage.

Prophylactic use of prostaglandins, both injectable carboprost and oral misoprostol, as an alternative to oxytocin or methylergonovine has been investigated. Prostaglandin administration during the third stage of labor appears to be effective in preventing postpartum hemorrhage, but data are insufficient to evaluate relative cost and safety. When using prostaglandins, the obstetrician must be cognizant of the systemic effects of these agents and any underlying medical condition of the patient. Side effects of diarrhea, hypertension, vomiting, fever, flushing, and tachycardia are common. Patients with significant cardiac or pulmonary disease will be at high risk should systemic side effects develop. Thus, prostaglandins should be used with extreme caution in these patients.

It may be beneficial to catheterize the bladder in cases of uterine atony. Catheterization also reduces the risk of bladder trauma during other maneuvers.

Condition Stable

Admit for conservative management with bed rest and intravenous antibiotics.

If bleeding does not settle after 24 hours of antibiotic treatment, consider surgical intervention (EUA and curettage).

Stabilization of Marked Bleeding

- Massage uterus to expel clots.
- Administer oxygen via face mask. Lay the woman on a flat surface. Secure two IV access using 16 gauge cannulae. Resuscitate with sodium chloride 0.9% or crystalloids. When using crystalloid, the ratio of resuscitative IV fluid required to blood lost is 3:1.
- To resuscitate quickly, administer IV fluids using a pressure infusion device. Use of blood warmer and hot air blanket avoids hypothermia.
- Pulse, blood pressure, respiration, SpO_2, capillary refill and urine output should be observed closely.

Surgical Management

Surgical management may include any of the following:
- Examination under anesthetic
- Under ultrasound guidance: Dilatation and evacuation of products of conception and gentle suction curettage
- Ligation of internal iliac arteries if interventional radiology is not readily available
- Hysterectomy.

Examination under anesthesia (EUA) and dilatation and suction curettage is indicated for retained products of conception if detected on ultrasound.

EUA with curettage should be performed by a senior obstetrician to minimize the risk of uterine perforation and Asherman's syndrome.

Concurrent ultrasound guidance may assist in the avoidance of uterine perforation during dilatation and suction curettage and therefore, minimize myometrial abrasion.

If dilatation and suction curettage is required, administer antibiotics for 6 to 12 hours before the procedure to guard against bacteremia, unless heavy bleeding mandates urgent intervention.

It is important to avoid over vigorous curettage as this can result in Asherman's syndrome (more common with late curettage, i.e. 2–3 weeks postpartum, than earlier on).

Tissue should be sent for histopathology to exclude trophoblastic disease and to confirm diagnosis.

If bleeding continues after curettage, there is need for further intervention (e.g. ligation of internal iliac arteries, hysterectomy or angiography with embolization of the uterine arteries).

If hemorrhage is persistent and severe in the presence of uterine arteriovenous malformation, a planned uterine artery embolization may reduce the need for hysterectomy.

3–5 % of women require hysterectomy to control bleeding.

It may be beneficial to catheterize the bladder in cases of uterine atony.

Catheterization also reduces the risk of bladder trauma during other maneuvers.

Repair Lacerations

A careful visual and manual examination of the perineum, vagina and cervix is carried out. Brisk bleeding may occur from an episiotomy in the absence of other lacerations or extensions. Vaginal sidewall lacerations may bleed profusely and should be repaired carefully. Repair of vaginal lacerations, as with episiotomy, must extend above the apex of the laceration because vessels can retract and cause a late hematoma. Small cervical lacerations need not be repaired unless they are bleeding. When necessary, repair of cervical lacerations should also begin with a deep suture above the apex of the laceration to reduce bleeding and to provide adequate control of the cervix for the repair.

Manual Removal of Placenta and Uterine Exploration

Signs of placental separation (lengthening of the umbilical cord, a show of blood, and a change of shape of the uterine fundus) are well known to obstetricians. Increased bleeding without evidence of placental separation suggests the need to remove the placenta manually. Anesthesia or analgesia may be necessary to allow adequate exploration of the uterus. Aseptic surgical technique is important to reduce the risk of infection. Placental delivery is performed using the following technique:

- With the nondominant hand grasping the fundus through the abdominal wall, use the other hand explore the uterine cavity to find the edge of the placenta
- Break through the membranes and enter the decidual plane
- Sweep the hand over the placental surface to separate it from the uterine attachment
- Grasp the entire placenta and withdraw it
- Carefully remove remaining membranes using a ring forceps.

If placental fragments cannot be removed manually, curettage with a large curette should be performed. Postpartum curettage must be performed with extreme caution because of the risk of perforating the soft postpartum uterus.

Prevent or Treat Shock

If initial attempts at control of hemorrhage by a uterotonic and inspection and repair of lacerations are unsuccessful, the obstetrician should ascertain that adequate blood replacement is available. Anesthesia personnel should be available in the event that surgical treatment is necessary. Vital signs must be monitored regularly. The first sign of impending shock is tachycardia; it is only when this compensatory mechanism cannot maintain adequate perfusion that the blood pressure will drop.

Coagulation Studies

If uterine bleeding persists, coagulation studies should be performed. Coagulation disorders are treated by specific factor replacement (e.g. platelet transfusion, cryoprecipitate).

Uterine Packing

Packing of the uterus can be considered if one is trained and experienced in this technique, else it is not recommended.

The use of a large Foley catheter has been reported to control PPH.

NON-PNEUMATIC ANTI-SHOCK GARMENT

The non-pneumatic anti-shock garment (NASG) has received attention for its use in gynecologic and obstetric hemorrhage. The NASG exerts its effect by returning more peripheral vascular blood supply to the central circulation owing to a direct pressure effect on the vessels within the garment, as well as controlling uterine hemorrhage by direct pressure on the uterus. The suit does appear to increase blood pressure dramatically when it is applied and to control hemorrhage by decreasing the rate of bleeding. The use of the NASG may control bleeding to the extent that surgery is not necessary. Use of the NASG depends on availability and familiarity with its use. The reports on its use are encouraging, and as obstetric units obtain more experience with this suit it may become not only readily available but also an important addition to the armamentarium of the obstetrician.

Arterial Embolization

As interventional radiology techniques become more widely available, arterial embolization is a reasonable choice for control of continued hemorrhage when lacerations have been excluded or repaired and uterotonics are not effective. This approach has also been effective in situations of continued hemorrhage after hypogastric artery ligation or hysterectomy.

Surgery

When uterotonic agents have failed, a decision must be made either to proceed with arterial embolization or to perform laparotomy.

The abdomen should be entered rapidly and the uterus compressed within both hands and elevated on traction. Upward traction on the uterus, as well as the bimanual pressure, decreases blood loss and allows for some stabilization of the patient. Should the patient be unstable or the blood loss rapid, aortic compression may be beneficial.

UTERINE ARTERY LIGATION

Uterine artery ligation is well described by O'Leary and O'Leary. This technique uses a large Mayo needle with one chromic suture. The needle is passed into and through the myometrium from anterior to posterior 2 to 3 cm medial to the uterine vessels and brought through the avascular area of the broad ligament lateral to the artery and the vein. This appears to be effective by reducing the pulse pressure to the uterus, because approximately 90% of the blood flow to the uterus is from the uterine artery. Uterine artery ligation was originally described at the time of cesarean section; the procedure failed in only 9 of 90 patients. It is technically less difficult than hypogastric artery ligation, and the risk of venous bleeding in the retroperitoneal space is avoided.

HYPOGASTRIC ARTERY LIGATION

The reported success rate of hypogastric artery ligation varies from 40% to 80%. It works by reducing pulse pressure and not by absolute control of blood flow; it decreases ipsilateral blood flow by approximately 50% and decreases pulse pressure by approximately 85%. If the operator is not familiar with this operation and assistance is not readily available from someone accomplished in the operation, proceeding directly to hysterectomy may be the more prudent course of action.

UTERINE COMPRESSION PROCEDURES

A few small case reports have appeared describing alternative surgical approaches for postpartum hemorrhage. The B-Lynch suture mechanically compresses the uterus to treat hemorrhage resulting from intractable atony. Multiple through-and-through square sutures have been described as an alternative to the B-Lynch technique. The safety and efficacy of these approaches cannot be evaluated on the basis of the few cases reported, and they are not recommended for general use.

Replacement of a Uterine Inversion (Figs 1A to D)

Uterine inversion may present as the uterine fundus protruding through the cervix and vaginal introitus (complete inversion) or as only a depression of the uterine fundus into the endometrial cavity (partial inversion). The uterus can usually be replaced by steady pressure against the fundus or by gradually replacing the uterus from the edges with pressure from the fingertips. Replacement of the uterus may be facilitated by tocolytic drugs, (B-sympathomimetics, or magnesium sulfate). Use of tocolytic agents for uterine relaxation may obviate the need to induce deep halothane anesthesia.

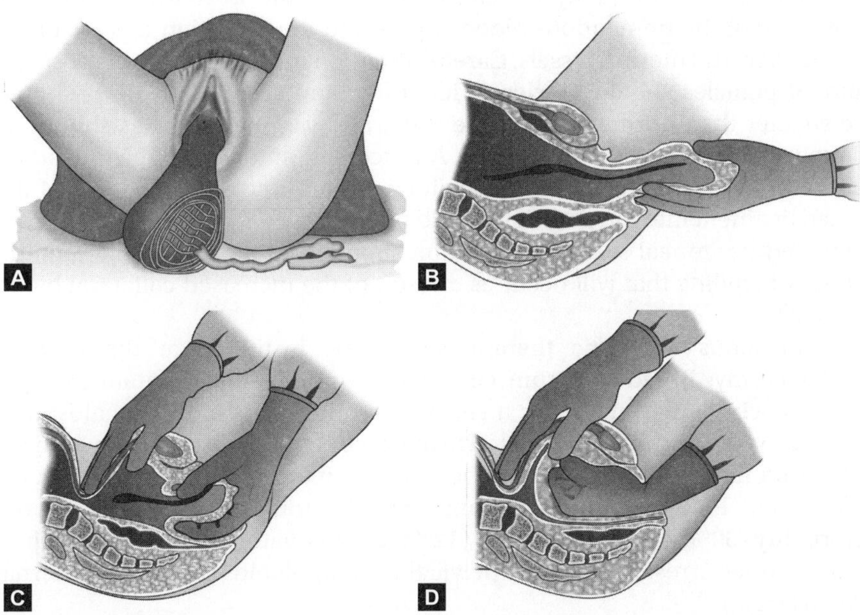

Figs 1A to D: Complete uterine inversion. Reduction by taxis. (A) Uterine inversion complete, with placenta attached. (B) First step in the reduction of the inverted uterus by taxis. (C) Second step in the reduction of the inverted uterus by taxis. (D) Third step in the reduction of the inverted uterus, showing organ restored to normal configuration, with one hand compressing the abdominal wall and the other within the uterine cavity. A uterotonic agent should be administered to promote uterine contraction

Once the uterus is replaced, it should be held firmly with bimanual compression until uterine tone develops. An oxytocin infusion is helpful; carboprost may also be beneficial. The obstetrician should be aware of the potential for spontaneous re-inversion of the uterus. In this situation, immediate replacement and adjuvant use of uterotonics are indicated.

In rare instances, vaginal replacement of the inverted uterus is not possible. In this case, laparotomy should be performed for reposition the uterus. The uterus is grasped within the contraction ring with Allis forceps, and gentle traction is applied. As the uterus is gradually restored to normal position, the forceps are advanced on the fundus. In some cases, an incision may be made through the contraction ring on the posterior side of the uterus to reduce constriction and a combined abdominal-vaginal repositioning may be performed. Although other surgical approaches, such as Spinelli's vaginal procedure, have been described, the rarity of this condition precludes an evaluation of the merit of these approaches.

HYSTERECTOMY

The choice of total versus subtotal (supracervical) hysterectomy is dictated by the patient's status at the time of operation, as well as by the difficulty of the procedure.

When performing a hysterectomy for PPH, the obstetrician must be cognizant of the tremendous blood supply and the dilatation that occurs in the ovarian and uterine vessels. Careful attention must be paid to hemostasis, and all pedicles should be clearly identified and secured. Pedicles should be smaller than normally would be used, and vascular pedicles should be doubly clamped and doubly ligated. An excessive amount of skeletonization in the broad ligament should be avoided. Incorporating both leaves of the broad ligament into the pedicles should be attempted to prevent oozing from denuded peritoneal surfaces. Attention should also be paid to the amount of back bleeding that will occur as a result of the increased collateral blood supply.

Intravenous antibiotic therapy should be instituted at the time of hysterectomy. Broad-spectrum coverage with ampicillin, gentamicin, and clindamycin is reasonable, or a second or third generation cephalosporin may be used. The morbidity related to hysterectomy for obstetric hemorrhage is considerable; however, it must be borne in mind that this is a life-saving operation. Potential complications include transfusion (96%), febrile morbidity (50%), wound infection (12%), coagulopathy (6%), ureteral injury (4%), cardiac arrest (4%), septic pelvic thrombophlebitis (3%), and maternal death (1%).

CONCLUSION

Once a postpartum hemorrhage has successfully been treated, the patient is still at risk of complications related to blood loss, the therapy, or both. It is important for the obstetrician to critically assess the patient for general organ complications. These complications include hypoperfusion injuries to the brain, heart and kidneys infection, coagulopathy, acute lung injury due to massive transfusion requirements, and pituitary necrosis. By being aware of these potential complications, the physician can ensure that proper post-hemorrhage care and consultation is available in time so that further morbidity can be avoided.

Morbidity Adherent Placenta

Rita Sinha, Hemali Heidi Sinha

DEFINITION

Abnormally firm attachment of the placental villi to the uterine wall with the absence of the normal intervening decidua basalis and Nitabusch's layer is known as morbidly adherent placenta (MAP). There is no clear plane of cleavage between the placenta and the underlying uterus.

Depending on the extent of adherence and invasion of the placenta, it is classified into three types as:

1. Placenta accreta—chorionic villi adherent to superficial myometrium.
2. Placenta increta—chorionic villi reach into myometrium.
3. Placenta percreta—chorionic villi penetrate full thickness myometrium and involve the serosa.

Morbidly adherent placenta (MAP) can also be classified as:

1. Focal adherence—when part of the cotyledon is involved.
2. Partial adherence—when more than one cotyledon is involved.
3. Total adherence—when whole placenta is involved.

MAP IS A LIFE-THREATENING COMPLICATION OF PREGNANCY

The incidence of MAP has increased 10 fold in the past 50 years and now occurs with a frequency of 1 per 2500 deliveries, as it is supposed to be associated with previous cesarean section delivery and rate of cesarean section has increased worldwide.

Benirrchke et al suggested that MAP results as a consequence of failure of reconstitution of the decidua basalis after repair of cesarean incision, resulting in absence of intervening decidual tissue between the invading trophoblast and myometrium.

It has also been proposed that the abnormality of placental uterine interface leads to leakage of fetal alpha fetoproteins into the maternal circulation resulting in elevated levels of maternal serum alpha fetoproteins.

During pregnancy MAP may be asymptomatic or may present as antepartum hemorrhage, abdominal pain and acute abdomen, while intrapartum; it may be retained associated with postpartum hemorrhage and uterine rupture.

Maternal risk is greatest at attempts to separate the placenta resulting in torrential hemorrhage, DIC, need for massive blood transfusion, emergency hysterectomy. Sometimes even death can occur.

Risk also increases in emergency without proper planning and absence of multidisciplinary team.

RISK FACTORS FOR MAP

- Previous uterine surgery—myomectomy, dilatation and curettage, placenta previa following previous cesarean section
- Placenta percreta is associated with a maternal mortality as high as 10% and significant maternal morbidity
- In mid trimester, MAP may present with uncontrollable vaginal bleeding or uterine rupture causing intraperitoneal bleeding
- Involvement of urinary bladder is associated with higher morbidity such as massive hemorrhage and need for bladder resection
- Even though there is bladder involvement, most common presenting symptoms are premature onset of labor and vaginal bleeding.

DIAGNOSIS

Antenatal diagnosis is the single most important factor is improving the outcome in MAP.

USG

First line investigation for suspected placental invasion of the myometrium. The two most used diagnostic criteria are:

1. Presence of irregular lacunae within the placenta.

   These lacunae may give the placenta a moth eaten or Swiss cheese appearance. The risk of MAP increases with the rise in the number of lacunae.

2. The second diagnostic criteria is thinning or absence of the myometrium overlying the placenta bladder interface and protrusion of the placenta into the bladder.

   The presence of at least two of these features has a positive predictive value of 86%.

Management of morbidity adherent placenta in the presence of risk factors includes:

- Previous LSCS/uterine surgery
- Anterior low lying placenta

Certain investigations are necessary:

- Ultrasonography (USG)
- Magnetic resonance imaging (MRI)
- Cystoscopy, if bladder invasion is suspected

- Multidisciplinary approach involving anesthetists, urologists, radiologists, hematologist, and blood bank team is required.
  - Decisions on treatment options should be taken in the antenatal period (radical surgery vs conservative treatment).
  - Consider placental mapping, ureteric stenting, uterine artery balloon occlusion.

Preplan

- Mid line incision vs pfannensteil incision
- Uterine incision/intraoperative placental mapping
- Avoid disturbing the placenta as much as possible.

Radical Surgery

- Cesarean hysterectomy
- Uterine artery embolization (UAE)/internal iliac artery ligation to minimize blood loss
- There is limited evidence for placental site excision and wedge section.

Conservative Approach

- Cut the cord short
- Repair the uterine incision
- Antibiotics/ecbolics
- Observation

Plan for Follow-up

- Methotrexate
- Serum β-hCG and USG
- Leave the placenta to resorb/expel/subsequent manual removal.

MRI

Effectively used for the investigation of placental invasion.

Although most studies have shown reasonable diagnostic accuracy, it appears that MRI is no more sensitive than USG.

However, MRI achieves better images than USG in posteriorly sited MAP and in patients with prior myomectomy because the ultrasound beam is impeded by the fetal head in the former and by the scar tissue in the latter. There are three significant MRI features for the detection of MAP.

1. Abnormal uterine bulging of the normal pear shaped gravid uterus
2. Heterogenecity of the signal intensity of the placenta on T2 weighted image.
3. Presence of T2 weighted dark linear bards in intraplacental signal intensity extending from the basal plate to the placental surface.

Other Diagnostic Features

1. Loss of myometrial contour in the lower uterine segment.
2. Thinning or irregularity of the myometrium transmural extension of signal abnormality through the myometrium, irregularity or disruption of the normal bladder wall architecture and invasion of local structures.
3. Attenuation and nonvisualization of the uterine wall, interruption of the uterine wall, interruption of the tissue plane between the myometrium and bladder wall by irregular masses and invasion of the myometrium by the placenta.

Cystoscopy

In cases of placenta accreta, where involvement of the bladder is suspected, cystoscopy is useful but biopsy should be avoided as it may precipitate severe hemorrhage. Placing ureteric stents during cystoscopy helps in intra-operative identification of the ureter.

TREATMENT OF MORBIDITY ADHERENT PLACENTA

Multidisciplinary approach is required to reduce morbidity and mortality associated with MAP

Particular consideration should be given to anticipation and management of massive hemorrhage, including availability of packed cells, platelets, frozen plasma, cryoprecipitate and activated factor VII.

Uterine Incision

It is best to avoid cutting through a MAP because of the possibility of massive hemorrhage. Various modifications of the uterine incision to avoid the placenta have been reported. These are classical incision, high transverse incision, fundal transverse incision have all been used to deliver the fetus.

➲ If hysterectomy is not planned, the risk of uterine rupture in a future pregnancy should be considered and explained to the patient in cases where non-lower segment incision is planned.
➲ Preoperative and/or intraoperative ultrasound mapping to delineate the area of the uterus overlying the placenta prior to uterine incision is useful.

Hysterectomy

Traditional management of MAP is cesarean hysterectomy, which results in various postoperative complications and loss of fertility. However, prompt hysterectomy has led to a reduction of maternal mortality to less than 2%.

It is essential to perform surgery under elective controlled conditions rather than as an emergency without adequate preparations.

The ideal abdominal incision is debatable.

A midline incision will facilitate better exposure especially if placenta percreta is suspected.

Leaving the placenta undisturbed until completion of hysterectomy would prevent unnecessary hemorrhage.

In cases where MAP is associated with placenta previa, total hysterectomy is preferred to a subtotal hysterectomy.

Devascularization of the Pelvis

Catheter occlusion of pelvic vessels or selective arterial embolization decreases blood flow to the uterus and makes it possible to perform surgery under easier and more controlled circumstances.

There are two different approaches for reducing chances of hemorrhage.

1. *In one approach:* Occlusive balloon catheters are placed preoperatively in the internal iliac arteries. These are inflated after the delivery of the baby and deflated after completing the hysterectomy.
2. *In other approach:* Catheters are placed preoperatively in the internal iliac arteries and embolisation of the uterine vessels performed after delivery of the fetus but before hysterectomy.

Bilateral internal iliac artery ligation is performed prior to peripartum hysterectomy in an attempt to reduce operative blood loss. This is especially important in situations where interventional radiology is not available.

Other Surgical Options

Sometimes placental site is excised by inverting the uterus to provide good access to the placental site. If the area of placental attachment is focal and majority of the placenta has been removed, then a wedge resection of the area can be performed.

SUGGESTED READING

1. Ellen AG, Porten TF, Soisson P, Silver RM. Optimal management strategies for placenta accreta. Br J Obstet Gynaecol. 2009;115:648-54.
2. Giel Chinsky Y, Rojansky N, Fasoulotes & T Ezra Y placenta accreta summary of 10 years, a survey of 310 cases placenta. 2002;23:210-4.
3. Oyelase simulian JC placenta preavia placenta accreta and vase previa, Obstet Gyecol. 2006;107:927-41.
4. Ramos Ga, Kelly TF, Moov TR. The important of preoperative evolution in patients with risk factors for placenta accreta. Obstet Gynaecol. 2007;109:75.
5. Sri Lanka Journal of Obstetric and Gynaecology. 2011;33:39-44.
6. Wong HS, Zuccollpgy, Straw L, et al. The use of ultrasound in assessing the extent of myometrial involvement in parting placenta accreta ultrasound. Obstet Gynaecol. 2007;30:277-30.
7. Yapyy, Pervin LC, Pain SR, Wong SF, Chan FY. Mannual removal of suspected placenta accreta at caesarean hysterectomy. Int of Gynecol Obstet. 2008;100:186-7.

PART-II

GYNECOLOGY

Chapter 26
Evaluation of the Infant with Ambiguous Genitalia

K Aparna Sharma, Alka Kriplani

Individuals with congenital discrepancy between external genitalia, gonadal and chromosomal sex are classified as having a Disorder of Sexual Differentiation (DSD). Some DSDs present with a genital appearance that does not permit gender declaration at birth, and the physical appearance is termed ambiguous genitalia.

The birth of an infant with ambiguous is distressing for any parent and needs immediate sensitive and professional counseling. Apart from this, one of the most common conditions resulting in genital ambiguity (congenital adrenal hyperplasia) can be life-threatening requiring urgent attention.

To understand the abnormalities of sexual differentiation, it is important to understand the normal process of sexual differentiation in a male and female.

NORMAL DEVELOPMENT

The fetus exists in an ambisexual state with bipotential gonads till 7 weeks of conception. After that period, the fetuses with a Y chromosome go on to develop the testes. Further gonadal development and function determines the genital phenotype.

Gonads

Many genes are involved in gonadal development like: **SRY** (testis formation), SOX9, SF1, DHH, DAX1/NROB1, Wnt4 and Wnt7a. Mutations in SRY affect gonads, reproductive structures but defects of other factors such as DAX1 lead to syndromic phenotypes.

Internal Genitalia

Wolffian and Müllerian ducts develop in both sexes. In males, the Sertoli and Leydig cells in the testes secrete anti-Müllerian (AMH) and testosterone, respectively. The AMH causes regression of the Müllerian duct and testosterone leads to the development of the Wolffian structures—epididymis, vas deferens and seminal vesicles. In females, the lack of AMH leads to development of Müllerian ducts maturation and regression of Wolffian regression.

External Genitalia

Dihydrotestosterone (DHT) is formed from testosterone by the action of 5α-reductase. At 9 weeks of period of gestation, by the action of DHT, there is posterior fusion of genital folds and the growth of a phallus from the genital tubercle. The male external genital morphogenesis is completed by 12 to 16 weeks.

Evaluation of an infant with ambiguous genitalia starts initially with the identification of the infants who can be considered to have ambiguous genitalia.

The presence of the following features in a newborn should initiate an evaluation:

- Bilaterally nonpalpable testes
- Microphallus (< 2.5 cm)
- Perineal hypospadias with bifid scrotum
- Clitoromegaly (width >6 mm or length >9 mm)
- Posterior labial fusion (anogenital ratio >0.5)
- Gonads palpable in the labioscrotal folds or inguinal region
- Hypospadias and unilateral nonpalpable gonad (undescended testis)
- Discordant genitalia and sex chromosomes.

The conditions which result in ambiguous genitalia can be broadly divided into three categories:

  I. XX DSD
 II. XY DSD
III. Sex chromosome DSD

I. 46,XX—DISORDER OF SEXUAL DIFFERENTIATION

- Disorders of ovarian development
    - Ovotesticular
    - Testicular
    - Gonadal dysgenesis
- Fetal androgen excess
- Others

Disorders of Ovarian Development

Ovotesticular

This disorder is characterized by the presence of both ovarian and testicular tissue which could be in the form of bilateral ovotestis or one ovotestis and contralateral ovary/testis. The majority have 46,XX karyotype, however, 7% can have XY and 10–40% can have mosaicism.

Clinical Features

Gonads: Testes are usually onthe right and ovaries are found on the left.
Internal genitalia: Both Müllerian and Wolffian structures are present on the side corresponding to the adjacent gonad. Most have vagina, and uterus may be normal, hypoplastic, vestigial or absent.

External genitalia: Depends on the level of androgen production. They can vary from ambiguous genitalia to isolated hypospadias.

Gynecomastia occurs in 3/4th of the patients out of which 50% menstruate.

Testicular DSD (Sex Reversal)

It is a rare disorder in which the chromosomal sex is 46,XX and gonads are testes. It can be either SRY positive or SRY negative.

It happens due to abnormal recombination between distal portion of short arm of the X and Y chromosomes and transfer of SRY from Y to X chromosome during division.

Androgen Excess

Fetal Origin (Virilizing Congenital Adrenal Hyperplasia)

Pathophysiology: Congenital adrenal hyperplasia (CAH) is a genetic disorder caused by enzyme defects leading to decreased cortisol production from the adrenals. This results in a rebound increase in pituitary ACTH secretion and adrenal hyperplasia. Consequently, there is an increased production of steroid hormones proximal to the block and increased androgen synthesis (Table 1).

Inheritance: All CAH have an autosomal recessive inheritance.

Diagnosis:
- Diagnosis is confirmed by doing 17-OHP levels (>3500 ng/dL in 21-hydroxylase deficiency)
- To rule out other enzyme defects, the levels of 11-deoxycortisol (11-β-hydroxylase deficiency) and 7-β-hydroxypregnenolone [3-β-hydroxysteroid dehydrogenase (3β-HSD) deficiency] are tested.

Maternal Origin: Gestational Hyperandrogenism

This is a rare cause of fetal virilization having an XX karyotype and a normal female internal anatomy. It occurs due to ingestion of drugs (danazol, arogestogen which binds to androgen receptors). In other conditions like maternal luteoma or theca lutein cyst virilization can occur. However, the diagnosis should be considered when the pregnant women show signs of rapid masculinization.

Fetoplacental Origin

The deficiency of placental aromatase and P450 oxidoreductase deficiency differs from the other classical forms of CAH in that it affects both the fetus and the placenta leading to fetal virilization as well as maternal hirsuitism (regresses after delivery).
- P450 aromatase deficiency: It presents with ambiguous genitalia at birth and hyperandrogenism at puberty and hypergonadotropic hypergonadism.
- P450 oxidoreductase deficiency (POR): It affects the activity of all of the P450 enzymes involved in steroidogenesis, to varying degrees, resulting in varying patterns of abnormal steroid hormone production.

Table 1: Differential diagnosis of virilizing CAH			
Deficiency of enzyme	*21-hydroxylase (90%): Most common endocrine cause of neonatal death*	*11-β-hydroxylase (5–8%)*	*3-β-hydroxy steroid dehydrogenase (type II) (<5%)*
Types	Classical: ❖ Salt wasting (2/3) ❖ Simple virilizing (1/3) ❖ Nonclassical	❖ Severe salt wasting ❖ Simple virilizing ❖ Mild late onset	❖ Salt wasting ❖ Nonsalt wasting
Gene	CXP21A2	CXP11B1	HSD3B2
Ambiguous genitalia	Occur in females	Occur in females Sexual precocity Hirsuitism/Menstrual irregularity	Mild in females May or may not occur in males
Addisonian crisis	+	Rare	+
HORMONES			
Glucocorticoids	Decreased	Decreased	Decreased
Mineralocorticoids	Decreased	Increased (11-DOC)	Decreased
Androgen	Increased	Increased	Increased
Estrogen	Decreased	Decreased	Decreased
PHYSIOLOGY			
Blood Pressure	Decreased	Increased	Decreased
Sodium balance	Decreased	Increased	Decreased
Potassium balance	Increased	Decreased	Increased
Acidosis	+	± alkalosis	+
Increased metabolite	17-OHP	11-deoxycortisol 11-deoxycorticosterone	DHEA, 17α OH pregnenolone

Phenotypic spectrum in patients with proven POR deficiency ranges from asymptomatic patients to virilized female infants. Diagnosis should be considered in virilized infants with low maternal serum estriol on triple screen.

II. 46,XY—DISORDER OF SEXUAL DIFFERENTIATION

46,XY DSD—Disorders of Testicular Development (Causing Genital Ambiguity) (Table 2)

Partial Gonadal Dysgenesis

This results from a wide variety of genetic mutations leading to abnormal gonadal development and function. The Müllerian structures may or may not be present and the external genitalia male/female/ambiguous.

Table 2: Etiology of 46,XY DSD	
Disorders of testicular development	**Disorders of androgen synthesis/action**
❖ Complete gonadal dysgenesis (Swyer Syndrome): No Ambiguity ❖ Partial dysgenesis: Possible Ambiguity ❖ Gonadal regression: No ambiguity ❖ Ovotesticular DSD: Possible Ambiguity	❖ Androgen synthesis defect: Genital ambiguity ❖ LH receptor defect: Genital ambiguity ❖ Androgen Insensitivity Syndrome: Genital ambiguity ❖ 5α-reductase deficiency: Genital ambiguity ❖ AMH disorders: No Genital ambiguity

Disorders of Androgen Synthesis

These result from the deficiency of enzymes or regulatory proteins involved in testosterone synthesis. These are quite rare and account for less than 5% of all the cases.

5 α-reductase Deficiency (Type 2)

This is characterized by an XY karyotype with a predominantly female external genitalia at birth and male internal genitalia. There is usually a severe perineal hypospadias and an incompletely closed urogenital opening resembling a blind vagina. The characteristic feature of this disorder is that the affected individuals virilize at puberty. Most are reared as females and assume a male gender and behavior at the time of puberty.

The supporting laboratory finding to establish the diagnosis would be a serum testosterone in the normal male range with the ratio of testosterone to DHT exceeding 10 in infants and 20 in adults.

Steroid Acute Regulatory (StAR) Protein Deficiency

This rarest and most severe form of CAH. There is deficiency of all adrenal and gonadal steroid hormones. Typically present very soon after birth or in early infancy with symptoms of severe adrenal insufficiency. Male infants usually have female external genitalia.

Disorders of Androgen Action

⮞ Complete androgen insensitivity syndrome (CAIS): No genital ambiguity
⮞ Incomplete androgen insensitivity syndrome (PAIS): Genital ambiguity may occur.

Complete Androgen Insensitivity Syndrome (AIS)

This is characterized by a 46,XY karyotype in a phenotypic female having an unambiguously female external genitalia, short blind vagina, normal female breast development, no axillary or pubic hair and abdominal or an inguinal testes.

Serum testosterone levels are those of normal adult male.

Incomplete Androgen Insensitivity Syndrome

The phenotype can present as ambiguous genitalia in infants, mild virilization in female or as fertile but undervirilized men (as summarized in Table 3).

LH Receptor Defects (Leydig Cell Hypoplasia)

It is an autosomal recessive disorder due inactivating mutations in the LH/hCG receptor leading to a decreased fetal testosterone production. The karyotype is 46,XY and the phenotype correlates with the level of residual LH/hCG receptor activity, ranging from completely female external genital development to ambiguous to nearly normal male genitalia. Müllerian duct derivatives are absent (normal action of AMH) and Wolffian duct development is impaired (reflecting decreased testosterone).

Serum LH concentration is elevated and testosterone levels are abnormally low.

III. SEX CHROMOSOME—DISORDERS OF SEXUAL DIFFERENTIATION

- ➲ No ambiguity
  - 45,XO
  - 47,XXY
- ➲ Ambiguity

45X,46XY (Mixed Gonadal Dysgenesis)

This is characterized by asymmetric reproductive anatomy and variable degrees of genital ambiguity. There can be poorly developed testicle on one

Table 3: Differential diagnosis of androgen insensitivity syndrome

	Complete	*Incomplete*	*Reifenstein*	*Infertile*
Inheritance	X-linked recessive	X-linked recessive	X-linked recessive	X-linked recessive
Spermatogenesis	Absent	Absent	Absent	Decreased
Müllerian	Absent	Absent	Absent	Absent
Wolffian	Absent	Underdeveloped	Male	Male
External	Female	Female (clitoromegaly)	Male (hypospadias)	Male
Breasts	Female	Female	Gynecomastia at puberty	Male (Gynecomastia)
Axillary/Pubic hair	Absent	Normal	Normal	Normal

side and the other is a streak absent altogether. There can be virilization at puberty depending on the degree of testosterone production.

46,XX/46,XY Mosaicism (Chimerism)

These are derived from two distinct zygotes rather than from a single zygote. Chimeras are not visibly different unless a developmental anomaly in one of the cell lines or sex discordance between the cell lines causes a visibly abnormal phenotype. Majority discovered by chance.

INITIAL EVALUATION

History

A history of prenatal exposure to androgens (progesterone, danazol, testosterone) and other endocrine disrupters like phenytoin and aminoglutethimide should be elicited. A history of maternal virilization in pregnancy would point towards a fetoplacental source of excess androgen.

The family history of infertility or amenorrhea could indicate the possibility of AIS while that of unexplained infant deaths could point towards CAH).

Examination

- **Penile length:** It should be measured from the pubic ramus to the tip of the penis (after completely depressing the suprapubic fat pad). At birth, the normal penile length is ≥2.5 cm while the diameter is ≥0.9 cm.
- **Gonads:** The scrotum, labia majora and the inguinal area should be palpated to identify the presence and position of the gonads.
- **Urethral opening:** The position should be ascertained and the findings must be confirmed by cystoscopy or vaginoscopy.
- **Clitoral size:** It is measured by pressing the shaft of the clitoris between the thumb and forefingers. A value of more than 9 mm is unusual.
  Clitoral index = length (mm) × width (mm)
  It is calculated to assess androgen exposure but it does not contribute much to the clinical assessment and management of infants with a DSD.
- **Virilization:** Various standards available:
  – Prader—degree of virilization of the urogenital sinus and external genitalia
  – Quigley scales—for children with DSD.

Anogenital Ratio

$$\frac{\text{Distance between the anus and posterior fourchette}}{\text{Distance between the anus and the base of the clitoris}}, \text{ if greater than 0.5—}$$

virilization with posterior labial fusion.

Laboratory Tests

- **Karyotype:** Can be done in peripheral leukocytes. At least 200 cells should be examined to rule out mosaicism.

- **Blood tests:** 17-hydroxyprogesterone should be measured to exclude congenital adrenal hyperplasia (CAH) due to 21-hydroxylase deficiency. Other forms of CAH: To detect 11-β-hydroxylase deficiency and 3-β-hydroxysteroid dehydrogenase deficiency, the following can be measured:
    - Dehydroepiandrosterone (DHEA)
    - 17-hydroxypregnenolone
    - 11-desoxycortisol

    Serum electrolytes should also be measured at least daily until 17-hydroxyprogesterone level makes it clear that it is not salt wasting due to 21-hydroxylase deficiency.
- **Evaluation for SRY gene** using fluorescence in situ hybridization (FISH) and with SRY-specific probes.
- **Imaging:** Ultrasound (USG) should be done to ascertain the presence and type of gonads and the presence of Müllerian structures.
- Laparoscopic visualization may be required in complicated cases.

DIFFERENTIAL DIAGNOSIS

I. 46,XX DSD

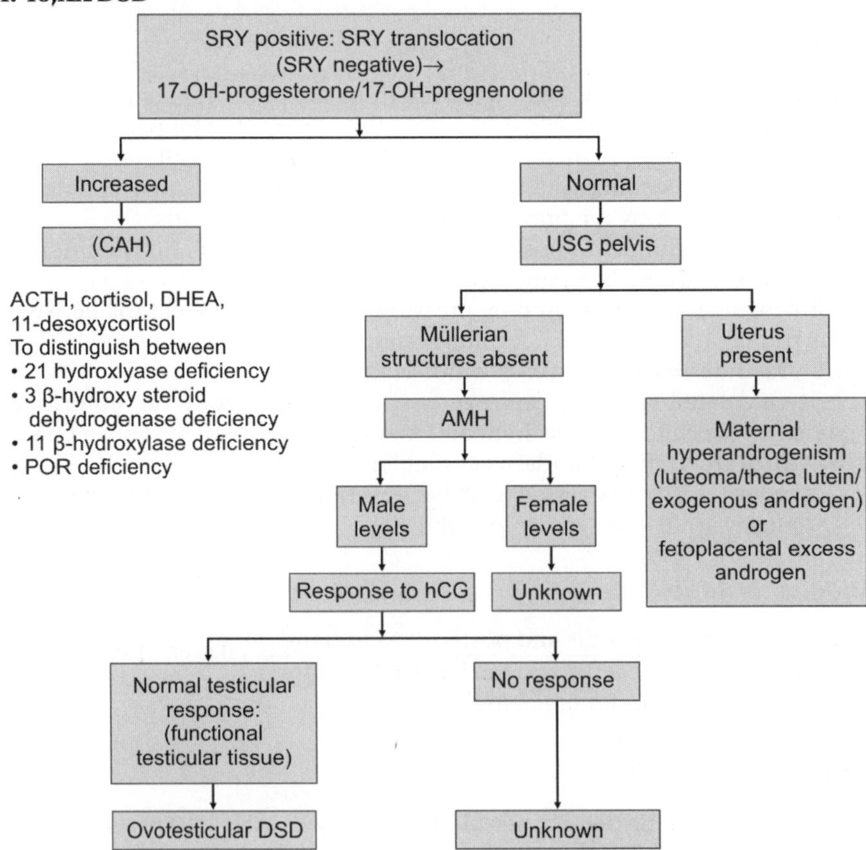

II. XY DSD

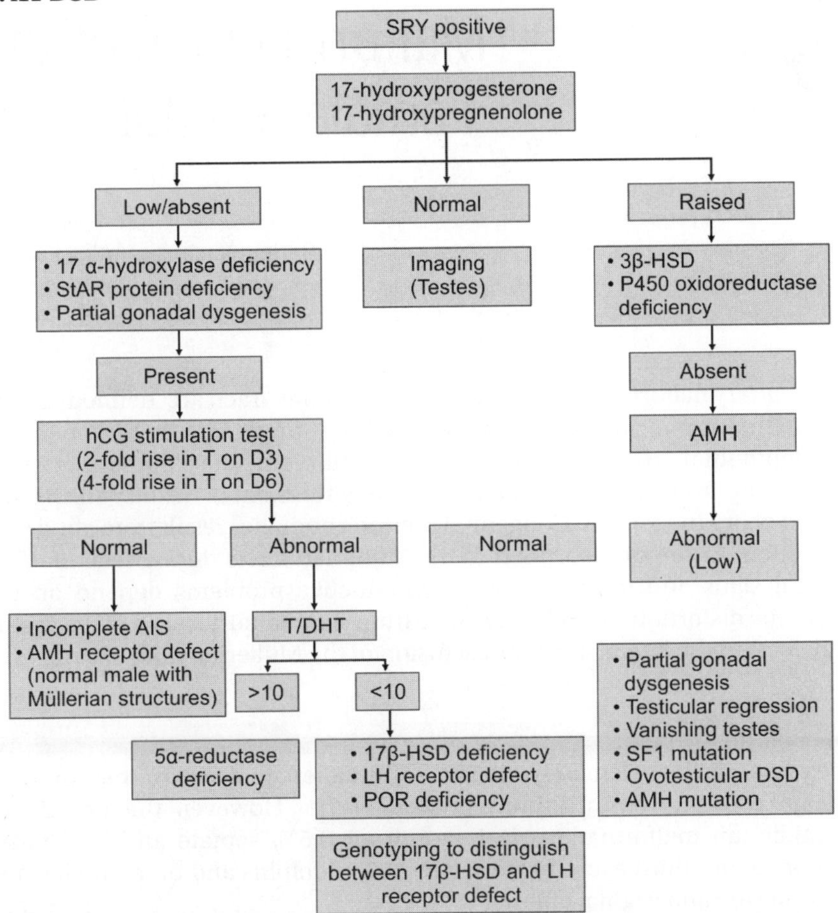

Abbreviations: LH, Luteinizing hormone; T, Testosterone; DHT, Dihydrotestosterone; POR, P450 oxidoreductase; AMH, Anti-Müllerian hormone; AIS, Androgen insensitivity syndrome; hCG, Human chorionic gonadotropin

SUGGESTED READING

1. Fritz MA, Speroff L. Clinical gynecologic endocrinology and infertility. 8th Edition.
2. Lee PA, Houk CP, Ahmed SF, Hughes IA. Consensus statement on management of intersex disorders and incollaboration with the participants in the international consensus conference on European Society for Paediatric Endocrinology Intersex organized by the Lawson Wilkins Pediatric Endocrine Society and the European Society for Paediatric Endocrinology. Paediatrics. 2006;118:e488-500.
3. Öçal G. Current Concepts in disorders of sexual development. J Clin Res Ped Endo. 2011;3(3):105-114. DOI: 10.4274/jcrpe.v3i3.22.

Malformations of the Female Genital Tract

Garima Kachhawa, Alka Kriplani

Congenital malformations of the female genital tract are defined as the deviations from normal anatomy resulting from mal-development or developmental arrest at a critical stage of embryonic development but may also result from genetic mutations or environmental insults during the period of organogenesis. Congenital uterine anomalies result from abnormal formation, fusion or resorption of the Müllerian ducts during fetal life. The clinical signs and symptoms and reproductive problems depend on the anatomic distortions, which may range from congenital absence of the vagina to defects in the lateral and vertical fusion of the Müllerian duct system.

INCIDENCE

The various forms of female genital tract anomalies represent a rather common benign condition with a prevalence of 4–7%. However, the prevalence of müllerian malformations is 1 in 200, or 0.5%, septate and bicornuate comprise one-third each, 10% arcuate, 10% didelphis and unicornuate, and < 5% uterine and vaginal aplasia.

Although nearly 57% of women with uterine defects have successful fertility and pregnancy, these anomalies have been associated with an increased rate of miscarriage, preterm delivery and other adverse fetal outcomes. Uterine anomalies comprise 5.5% of an unselected population, 8.0% of infertile women, 13.3% of those with a history of miscarriage and 24.5% of women with miscarriage and infertility. Arcuate uterus is the most common finding in the unselected population (3.9%), and its prevalence is not increased in high-risk groups. In contrast, septate uterus is the most common anomaly in high-risk populations. Correct diagnosis of the malformation is the most important part of its management but often very difficult.

DIAGNOSIS

Identification of symptoms is an important key to the diagnosis of an anatomical defect of the female genital tract. The presentation is typically at menarche, when obstruction at any level of flow of menses from the uterine cavity results in blood collection in the Fallopian tubes and finally in the peritoneal cavity. The symptoms include a history of amenorrhea or irregular bleeding with cyclic abdominal pain that gradually increases in frequency and duration to become a constant dull ache. There may also be difficulty in inserting or removing tampon. Physical examination reveals hymenal or vaginal anomalies and/or pelvic mass. In complicated cases, presence of pelvic masses can be detected by examination under anesthesia and laparoscopy, in addition to vaginoscopy, cystoscopy or hysteroscopy. Sonography is helpful in delineating detailed anatomy of abnormality as an essential prerequisite for appropriate planning of surgery. MRI is considered as the gold standard in complicated higher obstructive uterocervical anomalies. An HSG is uncomfortable unless done under anesthesia and should be reserved for adult women with infertility.

Owing to the close association of genital and urinary systems throughout fetal development, approximately 30–50% of patients have renal anomalies like renal agenesis, duplex collecting systems, duplication, malrotation and ectopic and horse shoe-shaped kidney. Intravenous pyelography is an essential investigation to detect renal anomaly. In some cases, skeletal, auditory or cardiac defects are also associated with vaginal agenesis.

HYMENAL DEFECTS

The normal hymen becomes patent during fetal life; however, failure of the hymen to perforate completely during the perinatal period can result in varying anomalies such as imperforate, microperforate, cribriform and septate hymen.

Imperforate hymen is the complete failure of the inferior plate of the vagina to canalize and is noted in approximately 1 in 2000 females. Although most cases occur sporadically, there are reports of familial occurrence.

Hymenal abnormalities are ideally recognized at birth as part of newborn examination or seen in childhood, but in our country owing to a large number of home deliveries and lack of awareness, it is not uncommon to see an adolescent girl presenting with severe pain due to trapped menstrual blood in the vagina.

In the neonatal period, it may present as hydrocolpos or mucocolpos, resulting from accumulation of mucus in response to maternal estrogens. It is usually asymptomatic and resolves spontaneously as the mucus is reabsorbed. Asymptomatic girls with an imperforate hymen can be monitored throughout the childhood and ideally surgery in these girls should be done after the onset of puberty (as evidenced by thelarche) but before menses.

However, more commonly, adolescents present after menarche when menstrual blood trapped in the vagina causes cyclical pain. After few months, the vagina distends greatly followed by cervix, uterus and tubes and allowing the formation of hematometra and hematosalpinx (Fig. 1).

Amenorrhea, cyclic abdominal pain and pain mimicking acute abdomen with difficulty in urination and defecation may be present. Retrograde menstruation may lead to the development of endometriosis.

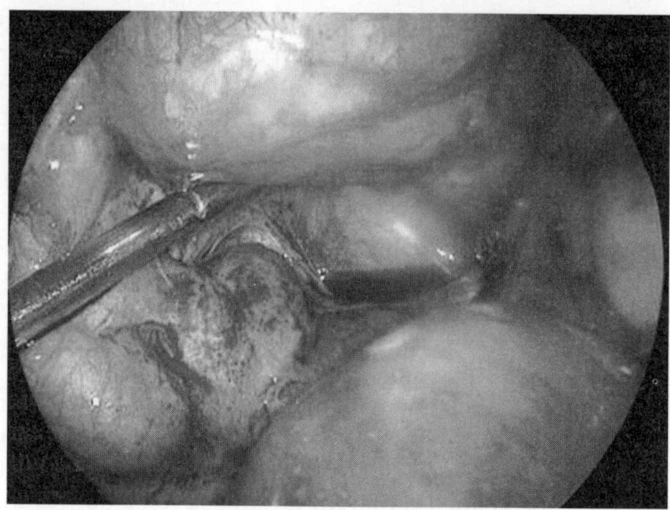

Fig. 1: Laparoscopic view showing hematometra, hematosalpinx and endometriosis
(*Courtesy:* Dr Alka Kriplani)
(*For color version, see Plate 1*)

These girls have an acute presentation with severe pain in lower abdomen and perineum. Definitive surgery should take place after appropriate evaluation of the external genitalia and a digital rectal examination that reveals bluish distended bulge at the introitus. Radiographic imaging may be required only to confirm obstruction at a higher level.

The goal of hymenotomy/hymenectomy is to open the hymenal membrane to allow the egress of menstrual flow, tampon use and eventually comfortable sexual intercourse.

VAGINAL SEPTUM

Transverse vaginal septum is believed to be due to failure in vertical fusion and/or canalization of the vaginal plate between urogenital bulbs and the Müllerian ducts. On the other hand, longitudinal vaginal septum results from defective lateral fusion and/or incomplete reabsorption of the paired Müllerian ducts.

Transverse vaginal septum is uncommon with a reported incidence of 1 in 80,000 females. It can occur at various levels in the vagina but appears to be more common in the upper part (46%), followed by middle (35%) and lower part (19%) of the vagina. The thickness of the septum is usually 1 cm but varies up to 5 cm, if present at higher level near the cervix.

Longitudinal vaginal septum is often associated with complete uterine septum, uterine didelphys and rarely bicornuate uteri. In addition to ipsilateral renal agenesis, associated anorectal anomalies like imperforate anus with rectovestibular fistula may be present. Septa may be partial or extend the complete length of the vagina.

In neonates and infants, it may go unnoticed but may be associated with mucus accumulation resulting in central pelvic mass leading to compression and rarely ascending infection in form of pyomucocolpos, pyometra and pyosalpinx.

The diagnosis of transverse septum is suspected when a foreshortened vagina with inability to visualize cervix and presence of hematometra is encountered. In longitudinal vaginal septum, a bulge on one side of vagina extending upward toward the pelvis is noted.

An adolescent with longitudinal septum may presents with normal menarche with mild unilateral lower abdominal and vaginal pain that gradually progresses to severe constant pain over a period of time. On examination, a patent vagina and cervix is noted, but a unilateral vaginal and pelvic mass due to obstructed hemivagina is felt. Per vaginal examination with a speculum is usually adequate for visualization of septum; however, USG or MRI confirms the findings and in addition determine the thickness and depth of the septum. MRI is especially useful in identifying whether cervix is present, thereby differentiating a high transverse vaginal septum from cervical agenesis.

Wide excision of the vaginal septum is done after confirmation of findings and evaluation of renal system. Some distension of the upper vagina with menstrual blood before the development of significant hematometra may be advantageous as it allows the potential to increase the available amount of upper vaginal tissue for reanastomosis and may also decrease the thickness of the septum. Thin septum is resected followed by primary end-to-end anastomosis of upper and lower vagina. Thicker septa may require undermining and mobilization of vaginal mucosa. A common complication is scar contracture and restenosis. A circumferential 'Z' plasty technique allows for scarring along the suture line to contract the incision in a longitudinal fashion rather than a transverse one. If there is not enough vaginal mucosa to accomplish a pull through procedure and reanastomosis, a graft may be necessary to create a patent vaginal tract.

VAGINAL AGENESIS (MÜLLERIAN APLASIA)

Varying degree of Müllerian hypoplasia or agenesis affects one in every 5,000 women and is a common cause of primary amenorrhea. Vaginal atresia, distal or segmental vaginal agenesis with normally developed uterus, cervix and upper vagina are managed as transverse vaginal septum and vaginoplasty.

On the other hand, aplasia of the Müllerian ducts result not only from the absence of uterus and cervix but also from the upper vagina, leading to complete vaginal agenesis, also referred to as Mayer Rokitansky Küster Hauser syndrome (MRKH) (Fig. 2).

MRKH accounts for 10% cases of primary amenorrhea and usual presentation is failure to attain menarche with normally developed secondary sexual characteristics. On examination, normal breast and pubic hair development is present, the perineum is normal with normal secondary sex characters with a hymenal ring and a vaginal dimple or shallow pouch up to 1.5 inches deep with complete absence of uterus, cervix and upper vagina. MRKH with functional endometrium is present in 7–10% women and this

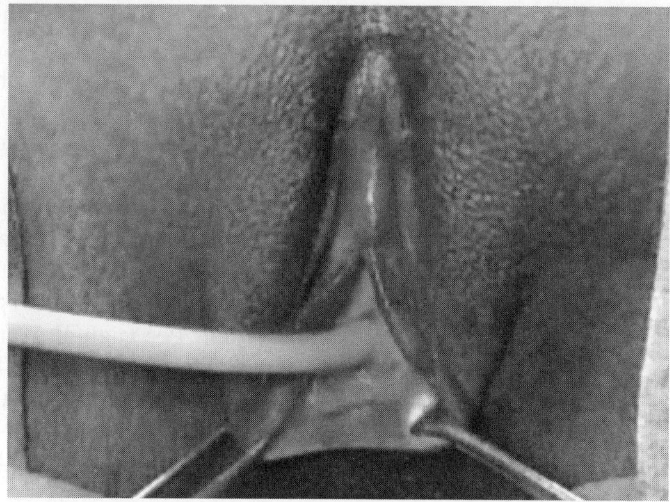

Fig. 2: Vaginal agenesis (Mayer Rokitansky Kustner Hauser syndrome)
(For color version, see Plate 2)

subgroup of patients may require excision of rudimentary horn due to cyclic pain after evaluation of upper reproductive organs by imaging.

In cases of Müllerian aplasia, conception is not possible, however, purpose can be achieved with the help of assisted reproductive technology (ART) and surrogacy.

The goal of treatment is development of a functional vagina for sexual intercourse that may be accomplished either conservatively or surgically. The non-operative approach attempts to use progressive invagination of the vaginal dimple and gradual dilatation to achieve adequate vaginal length and diameter. It involves the use of pressure against the vaginal dimple to create a progressive invagination of the mucosa with the use of graduated hard dilators. Although this technique is 85–90% successful, it may take months to create adequate vagina, thus proper counseling is important.

Surgical correction is considered as a more immediate solution but the patients must be counseled that success depends on maintaining postoperative dilatation of the neovagina to prevent restenosis. Most commonly used method is McIndoe vaginoplasty. A canal is created within the connective tissue between the bladder and rectum, which is lined by split thickness skin graft from buttocks or thighs. Modifications of the McIndoe procedure involve the use of human amnion, peritoneum, buccal mucosa or intercede absorbable adhesion barrier. Cutaneous and musculocutaneous flaps are also used to line the neovagina, e.g. Williams vaginoplasty.

CERVICAL ATRESIA/DYSGENESIS

Congenital agenesis of the uterine cervix is a rare Müllerian anomaly (Fig. 3), which is associated with both partial or complete vaginal aplasia and renal

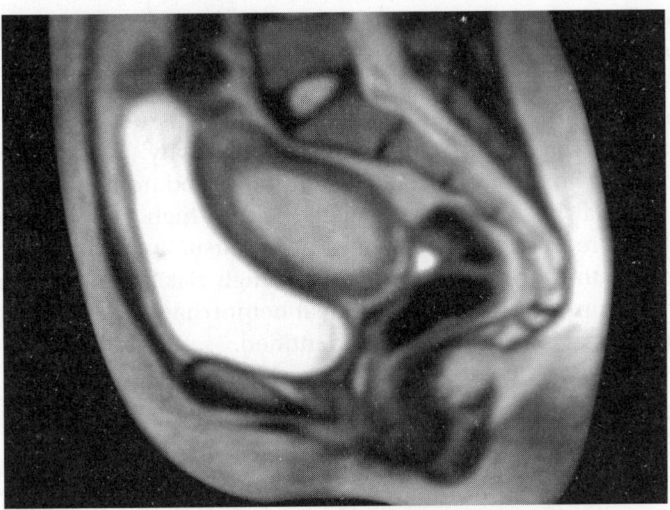

Fig. 3: T2-weighted MR imaging of sagittal view showing uterus with hematometra in a case of cervical agenesis
(*Courtesy:* Dr Alka Kriplani)

anomalies. Amenorrhea and severe rapidly progressive cyclic pain are the first symptoms with normally developed external sex organs, palpable vaginal recess, varying degrees of uterine enlargement and in some cases tubo-ovarian masses. Delayed diagnosis and treatment may result in extensive endometriosis, which in extreme cases cause irreversible damage to the reproductive potential. It is important to differentiate it from high transverse vaginal septum or segmental atresia. Traditionally, hysterectomy has been recommended due to high failure rate of canalization procedures, risk of serious and sometimes fatal ascending infection, and persistent low fertility. With the advancement in modern assisted reproductive facilities, the conservative management seems feasible but depends upon adequacy of cervix. These methods have included creation of neovagina and reconstruction of cervix around various stents, which is both challenging and controversial.

UTERINE DISORDERS

Unicornuate Uterus

Arrested development of one of the Müllerian duct results in unicornuate uterus also known as hemiuterus. It was present in 14% of a series of hysterosalpingography (HSG) cases during evaluation for infertility or bad obstetric outcome as a deviated banana shaped cavity with a single Fallopian tube. Transvaginal sonography with 3D or MR imaging is a key investigation for diagnosis and is considered even better than laparoscopy in differentiating a rudimentary horn with functional endometrium. Reproductive performance of unicornuate uterus is severely impaired with an increased incidence of dysmenorrhea, infertility and endometriosis. Preterm labor occurs in 20% of all pregnancies and live birth rate is 29%.

Unicornuate uterus is associated with rudimentary horn in 65% of cases (Fig. 4) and 31% contained endometrial tissue, and only half of these communicated with the main uterine cavity. Pregnancy in non-communicating horn may be conceived by intra-abdominal transit of sperm from the normal horn and is associated with a high incidence of uterine rupture. Rupture in rudimentary horn occurs usually before 20 weeks and in 80% prior to third trimester. Owing to the high-risk for maternal morbidity secondary to rupture and intraperitoneal hemorrhage excision of a cavitary rudimentary horn is indicated when identified.

Bicornuate Uterus

Incomplete lateral fusion of Müllerian ducts result in bicornuate uterus and the level of indentation of the fundus can be complete, partial or arcuate. Two separate but communicating endometrial cavities and a single cervix characterize it. Women with bicornuate uterus can expect a successful pregnancy outcome in 55–60% and only 14% of women with poor reproductive outcome had bicornuate uterus. As with other uterine anomalies, preterm delivery occurs in 20–60% and 28% have miscarriage.

HSG is usually the initial diagnostic modality, but confirmation is done by sonography or laparoscopy, which is especially useful to differentiate from septate uterus. Presently, no surgical reconstruction is recommended unless there is evidence of poor reproductive outcome and no other causative factors been identified. Strassman's technique of unification can be done abdominally and now via laparoscopy also. Although the actual benefit of

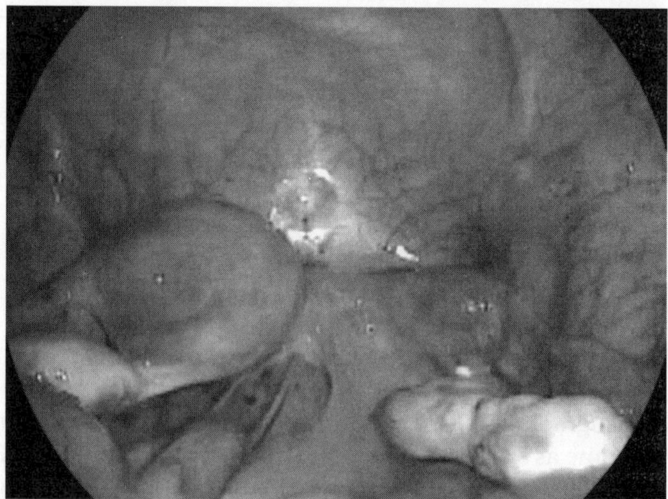

Fig. 4: Laparoscopic view showing unicornuate uterus (left horn)
with rudimentary horn (right horn)
(*Courtesy:* Dr Alka Kriplani)
(*For color version, see Plate 2*)

unification has not been proved, but improvement in pregnancy outcome has been observed in a few sporadic cases. Cesarean delivery is indicated after metroplasty due to high risk for uterine rupture.

Uterine Didelphys

Failed fusion of Müllerian ducts result in two separated uterine cavity each with a cervix known as uterus didelphys.

In most cases, a longitudinal vaginal septum runs between the two cervices, hence uterine didelphys should be suspected if longitudinal vaginal septum is present. The women has no menstrual symptoms, and infact of all the major anomalies, it has the best reproductive performance with fetal survival rate of 75% and a spontaneous abortion rate of 21%. Pregnancies are located more commonly (76%) in the right uterus. This anomaly is usually diagnosed incidentally on USG (ultrasonography) or HSG or dyspareunia due to the presence of vaginal septum. No surgical intervention is recommended unless repeated late trimester losses or premature delivery has occurred without any other cause.

Uterine Septum

Failure of resorption of the medial segment after lateral fusion of Müllerian ducts create a septum, which divides the uterine cavity in two halves. The septate uterus has a smooth but transversely broad outer surface on the fundus while the fibrous or fibromuscular septum in the endometrial cavity can be minimal only at the fundus or can extend half-way in the cavity or a complete uterine septum up to the internal os (Fig. 5). Septate uterus is associated with a significantly more pregnancy loss rate (88%) and first

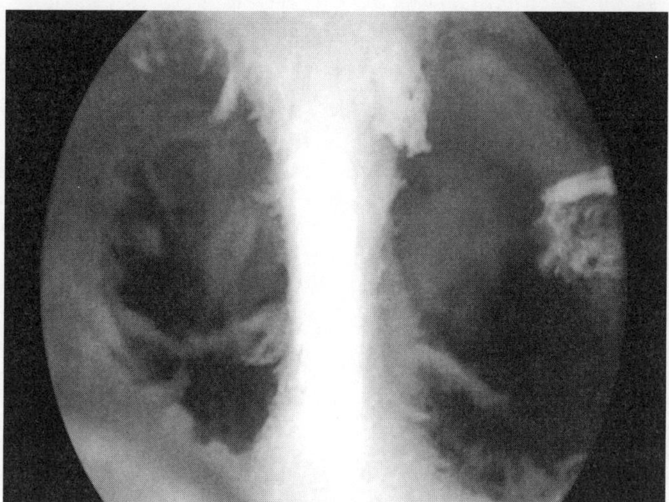

Fig. 5: Hysteroscopic view of a complete uterine septum
(*Courtesy:* Dr Alka Kriplani)
(*For color version, see Plate 2*)

trimester abortion rate (42%) than bicornuate uterus. Diagnosis is made on HSG and confirmed on sonography and laparoscopy. Traditionally, abdominal metroplasty was done to remove septum, but recently with the advent of endoscopy, hysteroscopic septal resection under laparoscopic guidance is an effective and safe alternative. Apart from being less invasive, hysteroscopic septoplasty showed improved reproductive outcome, reduced risk of pelvic adhesions and obviates the mandate for ceasarian section.

SUGGESTED READING

1. American Fertility Society. The AFS classification of adnexal adhesions, distal tubal occlusion, tubal occlusion secondary to tubal ligation, tubal pregnancies, Müllerian anomalies and intrauterine adhesions. Fertil Steril. 1988;49:944-55.
2. Brucker SY, Rall K, Campo R, Oppelt P, Isaacson K. Treatment of congenital malformations. Semin Reprod Med. 2011;29:101-12.
3. Buttram VC, Gibbons WE. Müllerian anomalies: A proposed classification (an analysis of 144 cases). Fertil Steril. 1979;32:40-6.
4. Chan YY, Jayaprakasan K, Zamora J, Thornton JG, Raine-Fenning N, Coomarasamy A. The prevalence of congenital uterine anomalies in unselected and high-risk populations: A systematic review. Hum Reprod Update. 2011;17:761-71.
5. Giannesi, Marchiole P, Benchaib M, Chevret-Measson M, Mathevet P, Dargent D. Sexuality after laparoscopic Davydov in patients affected by congenital complete vaginal agenesis associated with uterine agenesis or hypoplasia. Hum Reprod. 2005;10:2954-7.
6. Lin PC, Bhatnagar KP, Nettleton GS, Nakajima ST. Female genital anomalies affecting reproduction. Fertil Steril. 2002;78:899-915.
7. Rackow BW, Arici A. Reproductive performance of women with Müllerian anomalies. Curr Opin Obstet Gynecol. 2007;19:229-37.

Precocious Puberty

Shobha Chakraborty

Puberty in girls is the period which links childhood to adulthood.

It is the period of gradual development of secondary sexual characters. Precocious puberty is the appearance of signs of pubertal development at an abnormally early age in girls, this has traditionally been considered to be 8 years, although guidelines from the USA have recommended that puberty be considered precocious only with appearance of breast development or pubic hair before age 7 in white girls and before age 6 in black girls. Precocious puberty is often a benign central process in girls. Thelarche is the beginning of breast development and pubarche is the first appearance of pubic hair. Early appearance of these characteristics is more common than true precocious puberty.

ENDOCRINOLOGY FOR PUBERTY

Cause of Puberty

- **Central mechanism:** Negative feedback of estrogen to the hypothalamic pituitary system (Gonadostat). The Gonadostat remains very sensitive to the negative feedback effect, even though the level of estradiol is very low (910 pg/mL). As puberty approaches, this negative feedback effect of estrogen is gradually lost.
- **Kisspeptine:** Kisspeptine is neuropeptide (enclosed by kiss 1 gene) that signals via the G-Protein coupled receptor; GPR-54 (enclosed by kiss1R gene). Neurons expressing kiss1 are located in the arcuate nucleus, where gonadotropin-releasing hormone (GnRH) neurons also express GPR-54. Observation indicates that hypothalamic kisspeptine GPR-54 is a key component of the neurobiologic mechanism that triggers the onset of puberty. Kisspeptine neurons may provide the fuel for the hypothalamic GnRH pulse generator.
  - Data from the USA indicate that 1 in 5,000 children are affected and that it is ten times more common in girls. Girls in the USA are generally maturing at an earlier age than they did 30 years ago.[1]
  - Racial differences are significant. An analysis of the National Health and Nutrition Examination Survey (NHANES) from the USA showed

that black girls enter puberty earliest followed by Hispanic and then white girls[2]
- Obesity also contributes to earlier puberty[2]
- In Europe also earlier puberty has been reported, particularly in warmer climates. Reports also suggest higher incidence of precocious puberty in girls adopted in Western Europe from underdeveloped countries.[3]

Causes of Precocious Puberty

- Gonadotropin-dependent precocious puberty [central precocious puberty (CPP)]: There is premature activation of the hypothalamic-pituitary-gonadal (HPG) axis. Most children (especially girls) suspected of having CPP do not have any specific abnormality but lie at one end of the normal distribution curve.
- Idiopathic (sporadic or familial).
- Abnormalities of the central nervous system (CNS) include:
  - Tumors, including gliomas, astrocytomas, hamartomas, pineal tumors and human chorionic gonadotropin (hCG)-secreting germ cell tumors
  - CNS trauma or injury (causes include infection, radiation, surgery)
  - Hamartomas of the hypothalamus
  - Congenital disorders such as hydrocephalus and arachnoid cysts.
- Where no such CNS abnormalities are found, the causes of an early, normal puberty include:
  - Genetic—often early puberty is familial and autosomal dominant in inheritance; Russell-Silver's syndrome, McCune-Albright's syndrome (MAS)
  - Hypothyroidism.
- Obesity: In girls, early puberty is associated with increased body mass index (BMI). This is particularly the case in white girls.
- Gonadotropin-independent precocious puberty (or precocious pseudopuberty): These accounts for about 20% of cases of precocious puberty, and some of the specific types are rare. The normal pattern of puberty is absent. The gonad matures independently of GnRH stimulation and levels of estradiol. Luteinizing hormone (LH) and follicle stimulating hormone (FSH) are usually at pubertal levels (in the absence of gonadotropin pulsatility). There is a flat GnRH response and no response to treatment with gonadotropin-releasing hormone (GnRH) analog. Causes include:
  - Congenital adrenal hyperplasia (CAH)
  - HCG-secreting tumors in the liver (hepatomas, hepatoblastomas), choriocarcinomas (of gonads, pineal gland, mediastinum, etc) and adrenal tumors (rare)
  - Ovarian tumors may cause either masculinization or feminization
  - Hypothyroidism or Van Wyk-Grumbach syndrome. Growth is arrested (unusual with precocious puberty) rather than accelerated.

Precocious puberty may be GnRH and gonadotropin dependent or may be independent being caused by the peripheral secretion of sex steroids. In 80% of cases, no organic abnormality is found and the precocity appears to be merely an individual characteristic.

Sexual precocity has been seen in a few cases of primary hypothyroidism, perhaps by stimulation of FSH receptors by the increased levels of thyroid stimulating hormone (TSH).

A variety of lesions of midbrain, hypothalamus and pituitary result in precocious puberty. Congenital defects, e.g. hamartomas, hydrocephalus, craniopharyngioma; tumors, e.g. astrocytomas, gliomas, neurofibromas; non-tumor conditions, e.g. encephalitis, meningitis, Von Recklinghausen's disease, Albright's syndrome and cranial trauma, all result in precocious puberty. The pathophysiology is unclear but most lesions are associated with increased intracranial pressure and are located in the region of the hypothalamus. This stimulates the output of hypothalamic releasing factors and/or gonadotropins.

Precocious puberty is seen in patients with estrogen producing ovarian tumors such as granulosa and theca cell tumors. However, malignant teratomas, ovarian cysts and cystadenomas have also been reported as causes of precocious puberty. Menstruation is not regular in time or duration and is not accompanied by ovulation. The breasts are enlarged but there is little body hair because adrenal function is not mature.

The precocity in cases of adrenal cortical tumors is usually heterosexual; females show precocious virilism.

Androgenic tumors of the ovary, e.g. gonadoblastomas and lipoid cell tumors are associated with heterosexual precocity. Ectopic gonadotrophin secretion is rarely seen in hepatoblastomas, dysgerminomas and choriocarcinomas.

A flow diagram for diagnosis of precocious puberty is given in Flow chart 1.

Flow chart 1: Flow diagram for precocious puberty

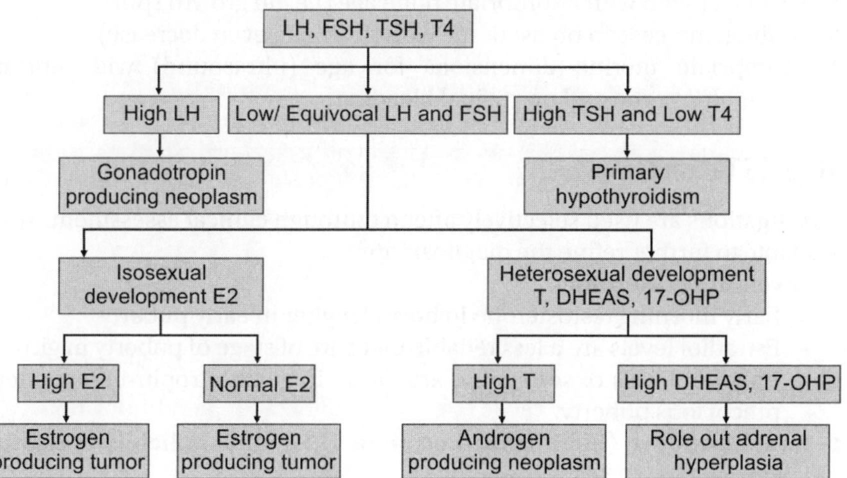

DIFFERENTIAL DIAGNOSIS

Premature Pubarche

There is early appearance of pubic (with or without axillary hair) but without other signs of puberty. Pubic hair may present in both boys and girls aged <7 years due to adrenal androgen secretion in middle childhood. Causes of premature pubarche may be:

- Weak androgens from adrenal glands (premature adrenarche). Temporarily the pubic hair development is in advance of breast development and other changes. This is usually benign.
- Signs of severe androgen excess (including clitoral enlargement, growth spurt) may be due to:
  - Congenital adrenal hyperplasia
  - Virilizing tumors—For example, in the adrenal glands, the ovary or a dysgenetic testis
  - Cushing's syndrome.
- Exogenous androgens could also cause these changes (e.g. contact with topical androgen preparations).
- Androgen activity in a pubertal girl may be evidence of polycystic ovarian syndrome.

Premature Thelarche

Breast development may occur in girls aged <3 years, and can then spontaneously regress. This is often seen in girls under the age of 3 years and is caused by maternal estrogens in the early months. There is fairly static breast development before true puberty eventually occurs at the normal time. It is a benign condition confirmed by:

- Absence of any other signs of puberty
- Normal growth with appropriate bone age (i.e. no growth spurt)
- Minimal increase in breast tissue with time (can even decrease)
- Appropriate uterine dimensions for age (ultrasound) with normal endometrial echo and no vaginal bleeding.

INVESTIGATIONS

Investigations are used selectively after a thorough clinical assessment. Tests available to further refine the diagnosis are:

- **Levels of sex steroid:**
  - Early morning testosterone in boys is higher in early puberty
  - Estradiol levels are a less reliable measure of stage of puberty in girls
  - Pubertal levels of sex steroid are found in gonadotropin-independent precocious puberty.
- **Gonadotropins (luteinizing hormone (LH) and follicle-stimulating hormone (FSH):**
  - A random LH is a useful initial test for central precocious puberty (CPP)

- A random FSH will not distinguish prepuberty from puberty
- Low or prepubertal levels with high sex steroid levels are found in gonadotropin-independent precocious puberty.

➲ **Thyroid function tests (TFTs):**
- Adrenal steroid precursors if congenital adrenal hyperplasia (CAH) is suspected
- HCG when HCG-secreting tumors are suspected
- Urinary 17-ketosteroids to quantify the amount of adrenal androgens being produced.

➲ **Diagnostic imaging:**
- Ultrasound:
  - Pelvic ultrasound is essential in gonadotropin-independent precocious puberty (precocious pseudopuberty) to detect ovarian tumors or cysts. Although not required in CCP, it will demonstrate changes in ovaries and uterus
  - Other ultrasound: Testicular and adrenal ultrasound can help to establish diagnosis of tumors, but much better imaging is ultimately achieved with MRI for adrenal tumors.
- Hand and wrist X-rays for bone age:
  - If bone age is within one year of chronological age, either puberty has not started or has only just started
  - If the bone age is two years advanced then puberty has probably been present for at least a year or is progressing rapidly.
- Bone scan is not routinely required but is useful with suspected McCune-Albright's syndrome (MAS).
- Brain MRI to exclude CNS abnormalities associated with CPP. MRI should be performed in all females with sexual precocity and in patients with neurological signs or symptoms.
- Pelvic MRI can be useful in girls to assess the uterus and ovaries.

➲ **Other tests:**
- Gonadotropin-releasing hormone (GnRH) stimulation test: LH and FSH levels are measured sequentially after GnRH is given. The gonadotropin stimulation test is useful in the assessment of precocious puberty.[4] There is a flat response in gonadotropin-independent precocious puberty[5]
- Leuprolide acetate stimulation testing is an alternative and can accurately predict puberty progression.[6]

Children presenting with vaginal bleeding before the age of 8 years should be examined for evidence of secondary sexual characters. If these are not present, the bleeding is probably not menstrual and a local organic cause in the uterus or vagina should be looked for.

If secondary sexual characters are present, then examination and investigations should be done to exclude an intracranial, ovarian or adrenal lesion. Measurements of serum estradiol, progesterone, 17-hydroxyprogesterone, testosterone and dehydroepiandrosterone sulfate (DHEAS), as indicated by the history and physical findings, along with basal FSH and LH levels are helpful. Any abnormality on neurological examination, CT or MRI brain suggests a cranial cause.

The management depends on whether it is gonadotropin-dependent or gonadotropin-independent tumor. The first test should be the measurement of basal gonadotropin level. Thyroid function should also be evaluated to rule out primary hypothyroidism. High levels of LH suggest a gonadotropin secreting tumor, most often a pinealoma (ectopic germinoma). Increased estradiol level suggests an estrogen secreting neoplasm, probably of ovarian origin.

Increased testosterone levels suggest androgen producing neoplasm of the ovary or the adrenal gland. Increased 17-hydroxyprogesterone levels are diagnostic of congenital adrenal hyperplasia (i.e. 21-hydroxylase deficiency).

Bone age should always be assessed in evaluating an individual with sexual precocity. The management with GnRH agonist therapy initially causes a flare up effect (increasing circulating gonadotropin and estradiol concentrations for a short period).

Chronic therapy is associated with suppression of pulsatile gonadotropin secretion. Suppression is best monitored with GnRH challenge tests. The various effects like cessation of menses, regression in physical pubertal signs (breast size and pubic hair), and diminution of uterine and ovarian size usually occur within the first six months of therapy.

Feminizing adrenal tumors are associated with an elevated DHEAS and estradiol and low gonadotropins. Virilizing ovarian tumors may result in elevated serum DHEAS or androstenedione levels. Both can be detected by ultrasonography or CT or MRI, and both should be surgically resected.

Precocious puberty with delayed bone age suggests primary hypothyroidism (increased serum TSH and low T4). All values return to normal with treatment.

The management of true precocious puberty requires attention to maximizing height, arresting further maturation and attenuating precocious features. In the past, medroxyprogesterone acetate, cyproterone acetate and danazol were used with some success. The use of GnRH analogs has significantly improved the results of treatment. The goal of therapy is to maintain the serum estradiol level below 10 pg/mL. Treatment has to be continued till pubertal and chronogical age matches. The final bone height is increased depending on how early treatment is instituted.

MANAGEMENT

For cases of central precocious puberty (CPP) with no underlying brain pathology and no psychosocial complications, treatment for the pubertal changes alone may not be required. Puberty can be arrested and growth hormone given if the height prognosis is poor. Examples of treatment include:
- Surgery: Tumors may require resection but resection rarely causes regression of the pubertal changes.[1]
- Medical treatments include:
  - Gonadotropin-releasing hormone (GnRH) agonists are used in CPP, as well as for other etiologies including McCune-Albright's syndrome (MAS)

- Glucocorticoids are used for congenital adrenal hyperplasia (CAH)
- Cyproterone acetate may be used for anti-androgen action. Flutamide is also used to counter androgen excess
- Medroxyprogesterone (a progesterone analog) has also been used.

COMPLICATIONS

- Psychological difficulties including feeling stressed and becoming withdrawn because of the early physical changes; bullying
- Behavioral and emotional problems
- Early puberty accelerates growth but bone maturation is also accelerated and so adult height is reduced.

PROGNOSIS

With proper treatment and care, most children with this disorder will ultimately experience a normal and happy adolescence.

GONADOTROPIN-INDEPENDENT PRECOCIOUS PUBERTY

This depends on the etiology. The possible diagnoses already discussed, cover a range of possible outcomes. With early recognition and treatment, the prognosis can be excellent.

Drugs used in the management of precocity (Constitutional/idiopathic):

- GnRH agonist therapy—drug of choice
  Dose: Buserelin nasay spray—100 µg/day
  Goserelin/ Leuprolide—once a month doses
- Medroxyprogesterone acetate: 30 mg/day orally OR 100–200 mg IM weekly. Can suppress menstruation and breast development but cannot change the skeletal growth rate
- Cyproterone acetate: 70–100 mg/day orally for 10 days starting from the 5th day of cycle
- Danazol: Produces amenorrhea and arrest breast development. But there is no change in skeletal growth. Used up to 11 years of age
  Individualization should be done.

  Puberty is a period of transition where precocity plays havoc in an adolescent's life.
- Timely intervention and management relieves the agony of the child and parents.

REFERENCES

1. Herman-Giddens ME, Kaplowitz PB, Wasserman R. Navigating the recent articles on girl's puberty in Pediatrics: What do we know and where do we go from here?. Pediatrics. 2004;113(4):911-7.

2. Kaplowitz PB, Slora EJ, Wasserman RC, et al. Earlier onset of puberty in girls: relation to increased body mass index and race. Pediatrics. 2001;108(2):347-53.
3. Parent AS, Teilmann G, Juul A, et al; The timing of normal puberty and the age limits of sexual precocity: variations around the world, secular trends, and changes after migration. Endocr Rev. 2003;24(5):668-93.
4. Kandemir N, Demirbilek H, Ozon ZA, et al. GnRH Stimulation Test in precocious Puberty. Single Sample is Adequate for J Clin Res Pediatr Endocrinol. 2011;3(1):12-7. Epub 2011 Feb 23.
5. Ng SM, Kumar Y, Cody D, et al. The gonadotropins response to GnRH test is not a predictor of neurological lesion in girls with central precocious puberty. J Pediatr Endocrinol Metab. 2005;18(9):849-52.
6. Sathasivam A, Garibaldi L, Shapiro S, et al. Leuprolide stimulation testing for the evaluation of early female sexual Clin Endocrinol (Oxf). 2010;73(3):375-81. Epub 2010 Feb 23.

Chapter
29

Primary Amenorrhea

N Palaniappan, Pankaj Desai

DEFINITION

Primary amenorrhea is defined as absence of menstruation by the age of 15–16 years. The conflict of definition continues as menarche involves a compendium of events. Therefore, failure of development of any secondary sexual characteristics by 14 years should be investigated and failure to menstruate by 16 years with secondary sexual characters should arouse concern.

NORMAL PUBERTY

The famous five classical changes that happen as secondary sexual characteristics are:

- Breast growth (Thelarche): Breast growth has 5 stages as described by Tanner.[1] The onset begins by 9 years and full development is complete within 5 years.
- Axillary hair: It has 3 stages and this tends to occur at around 13 years.
- Growth spurt: The peak height velocity of growth reaches 11 cm/year between the 10th and 14th year of age.[2]
- Pubic hair growth (Pubarche): It occurs in concurrence with breast development and has 5 stages.
- Menarche: Menstruation occurs in most girls by the age of 13 though this may be influenced by variables such as nutrition, genetic and racial factors.[3]

ETIOLOGY

- Normal secondary sexual characteristics
  - Imperforate hymen
  - Transverse vaginal septum
  - Absent vagina and non functioning uterus
  - XY female—androgen insensitivity
  - Resistant ovary syndrome
  - Constitutional delay

- ⊃ Absent secondary sexual characters
  - – Normal height
    - - Hypogonadotrophic-hypogonadism
      Congenital — Isolated GnRH deficiency
      — Kallmann's syndrome
      Acquired — Weight loss/Anorexia
      — Excessive exercise
      — Hyperprolactinemia
    - - Hypergonadotropic hypogonadism
      a. Gonadal agenesis
      b. Gonadal dysgenesis
      c. Turner's mosaic
      d. Ovarian failure
      e. Galactosemia
  - – Short stature
    - - Hypogonadotrophic hypogonadism
      Congenital — Hydrocephalus
      Acquired — Trauma
      — Empty sella syndrome
      — Tumors
    - - Hypergonadotropic hypogonadism
      Turner's syndrome
      Other X deletions/mosaics
- ⊃ Heterosexual development
  - – Congenital adrenal hyperplasia
  - – Androgen secreting tumors
  - – Partial androgen receptor deficiency
  - – 5 alpha reductase deficiency
  - – True hermaphrodite
  - – Absent Mullerian inhibitor factor

PRIMARY AMENORRHEA WITH NORMAL SECONDARY SEXUAL CHARACTERISTICS

Imperforate Hymen (Cryptomenorrhea)

The main complaint is cyclic abdominal pain, due to dysmenorrhea associated with collection of menstrual blood in the vagina, to produce a hematocolpos, and then in the uterus to produce a hematometra. The huge mass may produce pressure effects causing difficulty in micturition and defecation. A big collection can also present as an abdominal swelling (Fig. 1) and local examination of the introitus will reveal a tense, blue bulging membrane—the hymen (Fig. 2). Treatment should be restricted to hymenectomy by a cruciate incision on the hymen and allowing the altered menstrual blood to flow out. D and C is not required.

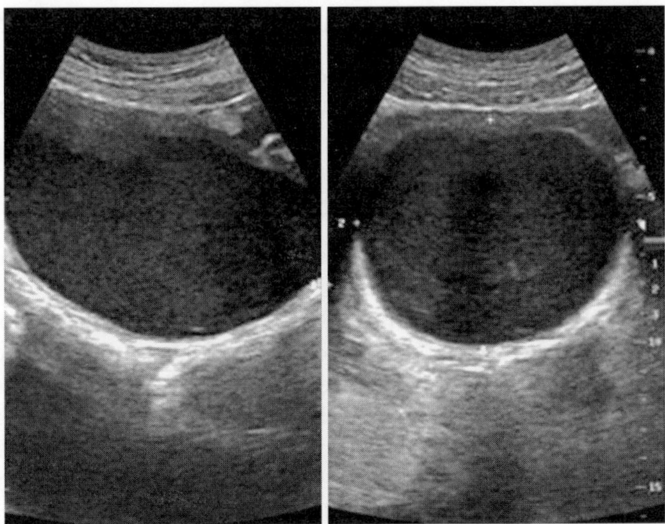

Fig. 1: USG picture—cryptomenorrhea

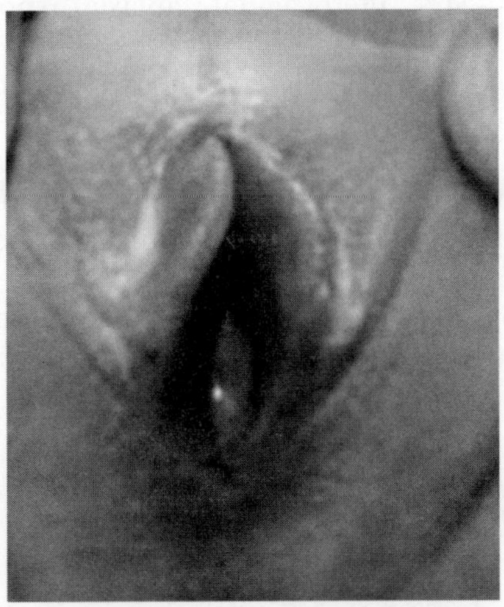

Fig. 2: Imperforate hymen with typical bluish discoloration behind the hymen
suggestive of collected blood
(For color version, see Plate 3)

Transverse Vaginal Septum (Cryptomenorrhea)

It may present similar to imperforate hymen, with cyclical abdominal pain, mass but inspection of the introitus may reveal a bulging membrane which is not blue in color. The vaginal septum may be at 3 levels—lower, middle or upper third. Excision of the septum is very difficult and help of a plastic reconstructive surgeon may be needed.

Absent Vagina and Functioning Uterus (Cryptomenorrhea)

These patients may have an absent cervix. Patients may present with cyclical abdominal pain without any mass but may have a uterus filled with blood—hematometra.

Absent Vagina and Nonfunctioning Uterus

This is Müllerian agenesis characterised by failure of the Müllerian ducts to develop, resulting in absent uterus and variable malformation of the upper vagina, called the Mayer-Rokitansky-Kustner-Hauser syndrome or MRKH syndrome. This is the second common method of presentation preceded by Turner's syndrome. These patients are hormonally normal, have normal development of secondary sexual characteristics including adrenarche and thelarche. They have 46XX chromosome pattern, normal ovaries and tubes. Vagina is blind and sometimes intercourse may be possible. Uterus, cervix and partial vagina are absent. They may have a variety of renal and musculoskeletal anomalies.

Typical MRKH—64% isolated uterovaginal aplasia/hypoplasia.

Atypical MRKH—24% uterovaginal aplasia/hypoplasia with renal malformations.

MURCS syndrome—12% Müllerian, renal, cardiac and skeletal malformations

Pelvic ultrasound (USG) may usually detect normal ovaries but may miss a uterus which can be rudimentary. Laparoscopy will confirm diagnosis and rudimentary uterus may be seen as a connecting cord between the normally developed adnexa (Fig. 3).

McIndoe's vaginoplasty with postoperative dilatation may allow patients to have normal sexual intercourse. Since ovaries are normal, ova can be retrieved

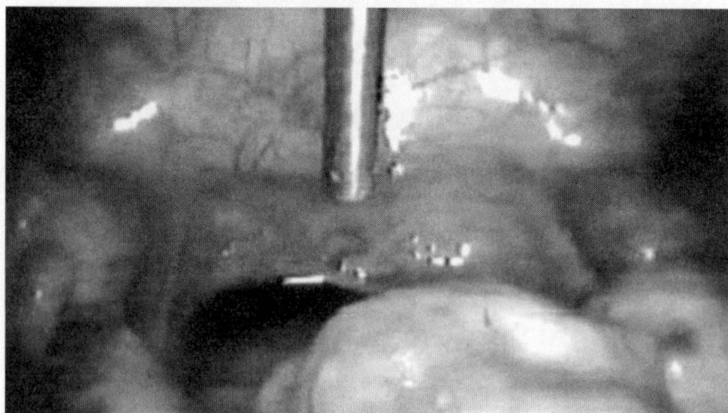

Fig. 3: Absent uterus in a subject with primary amenorrhea at laparoscopy
(For color version, see Plate 3)

and a child born through a surrogate mother. Uterine transplantation may be an option in future.

XY Female—Androgen Insensitivity

These patients have a XY karyotype due to:
- Failure of testicular development
- Enzymatic failure of the testes to produce androgens
- Androgen receptor failure.

They have good breast development due to peripheral conversion of androgen to estrogen and subsequent stimulation of breast tissue. Pubic hair is scanty, vulva is normal, vagina is short, uterus and tubes are absent. Testis would be found in the lower abdomen usually in hernial sacs in childhood which will alert the diagnosis. Serum testosterone levels are normal, chances of malignancy developing in the testis is about 20%, which warrants gonadectomy at 18 years to permit complete breast development and epiphyseal closure. They can be reared as female and can have sexual life but cannot procreate.

Resistant Ovary Syndrome

This is a very rare cause. In this, levels of gonadotropins are elevated in the presence of normal ovarian tissue. They have absence of FSH receptors and hence do not respond to FSH.

Constitutional Delay

This occurs due to delay in hypothalamic maturation of the pulsatile frequency or amplitude of GnRH. All sex characters are normal with no anatomical delay.

PRIMARY AMENORRHEA WITH ABSENT SECONDARY SEXUAL CHARACTERISTICS

Isolated GnRH Deficiency/Kallman Syndrome

Hypothalamus does not produce GnRH. Stimulation of pituitary with GnRH leads to normal release of gonadotropins (FSH+LH). Some patients may suffer from anosmia, called as olfactogenital syndrome/Kallmann's syndrome. It occurs due to a gene deletion.

Weight Loss/Anorexia

It is usually associated with secondary amenorrhea more than primary amenorrhea. These children have normal growth and secondary sexual characters, with a release of gonadotropin, due to the low body mass in the secretion of GnRH.

Excessive Exercises

This is usually seen in models, athletes and ballet dancers. Their percentage body fat is much reduced and hence there is suppression of GnRH release. Corrective dietary measures may reverse the condition and produce menstruation.

Hyperprolactinemia

This is usually associated with secondary more than primary amenorrhea. There may be recognizable prolactionoma but may not have an apparent lesion. CT of the pituitary fossa is worthwhile and treatment with cabergolin/surgery as per the size and prolactin levels may be the need.

Gonadal Agenesis

There is failure of development of the gonads. They may be 46XY, 45X/46XY. Absence of testicular determining factor (TDF) or its receptors may be the cause. It is an autosomal recessive disorder. All are phenotypically female since masculinization does not occur in absence of androgens. They have normal Mullerian structures—uterus, tubes and vagina. Since there is no hypothalamopituitary disorder, height is normal. Conception is possible with ovum donation and ART.

Galactosemia

Galactosemia occurs due to inborn error of metabolism due to the deficiency of galactose-1-phospate uridyltransferase. Its exact etiology remains unclear.

Gonadal Dysgenesis

The commonest condition is Turner's syndrome or single X chromosome. In Turner mosaicism, the higher percentage of 45X cells would produce features of Turner's syndrome. The presence of some normal 46XX means that there is a possibility of ovarian differentiation and associated secondary sexual characteristics. A few girls have conceived. Karyotype is essential to clinch the diagnosis.

Turner's Syndrome

In Turner's syndrome, ovarian development is normal till 20 years. Oocytes are found in the ovaries. Thereafter, these oocytes do not undergo further maturation, due to the lack of one X chromosome and become atretic until puberty. The ovary consists mostly of stroma and has no estrogenic potential. These patients will have normal female organ development due to the absence of Y chromosome. The loss of X-chromosome leads to short stature. There is webbed neck, wide spaced nipples, pectus cavum, short fourth metacarpal and heart disease. FSH level remains elevated. With the advances in artificial reproductive techniques, Turner's syndrome patients can become pregnant. The fetus may be at risk of heart disease. Growth hormone, either alone or with a low dose of androgen, will increase growth and adult height will be achieved.[4] Estrogen has been used to promote the development of secondary sexual characters.[4]

Algorithms for approach to subjects with primary amenorrhea are shown in Flow charts 1 and 2.

Flow chart 1: Approach to primary amenorrhea with normal secondary sex characters

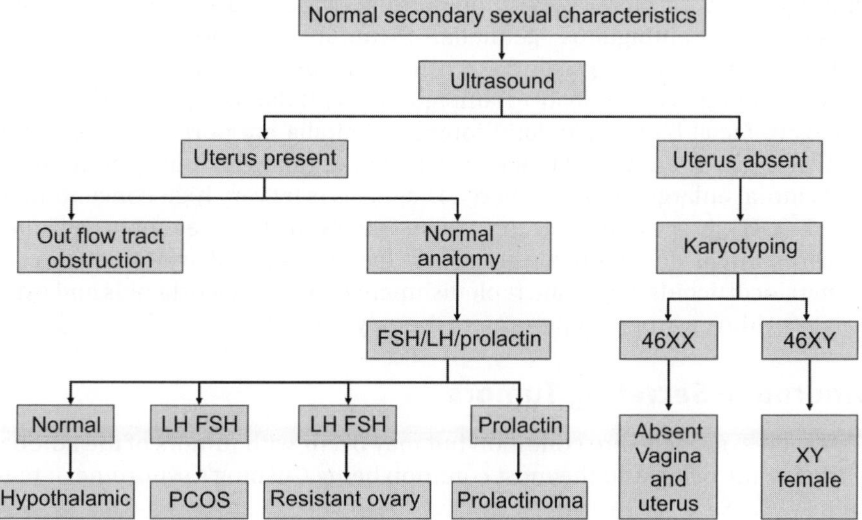

Flow chart 2: Approach to primary amenorrhea with poor or absent secondary sex characters

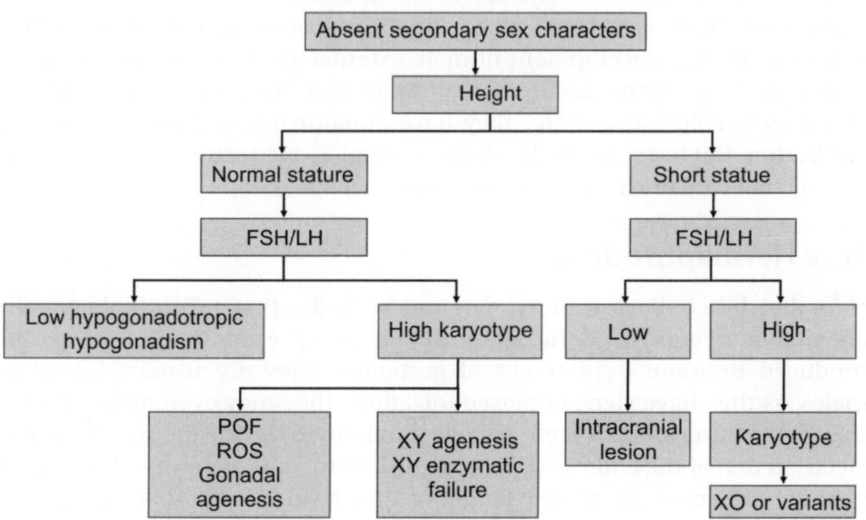

PRIMARY AMENORRHEA WITH HETEROSEXUAL DEVELOPMENT

Congenital Adrenal Hyperplasia

It most commonly presents at birth with heterosexual features. It can also present later at puberty with clitoral enlargement. It is autosomal recessive in nature, which leads to an enzyme deficiency of 21 hydroxylase, located on the short arm of chromosome 6. Failure to produce cortisol leads to elevated ACTH and high level of cortisol precursors, which in turn gets converted to androgens via 17 alpha (OH) progesterone, which leads to masculinizing features and ambiguous genitalia. Symptoms include vomiting and dehydration due to salt wasting as a cause of inadequate mineralocorticoids. Excess androgens may lead to ambiguous genitalia, early pubic hair, and excessive facial hair. Vagina and internal genitalia are normal, but external genitalia vary from fused labia to a stenosed vagina with a urogenital sinus, and clitoral enlargement at puberty. Diagnosis is by very high concentration of 17 (OH) progesterone (more than 242 nmol/L). Treatment includes replacement of glucocorticoids to reduce hyperplasia and over production of mineralocorticoids, adequate replenishment of mineralocorticoids and extra salt, providing estrogen replacement therapy at puberty.

Androgen Secreting Tumors

This is an extremely rare condition but may occur with tumors of the adrenal cortex or the ovary and the most common being Cushing's syndrome. It may mimic PCOS.

5-α-Reductase Deficiency

This is an autosomal recessive intersex condition, which lacks the enzyme that converts testosterone to 5 alpha dihydrotestosterone, a potent androgen, necessary for the development of male external genitalia in utero. Patients have a male karyotype, no uterus and tubes and male gonads, but they are raised as females. At puberty they have amenorrhea and may experience virilization. But testosterone levels are normal. Gonadectomy due to the risk of testicular cancer should be considered.

True Hermaphrodites

Here the child is born with ovarian and testicular tissue. External genitalia are often ambiguous and the degree depends on the amount of testosterone produced between 8–16 weeks of gestation. They are usually reared as males, as they have signs of masculinization. They may even menstruate at puberty, putting an extremely difficult situation to decide the sex of rearing. Decision to rear the child should be made before puberty by determining the gonadal sex, structure, phallic length of 1.5 cm (for male). This is done by a multidisciplinary approach.

REFERENCES

1. Tanner JM. Growth at adolescence. Oxford. Blackwell Scientific Publications, 1962.
2. Marshall WA, Tanner JM. Variation in the pattern of pubertal changes in girls. Arch Dis Child. 1969;44:291.
3. Marshal WA. Growth and secondary sexual characteristics and related abnormalities. Clin Obstet Gynecol. 1974;1:593.
4. Turner syndrome society of the United States. FAQ. 6. What can be done? Retrieved 2007-05-11.

Chapter 30

Secondary Amenorrhea

Alokendu Chatterjee, Partha Mukherjee

INTRODUCTION

Menstruation needs a complex hormonal interaction from hypothalamus to ovary. Finally, development of an ovarian follicle and ovulation occurs. Before ovulation, a functional ovarian follicle secretes estrogen and after ovulation, progesterone is secreted from corpus luteum, in addition to estrogen. These hormones stimulate endometrial development. Estrogen and progesterone secretion decreases, if pregnancy docs not occur and menstruation begins. If there is dysfunction and nonfunctioning of any of the components from hypothalamus to outflow tract, menstruation does not occur.

Absence of menstruation for three normal menstrual cycles in a woman who previously menstruated[1] or no menses for 6 months is defined as secondary amenorrhea.

ETIOLOGY

Uterine Factors

- Destruction of endometrium due to tubercular infection or radiation
- Surgical removal of uterus
- Uterine synechiae.

Ovarian Factors

- Polycystic ovarian syndrome (PCOS)
- Primary ovarian insufficiency (Premature ovarian failure)
- Resistant ovarian syndrome
- Loss of ovarian function due to radiation or removal
- Androgen producing ovarian tumor.

Pituitary Factors

- Trauma, tumor or infections inhibit secretion of growth hormones
- Prolactinoma

➲ Sheehan's syndrome
➲ Simmond's disease.

Hypothalamic Factors

➲ Trauma, tumor or infection
➲ Shock, stress, anorexia nervosa, strenuous exercise.

Adrenal Factors

➲ Congenital adrenal hyperplasia
➲ Adrenal tumor
➲ Cushing syndrome.

Other Factors

➲ Hyperprolactinemia
➲ Hypo- or hyperthyroidism
➲ Chronic nephritis
➲ Diabetes
➲ Drugs like contraceptive pills, psychotropic drugs and antihypertensive drugs.

A large number of patients of secondary amenorrhea have polycystic ovarian syndrome. Other common causes are hyperprolactinemia, hypothalamic causes and ovarian failure. A logical and systematic clinical approach is required to diagnose and manage these cases.

Polycystic Ovarian Syndrome

Polycystic ovarian syndrome (PCOS) is one of the most common causes of secondary amenorrhea. It is a common and complex endocrinopathy in reproductive age women presenting multiple clinical challenges. At a joint consensus meeting of the American Society of Reproductive Medicine (ASRM) and the European Society of Human Reproduction and Embryology (ESHRE), held in Rotterdam in May 2003, a refined definition of PCOS was agreed upon, namely the presence of any two of the following criteria: (a) Oligo and/or anovulation; (b) Clinical and/or biochemical evidence of hyperandrogenism; (c) Polycystic ovaries (presence of 12 or more follicles measuring 2–9 mm in diameter and/or increased ovarian volume >10 cc),[2] with exclusion of other etiologies. Criteria for the diagnosis of PCOS in adolescents differ from those used for older women of reproductive age. Diagnosing PCOS in the adolescents is challenging as many characteristics of PCOS are physiologic during puberty. On the basis of the current evidence, ESHRE/ASRM recently proposed requiring all of the three Rotterdam criteria for diagnosing PCOS in the adolescents.[3]

PCOS is a complex disease with a multifactorial cause. The etiology of PCOS remains unclear. The main determinants of PCOS are hyperandrogenemia, ovarian dysfunction and metabolic abnormalities. All appear to be involved in a synergistic way in the pathophysiology of PCOS. There are interactions between susceptible genes and environmental factors with known defects in pituitary secretion of the luteinizing hormone (LH). Hyperinsulinemi-potentiated gonadotropin-stimulated ovarian androgen production in women with PCOS.[4] The metabolic and reproductive abnormalities in PCOS are further exacerbated by obesity, which is also associated with insulin resistance.[5]

Dyslipidemia is also a common aberration in PCOS. Obesity is prevalent in women with PCOS, with more than 50% of women with PCOS being overweight or obese. Additionally women with PCOS tend to have an increased waist : hip ratio, indicative of increased rate of central (visceral) obesity. Obese women with PCOS have the most atherogenic lipid profiles.[6] Genetic, ethnic factors, hyperandrogenemia and obesity are also related with dyslipidemia in women with PCOS.[7]

Asherman Syndrome

Intrauterine adhesions may develop due to severe infection, vigorous curettage or radiation. Asherman syndrome cannot be diagnosed by physical examination. It is suspected when no withdrawal bleeding occurs after estrogen and progesterone administration. It can be diagnosed by hysterosalpingography, saline infusion sonography or hysteroscopy.

Hyperprolactinemia

Hyperprolactinemia is a common cause of secondary amenorrhea in up to 30% women.[8] Estimation of serum prolactin level is justified in all women with secondary amenorrhea. Elevated prolactin level suppresses gonadotropin-releasing hormone (GnRH) secretion and leads to anovulation. Causes of hyperprolactinemia may be pituitary adenoma, other central nervous system (CNS) lesion that disrupt transport of dopamine down the pituitary stalk, hypothyroidism and drugs like antipsychotics, metoclopramide, some antihypertensive and H_2-receptor blockers. Other rare causes are breast or chest wall surgery, cervical spine lesion and renal insufficiency.

Primary Ovarian Insufficiency (Premature Ovarian Failure)

It is defined as the presence of amenorrhea for 4 months or more accompanied by two serum follicle-stimulating hormone (FSH) levels in the menopausal range for a woman who is less than 40 years of age. Premature ovarian insufficiency (POI) is a heterogeneous disorder and may be caused by sex chromosomal disorders, mutation of single genes and by fragile X syndrome. Women with POI should be offered karyotype and testing for FMR1 mutation. POI may be caused by radiation and chemotherapy. The cause of POI may be a consequence of autoimmune disease but in majority cases cause remains unknown.

Abnormalities Affecting Release of Gonadotropin and Gonadotropin-releasing Hormone

Anorexia nervosa is an eating disorder. A criterion for diagnosis is refusal to maintain body weight up to 15% below normal. Patients try to maintain their low body weight by dieting, exercise and laxative. It may be a life-threatening disorder. Weight loss, high intensity training and stress may induce amenorrhea. There is decrease in the frequency of GnRH pulses resulting in hypoestrogenic state in patients. Synchronized secretion of GnRH and gonadotropin from hypothalamus and pituitary gland is essential for normal menstruation to occur. Tumors of pituitary or hypothalamus, like craniopharyngiomas, germinomas, tubercular or sarcoid granulomas may cause amenorrhea by preventing appropriate hormone secretion. Sheehan syndrome is associated with postpartum necrosis of the pituitary gland due to acute hypotensive episodes associated with severe postpartum hemorrhage (PPH). There may be features of pan-hypopituitarism. Patients with milder form have lactation failure, loss of pubic and axillary hair, lethargy and amenorrhea.

EVALUATION

Pregnancy must be excluded before the evaluation of secondary amenorrhea. A careful medical history and physical examination always provides valuable information regarding diagnoses. Thorough menstrual history is very important. Amenorrhea following curettage or sepsis indicates endometrial damage. History of chronic illness like diabetes, tuberculosis, renal disease or previous head injury should be enquired. History of weight gain or weight loss, intensity of exercise or evidence of hirsuitism, is important. Clinical assessment of estrogenic status to diagnose hypoestrogenic state should be done. Presence of hot flushes and vaginal dryness indicate hypoestrogenism. Serum estradiol level less than 40 pg/mL indicates less estrogen production. Presence of superficial cells in vaginal cytology indicates estrogen production. Height, weight and body mass index should be determined for management of PCOS.

Serum prolactin and serum thyroid-stimulating hormone (TSH) level estimation are important in evaluation of secondary amenorrhea because of their relatively common incidence. All possible causes of hyperprolactinemia including hypothalamic and pituitary mass should be evaluated.

Assessment of serum FSH level is important to determine whether the patient is normogonadotropic, hypogonadotropic or hypergonadotropic. Low estrogen production along with low serum FSH concentration (5–10 mIU/mL) indicates inadequate gonadotropin production. Magnetic resonance imaging (MRI) is required to exclude tumor of pituitary and to differentiate between pituitary and hypothalamic causes, in absence of other clear causes of hypogonadotropic hypogonadism like hyperprolactinemia, significant physical, mental and emotional stress. When no mass is revealed on imaging, the diagnosis is functional hypothalamic amenorrhea. FSH level more than 25–40 mIU/mL, indicates hypergonadotropic amenorrhea or ovarian insufficiency. Hormonally active ovarian tumor can be diagnosed by USG or CT scan along with clinical evaluation.

MANAGEMENT

Treatment of secondary amenorrhea is challenging due to variety and complexity of the disease. It varies widely according to cause. Underlying disorder should be treated first.

Polycystic ovary syndrome is a persisting challenge to the clinician as the presentation of the syndrome can vary widely. Clinicians treating women with PCOS have to remember that, because of the multifactorial spectrum of PCOS, a multifaceted therapeutic approach may be required.

Lifestyle modification with dietary changes and exercise is the first-line therapeutic approach for treating metabolic disease and reducing CVD risk in women with PCOS. Oral contraceptives (OC) and antiandrogens have been used in the treatment of PCOS for a long time. Oral contraceptives suppress LH secretion and lead to a decrease in ovarian androgen production. The estrogenic component increases the levels of sex hormone-binding globulin, which, in turn, results in a decrease in circulating free testosterone levels. The progestin in the pill can compete for 5 alpha-reductase at the level of the androgen receptor. A large number of patients have associated anovulation and infertility. Ovulation induction is generally the appropriate treatment in this condition.

Hyperandrogenemia may be one of the initiating factors of metabolic aberration. In women with PCOS, antiandrogens, such as cyproterone acetate, spironolactone or flutamide have been used for the treatment of hirsuitism. They are usually administered in combination with OC because of the hyper-additive synergism of these medications, to prevent pregnancy as there are risks of feminization in male fetuses and for minimization of irregular menses.

The strong pathophysiological association of insulin resistance with PCOS aberrations supports the therapeutic use of insulin sensitizers in the management of PCOS. Metformin is currently the main insulin sensitizer recommended for women with PCOS with prediabetes or type-2 diabetes (T2DM). Pioglitazone remains a reasonable first choice or as a second agent if metformin monotherapy is insufficient to reach treatment goals.

Statins are an emerging and promising new therapeutic option for women with PCOS. They act by selective inhibition of 3-hydroxy-3-methylglutaryl-coenzyme A (HMG-CoA), the rate-limiting enzyme in the cholesterol biosynthesis pathway.[9] In a randomized double blind trial of atorvastatin versus placebo in women with PCOS, atorvastatin improved lipid profile and reduced CRP and serum insulin levels.[10]

Clinical studies largely indicate a role of vitamin D deficiency in the pathogenesis of insulin resistance and T2DM in women with PCOS. Low levels of vitamin D are associated with obesity and insulin resistance, impaired β-cell function, IGT and metabolic syndrome, indicating a possible role of vitamin D in the pathogenesis of PCOS.[11] Further studies are warranted to establish the role of vitamin D in PCOS treatment.

Hyperprolactinemia is treated with discontinuation of contributing medicines. Treatment with dopamine agonists like bromocriptine or cabergoline is the first choice. In all cases of microadenoma and nearly all cases of macroadenoma, prolactin level can be normalized with dopamine agonist.[12] When associated with hypothyroidism, thyroxin should be given first. In patients with pituitary lactotroph adenoma not responding to dopamine agonist, surgery should be offered. Rarely surgery for very large macroadenoma is required in women who want to conceive, even when the tumor is responding to medical treatment. Thyroid disorders are treated with antithyroid drugs or thyroid hormone as appropriate.

Management of POI includes careful counseling and emotional support. It is important to start hormone replacement therapy after proper counseling about the risks and benefits of HRT. Gonadectomy is required when a Y cell line is present. Though it is reported that 5–10% women with POI may conceive,[13] only egg donation—IVF can increase the chance of pregnancy.

Ovarian tumor secreting hormones is surgically removed. Obesity, malnutrition, Cushing's syndrome and acromegaly are treated accordingly. Psychotherapy is required for stress induced amenorrhea. A multidisciplinary approach is required for the treatment of anorexia nervosa.

CONCLUSION

Secondary amenorrhea may be associated with a medical condition that may affect the overall health of the patient. Medical cause of amenorrhea should be established and treated first. An important part of evaluation of secondary amenorrhea is exclusion of pregnancy. Physical examination for obesity, malnutrition or evidence of hyperandrogenism is important. As PCOS is one of the most common causes of secondary amenorrhea, it should be evaluated first. Measurement of serum prolactin and TSH level are important, and assessment of FSH level should be done to differentiate between hypergonadotropic and hypogonadotropic amenorrhea. Chronic anovulation with PCOS may be treated according to desire of the patient. Ovulation induction is required when the associated problem is infertility. In all other cases, the endometrium should be protected with progesterone. Hormone replacement along with calcium should be given in hypoestrogenic individuals as in POI.

REFERENCES

1. The Practice Committee of the American Society for Reproductive Medicine. Current evaluation of amenorrhea. Feril Steril. 2008;90:S219-25.
2. Rotterdam ESHRE/ASRM-Sponsored PCOS Consensus Workshop Group. Revised 2003 Consensus on diagnostic criteria and long-term health risks related to polycystic ovary syndrome. Fertil Steril. 2004;81:19-25.

3. Zachurzok-Buczynska A, Szydlowski L, Gawlik A, et al. Blood pressure regulation and resting heart rate abnormalities in adolescent girls with polycystic ovary syndrome. Fertil Steril. 2011;96:1519-25.

4. Tosi F, Negri C, Perrone F, et al. Hyperinsulinemia amplifies GnRH agonist stimulated ovarian steroid secretion in women with polycystic ovary syndrome. J Clin Endocrinol Metab. 2012;97:1712-9.

5. Kahal H, Atkin SL, Sathyapalan T. Pharmacological treatment of obesity in patients with polycystic ovary syndrome. J Obes. 2011;2011:402052.

6. Castelo-Branco C, Steinvarcel F, Osorio A, et al. Atherogenic metabolic profile in PCOS patients: role of obesity and hyperandrogenism. Gynecol Endocrinol. 2010;26:736-42.

7. Economou F, Xyrafis X, Christakou C, Diamanti-Kandarakis E. The pluripotential effects of hypolipidemic treatment for polycystic ovary syndrome (PCOS): Dyslipidemia, cardiovascular risk factors and beyond. Curr Pharm Des. 2011;17(9):908-21.

8. Schlechte J, Sherman B, Halmi N, VanGilder J, Chapler F, Dolan K, et al. Prolactin-secreting pituitary tumors in amenorrheic women: a comprehensive study, Endocr Rev. 1980;1:295.

9. Sacks FM, Pfeffer MA, Moye LA, Rouleau JL, Rutherford JD, Cole TG, et al. The effects of pravastatin on coronary events after myocardial infarction in patients with average cholesterol levels. Cholesterol and Recurrent Events Trial investigators. N Engl J Med. 1996;335(14):1001-09.

10. Sathyapalan T, Kilpatrick ES, Coady A-M, Atkin SL. The effect of atorvastatin in patients with polycystic ovary syndrome: a randomized double-blind placebo-controlled study. J Clin Endocrinol Metab. 2009;94(1):103-08.

11. Wehr E, Pilz S, Schweighofer N, Giuliani A, Kopera D, Pieber TR, et al. Association of hypovitaminosis D with metabolic disturbances in polycystic ovary syndrome. Eur J Endocrinol. 2009;161(4):575-82.

12. Di Sarno A, Landi ML, Marzullo P, Di Somma C, Pivonello R, Cerbone G, et al. The effect of quinagolide and cabergoline, two selective dopamine receptor type 2 agonists, in the treatment of prolactinomas. Clin Endocrinol (Oxf). 2000;53:53.

13. Luborsky JL, Meyer P, Sowers MF, Gold EB, Santoro N. Premature menopause in a multi-ethnic population study of the menopause transition, Hum Reprod. 2003;18:199.

Premenstrual Syndrome

Jagdishwari Mishra, Rita Kumari Jha

INTRODUCTION

A universal definition of premenstrual syndrome (PMS) is yet to come. As it does not occur prior to puberty, after the menopause or during pregnancy, we can say that this syndrome does not occur if there is no ovarian function and this is a diagnosis of exclusion. It is also called ovarian cycle syndrome or perimenstrual syndrome.

It can be defined as a common cyclical disorder of young and middle aged women having wide range of distressing physical, psychological and behavioral symptoms which regularly occur only during luteal phase of the menstrual cycle and significantly regress or disappear during the remainder of the cycle, without any organic disease.[1]

It affects millions of women during their reproductive years. Upto 85% of menstruating women report having one or more premenstrual symptoms and 2 to 10% report disabling and incapacitating symptoms, when it is known as premenstrual dysphoric disorder (PMDD). Emotional/Mood symptoms are dominant in this severe variety.

HISTORICAL BACKGROUND

Hippocrates mentioned the condition as early as the fourth century BC, but it only became a medical epidemic in the nineteenth century. Frank was the first to introduce the term premenstrual tension in 1931, when he described 15 women with typical symptoms of PMS. Greene and Dalton extended the definition to premenstrual syndrome in 1953 recognising the wider range of symptoms. Growing public attention was given to PMS since 1980s.

EPIDEMIOLOGY

The number of women who experience PMS depends entirely on the stringency of the definition of PMS. The World Health Organization estimates that 199 million women have premenstrual syndrome as of 2010 (5.8% of the female population). While 80% of menstruating women have experienced at least one symptom that could be attributed to PMS, estimates of prevalence range from as low as 3% to as high as 30%.

Mood symptoms such as emotional lability are both more consistent and more disabling than somatic symptoms such as bloating. A woman who experiences mood symptoms is likely to experience these symptoms consistently and predictably, whereas physical symptoms may come and go. Most women find that physical symptoms related to PMS are less disruptive than emotional symptoms.

ETIOPATHOGENESIS

The exact cause of PMS is uncertain. As Magos showed there are an abundances of theories. The basic pathogenesis was summarized best by Studd[1,2] as:

- **Biological**
  - Female sex hormones—fluctuations of the level of sex hormone in luteal phase of menstrual cycle are the most important causes. These are as follows:
    - Estrogen excess, progesterone deficiency, altered estrogen/progesterone ratio, estrogen/progesterone withdrawal.
  - Neurotransmitters—decrease in serotonin, increase in catecholamines, glutamate level, and serum pseudocholinesterase
  - Fluid retention—sex hormones, renin-angiotensin-aldosterone axis, prolactin, vasopressin, dietary factors
  - Glucocorticoids
  - Androgens
  - Prolactin
  - Antidiuretic hormone
  - Vitamin deficiency—A, B_6
  - Reactive hypoglycemia
  - Endogenous hormone allergy
  - Prostaglandins—excess or deficiency
  - Endogenous opiate peptides—mid-luteal increase, premenstrual withdrawal
  - Menstrual toxin
  - Magnesium deficiency
  - Melatonin
- **Psychological**
- **Social and evolutionary**
- **Genetic:** Variants in the estrogen receptor alpha gene are associated with it. Association was also seen with a variant of another gene, catechol-o-methyltransferase also known as COMT, which is involved in regulating the function of the prefrontal cortex.

RISK FACTORS[3]

These are:
- High caffeine intake

- Stress
- Increasing age
- History of depression
- Family history
- Dietary factors—low level of certain vitamins in particular vitamin B_6, vitamin E and D and minerals like magnesium, manganese and zinc.

SIGNS AND SYMPTOMS[4,5]

More than 200 different symptoms have been associated with PMS. It could probably be stated that virtually any symptom affecting any system in the body can fluctuate and cause distress during the ovarian cycle. The most common symptoms were categorized into eight symptoms clusters with six being more important by Moos.

- Pain: Headache, cramps, muscle stiffness, backache, fatigue, general aches and pains
- Concentration: Difficulty in concentrating, accidents, forgetfulness, insomnia, confusion, lowered judgement, lowered motor coordination and distraction
- Behavioral change: Avoid social activities, lowered work or school performance, stay in bed, stay at home and decreased efficiency
- Autonomic reaction: Dizziness, faintness, cold sweats, nausea, vomiting and hot flushes
- Water retention: Breast tenderness, bloating, weight gain and skin disorders
- Negative affect: Depression, mood swings, irritability, restlessness, anxiety, tension, loneliness and crying.

A broader classification, would, therefore include physical, psycholosical, behavioral symptoms.

- **Physical symptoms:** The most common manifestations are breast tenderness and swelling, bloating, edema and weight gain. Other complains are pelvic discomfort, headache or migraine, change in bowel habit and reduced coordination
- **Psychological symptoms:** Depression, tension, irritability, anxiety and tiredness seem to be the most common complaints. Libido, sleeping and eating patterns could also be affected
- **Behavioral changes:** Many activities are reported to change during the menstrual cycle. Criminal behavior, suicide attempts, hospital admissions, absenteeism from work, decrease in cognitive function, reports of minor illness in children and increased proneness to accidents have all been associated with the menstrual cycle. These are, however, less common occurrences and therefore not so easy to include in any definition of this complex condition
- **Other medical conditions:** There are many medical problems that deteriorate in the week before the menstrual period. These include asthma, depression, epilepsy, rheumatioid arthritis, migraine and many

others. The severity of these medical conditions are also responsive to hormonal manipulation.

DIAGNOSIS[6]

There is no laboratory test or unique physical findings to verify the diagnosis of PMS. The three key features are:

- The woman's chief complaint is one or more of the emotional symptoms associated with PMS (most typically irritability, tension, or unhappiness)
- Symptoms appear predictably during the luteal (premenstrual) phase, reduce or disappear predictably shortly before or during menstruation, and remain absent during the follicular (preovulatory) phase of the menstrual cycle
- The symptoms must be severe enough to disrupt or interfere with the woman's everyday life.

To establish a pattern, a woman's physician may ask her to keep a prospective record of her symptoms on a calendar for at least two menstrual cycles. This will help to establish if the symptoms are, indeed, limited to the premenstrual time and are predictably recurring. A number of standardized instruments have been developed to describe PMS, including the calendar of premenstrual syndrome experiences, the prospective record of the impact and severity of menstruation and the visual analogue scales.

Although there is no universal agreement about what qualifies as PMS, two definitions are commonly used in research programs:

- The National Institute of Mental Health Research compares the intensity of symptoms from cycle days 5 to 10 to the six-day interval before the onset of menses. To qualify as PMS, symptom intensity must increase at least 30% in the six days before menstruation. Additionally, this pattern must be documented for at least two consecutive cycles
- The definition formulated at the University of California at San Diego requires both affective and somatic symptoms during the five days before menses in each of three consecutive cycles, and must not be present during the preovulatory part of the cycle. For this definition, affective symptoms include symptoms like depression, angry outbursts, irritability, anxiety, confusion, and social withdrawal. Somatic symptoms include symptoms like breast tenderness, abdominal bloating, headache, and swelling of hands and feet.

ALTERNATIVE VIEWS

Some medical professionals and other people believe that PMS might be a socially constructed disorder rather than a physical illness.

Another view holds that PMS is too frequently or wrongly diagnosed in many cases. A variety of problems, such as chronic depression, infections, and outbursts of frustration can be misdiagnosed as PMS if they happen to coincide with the premenstrual period. Tavris says that PMS is blamed as an explanation for rage or sadness.

MANAGEMENT[7-10]

Treatment goals for PMS are to ameliorate or eliminate symptoms, reduce their impact on activities and interpersonal relationships, and minimize adverse effects of treatment. Although numerous treatment strategies are available, few have been adequately evaluated in randomized, controlled trials.

Initially, all patients with PMS should be offered nonpharmacologic therapy. Medication should be offered to patients with persistent symptoms. Surgical treatment, principally hysterectomy plus bilateral oophorectomy, is controversial because it is irreversible and associated with significant risks. Surgery may be considered in severely affected patients who fail to respond to other therapies and also have significant gynecologic problems for which surgery would be appropriate.

Nonpharmacologic Therapy

Nonpharmacologic interventions for PMS include patient education, supportive therapy, and behavioral changes. Women who have been educated about the biologic basis and prevalence of PMS, report an increased sense of control and relief of symptoms.

The daily symptom diary may help patients identify optimal times for implementing behavioral and other changes to manage symptom exacerbations. Women report that maintaining a symptom diary helps them manage PMS.

Sleep disturbances, ranging from insomnia to excessive sleep, are common in women with PMS. A structured sleep schedule with consistent sleep and wake times is recommended, especially during the luteal phase.

Dietary restrictions and exercise may also be useful in patients with PMS. Sodium restriction has been proposed to minimize bloating, fluid retention, and breast swelling and tenderness. Caffeine restriction is recommended because of the association between caffeine and premenstrual irritability and insomnia. In epidemiologic and short-term prospective studies, women with PMS who practiced aerobic exercise reported fewer symptoms than control subjects.

Dietary Supplementation[11]

Dietary supplements that have been evaluated in women with PMS include vitamin (A, E and B_6), calcium, magnesium, multivitamin/mineral supplements, and evening primrose oil. Because most studies have been small or poorly designed, efficacy needs to be confirmed in large, well-designed clinical trials before evidence-based recommendations can be made.

Supplements of calcium carbonate in a dosage of 1,200 mg per day for three menstrual cycles resulted in symptom improvement in 48 percent of women with PMS, compared with 30 percent of placebo-treated women.

Magnesium in a dosage of 200 to 400 mg per day has shown minimal benefit in alleviating bloating. The ACOG recommends calcium supplementation but not magnesium supplementation.

Evening primrose oil, a prostaglandin precursor, has been studied in women with PMS, based on the theory of inadequate levels of prostaglandin. A systematic review of placebo-controlled trials of evening primrose oil suggested lack of benefit in PMS, although mild relief was demonstrated in women with breast tenderness.

Pharmacological Therapy

Nonpharmacologic measures should be monitored at least every three months. If symptoms are not adequately relieved, the addition of pharmacologic treatment should be considered. Medications are given to treat specific symptoms or alter the menstrual cycle. Treatment should be individualized to target the most troublesome symptoms in each patient.

Nonprescription Preparations

Several non-prescription products contain mild diuretics, analgesics, prostaglandin inhibitors, and antihistamines. Women should be cautioned about using combination products, which may provide inadequate doses of some ingredients and excessive doses of others. If nonprescription preparations are used, single-ingredient products are preferred.

Psychotropic Agents[12]

Because serotonin has been implicated in the pathogenesis of PMS, various SSRIs have been tested in these disorders.

In general, 20 mg of fluoxetine or 50 mg of sertraline taken in the morning is best tolerated and sufficient to improve symptoms. Benefit has also been demonstrated for the continuous administration of citalopram.

Fluoxetine is currently labeled for use as continuous therapy in a dosage of 20 mg per day. Sertraline, in a dosage of 50 mg per day, is labeled for continuous therapy or for use during the luteal phase. Administration only during the luteal phase decreases drug cost, minimizes drug exposure and side effects, and may be more acceptable to some women. For intermittent therapy, fluoxetine or sertraline can be given during the 14 days before the menstrual period, or treatment can be initiated just before the expected onset of symptoms.

Treatment using anxiolytic agents such as alprazolam is not recommended because of addictive potential, tolerance, and significant side effects.

Diuretics

Spironolactone, an aldosterone antagonist structurally similar to steroid hormones is the only diuretic that has been shown to effectively relieve PMS symptoms such as breast tenderness and fluid retention. In most studies, spironolactone was administered only during the luteal phase. Thiazide diuretics have not been found to be beneficial in the treatment of patients with PMS.

Prostaglandin Inhibitors

Most NSAIDs should be effective, but mefanamic acid and naproxen sodium have been the most studied. Mefenamic acid therapy given during the luteal phase is effective in relieving symptoms, but gastrointestinal toxicity prohibits its use. Naproxen sodium improves physical symptoms and headache in women with PMS. Overall, NSAIDs may alleviate a wide range of symptoms, but they do not appear to improve mastalgia. All NSAIDs must be used with caution in patients with underlying gastrointestinal or renal disorders.

AGENTS USED TO ALTER THE MENSTRUAL CYCLE[13,14]

Danazol, gonadotropin-releasing hormone agonists, estrogen, and progesterone have been studied in the treatment of PMS. Although efficacy has been demonstrated for some of these agents, their use is limited by significant adverse effects and treatment costs.

Danazol is an androgenic agent that inhibits gonadotropin release, thereby improving mastalgia. Continuous danazol therapy may also relieve other PMS symptoms. However, continuous therapy is limited by side effects such as masculinization (e.g. decreased breast size, deepening of the voice, weight gain), as well as adverse effects on liver function tests and serum lipid profiles.

GnRH agonists are synthetic analogs of naturally occurring GnRH and suppress ovulation by inhibiting the release of pituitary gonadotropin. GnRH agonists have been shown to be more effective than placebo in treating behavioral and physical symptoms of PMS. Side effects and cost may limit GnRH agonist therapy to patients with severe PMS.

The hypoestrogenic effects of GnRH agonists can lead to atrophic vaginitis, urinary tract symptoms, and a decrease in skin collagen content. Use of these agents for longer than six months can significantly increase the risk of osteoporosis. If treatment for more than six months is necessary, "add-back" therapy with estrogen and/or progesterone should be considered to minimize long-term adverse effects. Unfortunately, add-back therapy is often associated with a recurrence of PMS symptoms. Some improvement in premenstrual depression and irritability has been demonstrated for lower dosages of GnRH agonists.

Tibolone is an investigational synthetic steroid with weak estrogenic, progestogenic, and androgenic activity. Although this agent has primarily been studied in the treatment of menopause and osteoporosis, it has been shown to provide significant improvement in premenstrual symptoms compared with placebo and a multivitamin.

Limited evidence suggests that estrogen therapy is efficacious in alleviating PMS symptoms. The administration of estrogen late in the luteal phase (to minimize premenstrual decline in the women) relieves premenstrual migraine. For overall symptom management, estrogen must be given continuously to suppress ovarian activity. Because unopposed estrogen can promote endometrial hyperplasia and carcinoma, cyclic progesterone must be added. The progesterone may induce PMS symptoms, thereby limiting the efficacy of estrogen.

Although oral contraceptive pills (OCPs) are widely prescribed for the management of PMS, they have not been shown to be consistently effective. Any benefits are probably due to the estrogenic component; therefore, monophasic pills may be most appropriate. OCPs may improve physical symptoms such as bloating, headaches, abdominal pain, and breast tenderness, but they can also exacerbate these symptoms. Anecdotal reports indicate that women with PMS who take OCPs tend to have fewer physical symptoms than those who do not take them. However, the pills do not appear to have a positive effect on mood symptoms.

HYSTERECTOMY AND BILATERAL OOPHORECTOMY

It is well recognized that in some women all treatment options will fail or side effects may be unbearable. Some women are unlikely to want to continue with treatment that needs to be taken for many years until the menopause or in some cases concomitant pathology may co-exist. In all of these instances, it may be necessary to perform a hysterectomy and bilateral salpingo-oophorectomy. It is important to stress that the bilateral oophorectomy is the essential part of the surgery as this would remove all ovarian function. By removing the uterus at the same time, it would be unnecessary to administer progestogens postoperatively and thus potential side-effects are avoided.

PROGNOSIS

PMS is generally a stable diagnosis, with susceptible women experiencing the same symptoms at the same intensity near the end of each cycle for years. Treatment for specific symptoms is usually effective at controlling the symptoms. Even without treatment, symptoms tend to decrease in perimenopausal women, and disappear at menopause. Women who have PMS have an increased risk for clinical depression.

REFERENCES

1. Cronje WH, Hawkins AP, Studd JWW. Premenstrual Syndrome. In: Studd JWW (ed). Progress in Obstetrics and Gynecology. Churchill Livingstone, 2003;15:169-83.
2. www.always.com. Premenstrual Syndrome symptoms/what is Premenstrual Syndrome? Retrieved on 2007. 02. 11.

3. www.marins specialty surgery center.com. Risk factors for PMS. Amy Scholten, MPH Retrieved on 2008. 01. 10.
4. www.mayoclinic.com. Premenstrual Syndrome. Mayo Clinic Staff. Retrieved on 2007. 02. 02.
5. Wyatt K, Dimmock PW, O'Brien PM. Premenstrual syndrome. In: Barton S, ed. Clinical evidence. 4th issue. London: BMJ Publishing Group. 2000:1121-33.
6. Kessel B. Premenstrual syndrome. Advances in diagnosis and treatment. Obstet Gynecol Clin North Am. 2000;27:625-39.
7. Daugherty JE. Treatment strategies for premenstrual syndrome. Am Fam Physician. 1998;58:183-92,197-8.
8. Moline ML, Zendell SM. Evaluating and managing premenstrual syndrome. Medscape Womens Health. 2000;5:1-16.
9. ACOG Practice Bulletin. Clinical Management guidelines for obstetrician-gynecologists. Number 15, April 2000. Premenstrual syndrome. Obstet Gynecol. 2000;95:1-9.
10. Blake F, Salkovskis P, Gath D, Day A, Garrod A. Cognitive therapy for premenstrual syndrome: a controlled trial. J Psychosom Res. 1998;45:307-18.
11. Wyatt KM, Dimmock PW, Jones PW, O'Brien PM. Efficacy of vitamin B-6 in the treatment of premenstrual syndrome: systematic review. BMJ. 1999;318:1375-81.
12. Dimmock PW, Wyatt KM, Jones PW, O'Brien PM. Efficacy of selective serotonin-reuptake inhibitors in premenstrual syndrome: a systematic review. Lancet. 2000;356:1131-6.
13. Sundstrom I, Nyberg S, Bixo M, Hammarback S, Backstrom T. Treatment of premenstrual syndrome with gonadotropin-releasing hormone agonist in a low dose regimen. Acta Obstet Gynecol Scand. 1999;78:891-9.
14. Waytt K, Dimmock PW, Jones P, Obhrai M, O'Brien S. Efficacy of progesterone and progestogens in management of premenstrual syndrome: systematic review. BMJ. 2001;323:776-80.

Treatment and Prognosis of Dysmenorrhea

Pramila Modi, Charu Modi, Smriti Modi

INTRODUCTION

Dysmenorrhea is a medical condition of abdominal pain and discomfort during menstruation that interferes with routine activities as defined by American Congress of Obstetricians and Gynecologists (ACOG)[1] and others.[2] The intensity of pain during menstruation varies from person to person, can be described as mild, moderate, severe, sharp, throbbing and shooting. It can be associated with nausea, vomiting and GIT upset. Dysmenorrhea can precede the onset of menstruation by a week or may co-exist and usually the pain subsides as the menstrual flow tapers off. Sometimes, it is associated with excessive bleeding. The rough estimation of grading dysmenorrhea is useful for all practical purposes (Fig. 1). Before outlining the treatment it is necessary to know the etiopathology of dysmenorrhea.

TYPES OF DYSMENORRHEA

- Primary
- Secondary

Primary dysmenorrhea is pain during menstruation without any associated underline disease or pathology in the uterus or pelvic organs. It is

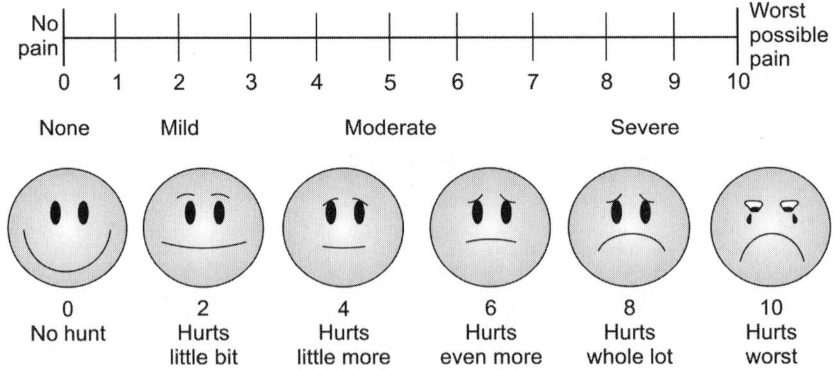

Fig. 1: Pain scoring system

characterized by crampy lower abdominal pain which may radiate to lower back or thighs. The pain usually starts few hours before or with the beginning of menstruation and is most intense on the first or second day of the cycle. It affects young girls, in teenage or late 20s. Pregnancy and child birth often results in relief in the majority.

Prostaglandins play a major role in etiology of dysmenorrhea by inducing painful uterine contractions (muscular) and constriction of the blood vessels (Fig. 2). Due to diminished blood circulation and oxygenation to the uterus, waste products like carbon dioxide and lactic acid accumulate which in turn aggravate the intensity of pain and discomfort. It has been observed that women with severe dysmenorrhea have higher level of prostaglandins. Research has shown that women who do not ovulate, do not suffer from dysmenorrhea and hence inducing an ovulation by oral contraceptive pills (OCPs) is an accepted method of treatment.

Secondary dysmenorrhea is always associated with some underlying pelvic pathology. The symptoms depend upon the cause. Hence, the treatment and prognosis also vary from case to case. This occurs in late 30s or 40s. It is less prevalent and is usually relieved after medical or surgical treatment.

The cause of secondary dysmenorrhea can be situated inside the cavity, in the muscle layer or outside the uterus.

- ➲ Extrauterine
  - – Endometriosis

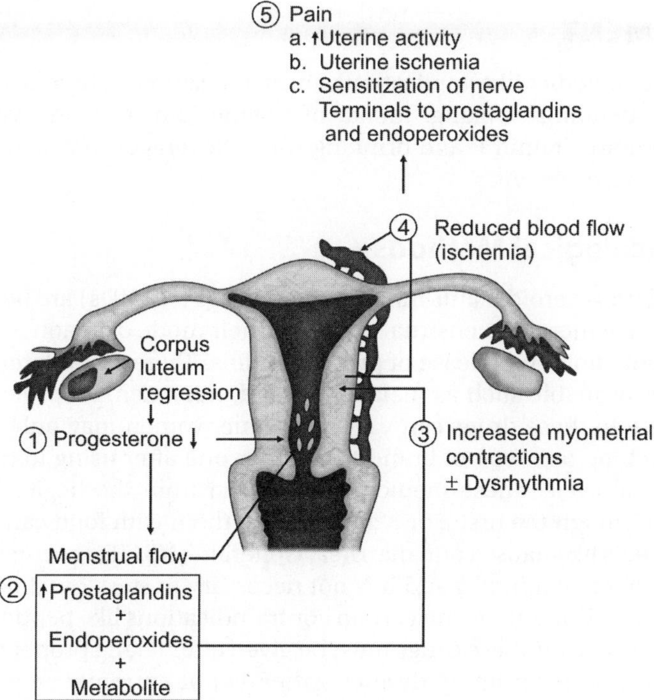

Fig. 2: Etiology of dysmenorrhea

- – Pelvic inflammatory disease
- – Adhesions
- – Structural abnormalities of the genital tract
- ➲ Intramural
  - – Adenomyosis
  - – Fibroids
- ➲ Intrauterine
  - – Submucous fibroids
  - – Polyps
  - – Intrauterine device
  - – Cervical stenosis
  - – Infection

The diagnosis is reached by taking a thorough history in general and menstrual history in particular, clinical examination and supportive investigations are as follows:

- ➲ Blood test for CBC, sugar estimation, culture for excluding sexually transmitted diseases like gonorrhea, syphilis or chlamydia
- ➲ Ultrasonography of pelvis (abdominal or transvaginal)
- ➲ Hysteroscopy with or without cervical dilatation for viewing the intrauterine environment
- ➲ Laparoscopy for evaluating the intra-abdominal status, looking for pelvic tumors, adhesions, endometriosis and presence of IUCD, etc.

TREATMENT

Household remedies like application of heat, relaxation techniques, exercises like waist bending, walking, intake of magnesium, calcium, vitamin B_1, vitamin B_6 and vitamin E and drinking warm beverages may help reducing the pain to some extent.

Pharmacological Methods

- ➲ Several non-steroidal anti-inflammatory drugs (NSAIDs) are beneficial in the management of menstrual cramps.[3] Their mode of action is inhibiting the production and release of prostaglandins. There are different types of NSAIDs available such as mefanemic acid, naproxen, ibuprofen and the response to these drugs can vary and some women may only find relief by switching one type of brand to another one after using in one or two menstrual cycle. These medicines are taken from the beginning of the period through the first 2 or 3 days. Taking them with food can minimize side effects like nausea and diarrhea. Generally, NSAIDs become effective within 30 to 60 minutes and it is not necessary to start 2 to 3 days before the period. Since, there are certain contraindications like peptic ulcer and others, advise for these drugs must be given after taking proper history
- ➲ Aspirin used for primary dysmenorrhea is not currently recommended since it is not enough in the normal doses to reach sufficient anti prostaglandin activity. This drug should not be used on long term basis

- ⊃ Oral contraceptives or commonly termed OCP are effective for treating primary dysmenorrhea. Their mode of action is inhibition of ovulation and reduction in menstrual flow. For women who suffer from primary dysmenorrhea and who require contraception, using OCP is the ideal and is the first line treatment
- ⊃ Other hormonal therapy that induce amenorrhea can be used such as intramuscular injectable depot medroxyprogesterone acetate (depo Provera) or the levonorgestrel releasing intrauterine system (Mirena).[4] However, these are rarely used in clinical practice for treating dysmenorrhea primarily
- ⊃ For secondary dysmenorrhea, medication is aimed at the underlying disease:
  - For pelvic inflammatory diseases, appropriate antibiotics are prescribed depending upon the detection of specific microorganisms in the culture specimen
  - For endometriosis, a number of drugs are available including NSAIDs to inhibit prostaglandin production by ectopic endometrium and continuous treatment with hormones.

Nonpharmacological Methods

- ⊃ Transcutaneous electrical nerve stimulation (TENS) is the use of a device placed over the skin which uses electrical current to stimulate nerves. This stimulate endorphins from the peripheral nerves and spinal cord which result in lower perception of painful uterine signals. High frequency TENS has to be found to be effective for dysmenorrhea but less utilized than the medication regimen
- ⊃ Complimentary or alternative medicine (e.g. acupuncture) is being used without evidence based support
- ⊃ Spinal manipulation offered by physiotherapists has not been found effective
- ⊃ Behavioral interventions include ways to alter women's perception and response to pain. Examples of these are hypnotherapy, relaxation techniques, coping strategies, etc. There is no evidence to prove their efficacy.

Surgery

This may be necessary in women who cannot obtain adequate pain relief or control, and is especially indicated in secondary dysmenorrhea to remove endometriotic cysts, polyps, adhesions and fibroids. There are various methods of surgery, depending on the underlying condition. This can be done either by laparoscopy, laparotomy (open incision into the abdomen) or hysteroscopy. A hysterectomy (surgical removal of uterus) may be indicated in cases of adenomyosis and large fibroids. Hysterectomy with or without the removal of the ovaries should be considered only as a last resort for endometriosis, as it is a condition which is situated outside the uterus (ectopic sites). Removing the uterus solely because of endometriosis will not guarantee relief of symptoms.

Interruption of the sensory nerves supplying the uterus can be performed by means of a presacral neurectomy or laparoscopic uterosacral nerve ablation (LUNA), meaning the cutting of nerves, which run in the uterosacral ligaments (in the ligaments from the uterus to the sacral bone of the pelvis). There is limited evidence that LUNA offers relief for primary dysmenorrhea. However, LUNA does not appear to be effective for women suffering from chronic pelvic pain and endometriosis. Presacral neurectomy has been found to be effective in those with midline abdominal pain but not in those with pain in the right and/or left sides of the pelvis. The benefits of LUNA and presacral neurectomy appear to decline with time and therefore are not routinely recommended. These operations are very rarely performed and only in patients with severe dysmenorrhea who did not respond satisfactorily to other medical and/or surgical treatment. These should only be performed by a highly experienced surgeon.

Flow chart 1 outlines the management options in dysmenorrhea.

PROGNOSIS

In secondary dysmenorrhea, the underlying cause needs to be treated. This may require medication such as the oral contraceptive pill or other hormone treatment, antibiotics or even surgery to remove any masses or repair any abnormalities. The incidence of primary dysmenorrhea decreases with age and the prognosis for primary dysmenorrhea is excellent. The prognosis

Flow chart 1: Management options in dysmenorrhea

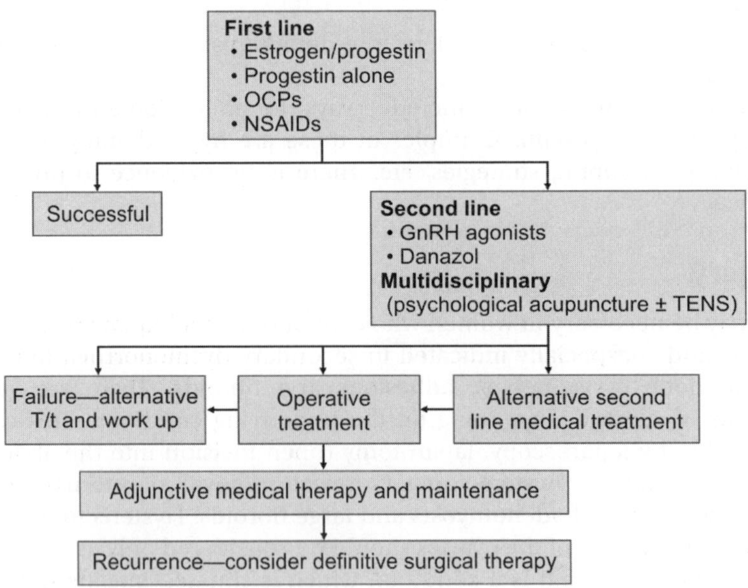

for secondary dysmenorrhea depends on the underlying cause. Effective treatment of the underlying cause may abolish this pain.

Prognosis depends on the type of dysmenorrhea and presence of any root cause which can be managed medically or surgically. In general, the prognosis of primary dysmenorrhea is quite good. It gets relieved naturally after few years of menarche due to the establishment of the proper hormonal balance.

Pregnancy and delivery result in cure of the primary dysmenorrhea. Secondary dysmenorrhea is relieved only after treating the cause either long medical treatment for the pelvic infection or removal of pelvic tumors by minimal invasive surgery like laparoscopy or hysteroscopy. Very rarely, the need for laparotomy arises.

SUMMARY

Many women never seek medical attention for dysmenorrhea. Self-medication with analgesics and non-steroidal anti-inflammatory drugs (NSAIDs) and direct application of heat are common effective strategies. Treatment of dysmenorrhea is aimed at providing symptomatic relief as well as inhibiting the underlying processes that cause symptoms. Grading dysmenorrhea according to the severity of pain and the degree of limitation of daily activity may help guide the treatment strategy. Medications used may include NSAIDs and opioid analgesics, as well as oral contraceptives (OCs). In addition to pain relief, mainstays of treatment include reassurance and counseling. Other therapies have been proposed, but most are not well studied.

REFERENCES

1. Patient Education Pamphlet: Dysmenorrhea By American Congress of Obstetricians and Gynecologists. Retrieved in January 2011.
2. The Free Dictionary > dysmenorrhea Citing: Jonas: Mosby's Dictionary of Complementary and Alternative Medicine. Copyright 2005.
3. Marjoribanks J, Proctor M, Farquhar C, Derks RS. "Non-steroidal anti-inflammatory drugs for dysmenorrhea". In Majoribanks, Jane. Cochrane database of systematic reviews (online). 2010;(1): CD001751. doi:10.1002/14651858.CD001751.pub2. PMID 20091521.
4. Gupta HP, Singh U, Sinha S. "Levonorgestrel intra-uterine system--a revolutionary intra-uterine device". J Indian Med Assoc. 2007;105(7): 380, 382-5. PMID 18178990.

Dysfunctional Uterine Bleeding

Pragya Mishra Choudhary, Kumari Mamta

Dysfunctional uterine bleeding (DUB) is a relatively common occurrence in women—most women suffer from it at some time or the other during reproductive years of their lives. Since it often gets corrected spontaneously, women often refrain from seeking medical attention. However, at times DUB can be persistent and affect the health status of an individual.

Novak has defined it as "an abnormal bleeding from the uterus unassociated with tumor, inflammation or pregnancy".[1]

The classification based on histopathological findings is essential not just to aid in the diagnosis but also to chart out the management.

DUB is classified into anovulatory and ovulatory bleeding.

OVULATORY DUB

The endometrial histology reveals various types of secretory endometrium.

- Irregular shedding of endometrium (Halban's disease): It is due to persistent corpus luteum. The menstruation comes on time, is not heavy, but is prolonged. Histopathology reveals a mixed picture of secretory and proliferative endometrium even on day 5–6 of menstruation
- Irregular ripening: In this condition, the endometrium receives inadequate support of progesterone due to deficient corpus luteum function, so breakthrough bleeding occurs before the actual menstruation in the form of spotting or brownish discharge. The endometrium reveals incomplete secretory changes.

ANOVULATORY DUB

In anovulatory DUB, the lack of progesterone results in a decrease in $PGF_2\alpha$ to PGE_2 ratio and a relative increase in vasodilator and antiplatelet aggregation factor PGE_2. This could be the reason for the increased blood loss. It also accounts for the absence of uterine contractions and painless periods, which are characteristic features of anovulatory menstruation. In anovulatory DUB, the endometrial histology could be of the following types:

- Proliferative endometrium
- Simple hyperplasia without atypia

- Complex hyperplasia without atypia
- Simple hyperplasia with atypia
- Complex hyperplasia with atypia

DYSFUNCTIONAL UTERINE BLEEDING WORK-UP

The diagnosis of DUB begins with a thorough questioning about the history, meticulous clinical examination including general as well as pelvic examination. Certain laboratory tests and gynecological investigations are done for the assessment of the patient and for differential diagnosis.

History

- Detailed menstrual history
- Any pregnancy related event recently
- Systemic illness
- Coagulopathy
- Anticoagulant
- Contraceptives (these days use of emergency contraception poses problems).

A Thorough General Examination

- Pallor
- Acne
- Obesity
- Galactorrhea
- Enlargement of thyroid.

Laboratory Tests

- Complete blood count
- Platelet count
- Coagulation factors
- hCG (Human chorionic gonadotropin)
- Coagulation profile
- Thyroid function tests
- Prolactin
- FSH, LH
- Testosterone, DHEAS
- TB IgM
- LFTs (Liver function tests).

All tests are not necessary in each patient. The tests should be ordered only after clinical evaluation and as per the clinical suspicion raised by the examination.

For example, a finding of hirsutism calls for testing the patient for androgens.

Pap smear—A Pap smear shows the presence or absence of inflammation or cancer of cervix. It is of great value in excluding this condition especially in the perimenopausal group. This age is vulnerable because of cancer of the endometrium and cervix as well as DUB occurring commonly in this age group.

The presence of atypical glandular cells has been associated with premalignant or malignant lesions of the cervix and the endometrium in 10–40% women. Unexplained bleeding with this type of smear may further call for invasive testing.[2]

Gynecological Investigations

Endometrial Evaluation

For the evaluation of endometrium, USG or sonohysterography should preferably be done when the bleeding has stopped and the endometrium is thin.

USG (Ultrasonography): USG is of great help in patients in whom pelvic examination is not possible or is unsatisfactory. It is useful in assessing the adnexa. For assessing endometrium, transvaginal sonography (TVS) is useful in both postmenopausal as well perimenopausal women.[3] Sonographic evaluation of uterine volume is useful. Larger the volume, lesser is the chance of success with medical treatment.[4]

Sonohysterography: It is inexpensive, simple and well tolerated as an OPD procedure. This can be used to detect endometrial polyp and submucous fibroid. It is useful in differentiating globally thickened endometrium from diffuse thickening.

Magnetic Resonance Imaging

MRI is expensive but it is valuable in diagnosing deep endometriosis, adenomyosis and pelvic masses. It helps in choosing between medical and surgical modalities of treatment.

Dilatation and Curettage

At present, its role is limited to stop bleeding in women who present with excessive bleeding. In this situation, it plays therapeutic as well as diagnostic role. It is also indicated in all perimenopausal and postmenopausal women, where hysteroscopy is not available. It is useful in cervical stenosis. In fact, it has been seen that this test may miss 2–6% of cancer or hyperplasia.[5]

Endometrial Biopsy

Being a blind procedure, it is an outdated modality of evaluation of DUB. Targeted biopsy using hysteroscopy or USG is a better approach. Instruments like Vabra curette and Pipelle have been used for collection. In comparison to Pipelle, which covers only 4%, the Vabra curette covers 40% of the endometrium. Endometrial biopsy in combination with sonohysterography has been used successfully for a precise evaluation of endometrium.[6] Endometrial biopsy should always be considered in women > 40 years of age with various risk factors for endometrial carcinoma.

Hysteroscopy

The development of 2–4 mm diameter hysteroscope has made it possible to use it as an office procedure, because cervical dilatation is not needed.[7] Hysteroscopic directed biopsy is superior to a blind biopsy or dilation (D) and curettage (C). Hysteroscopy should be performed on women in whom the ultrasound reports are not conclusive.

PRINCIPLES OF MANAGEMENT IN DUB

An important aspect in the clinical management of DUB is identification of the mechanism that is operating or responsible. Anovulatory bleeding can be effectively and confidently managed with medical treatment regimens based on proven physiologic concepts. The process of menstruation is a well-programmed one. It is self-limiting predominantly due to coagulation, thrombosis and platelet activation that follows at the basal layer during menstruation as well as due to well planned though complex hormonal interaction, which occurs *via* the hypothalamo-pituitary axis.

Options for medical care of dysfunctional uterine bleeding usually involves various protocols of estrogen or progesterone supplementation, yet there is no clear consensus on which exact regimen is most effective. Dysfunctional uterine bleeding associated with ovulatory cycles is much more difficult to manage in the long term.

OCPs (Oral contraceptive pills) suppress endometrial development, establish predictable bleeding patterns, decrease menstrual flow and lower the risk of iron deficiency anemia.

OCPs can be used effectively in a cyclic or continuous regimen to control DUB. Acute episodes of heavy bleeding suggest an environment of prolonged estrogenic exposure and build-up of lining. Bleeding is usually controlled within the first 24 hours, as the over grown endometrium becomes pseudodecidualized. If bleeding fails to decrease, seek alternate diagnosis. OCPs that contain drospirenone pose a higher risk of thromboembolic events compared to OCPs that contain levonorgestrel.

Estrogen

Estrogen alone is indicated in certain clinical situations. Prolonged uterine bleeding suggests the endometrial lining of the uterine cavity has become denuded over time. In this setting, a progestin is unlikely to control bleeding. Here use of estrogen will induce return to normal endometrial growth rapidly.

Hemorrhagic uterine bleeding requires high dose estrogen therapy. If bleeding is not controlled within 12–24 hours, D and C is indicated. Beginning progestin therapy shortly after initiating estrogen therapy, to prevent a subsequent bleeding episode from treatment with prolonged estrogen is wise.

Progestins

Progestins have a growth limiting activity on the endometrium predominantly by causing down regulation of the estrogen receptors, thus increasing the induction of the enzymes that aid in metabolism of estrogen, and down regulating the estrogen mediated oncogenes, hence chronic management of DUB requires episodic or continuous exposure to a progestin. In patients without contraindications, this is best accomplished with an OCP, given the many additional benefits including decreased dysmenorrhea, decreased blood loss, ovarian cancer prophylaxis and decreased androgens. In patients with a pill contraindication, cyclic progestin starting from day 15 or earlier till day 25 using medroxyprogesterone acetate (10 mg/day) or norethindrone acetate (2.5–5 mg/day) provides predictable withdrawal bleeding but not contraception. Cyclic natural progesterone (200 mg/day) may be used in women susceptive to pregnancy, but may cause more drowziness and does not decrease blood loss as much as a progestin.

Levonorgestrel Intrauterine System

Levonorgestrel intrauterine system has been approved for its use in patients with heavy menstrual bleeding and apart from that in women of reproductive age group, it also provides an added contraceptive benefit. It reduces abnormal bleeding in 75% of the women within 6 months.[8]

Androgens

Certain androgenic preparations have been used historically to treat mild to moderate bleeding, particularly in ovulatory patients with abnormal uterine bleeding. These regimens offer no real advantage over other regimens and might cause irreversible signs of masculinization in the patient. They are seldom used for this indication today.

GnRH Agonists

Act by reducing concentration of GnRH receptors in the pituitary *via* receptor down regulation and induction of post-receptor effects, which suppress gonadotropin release. After an initial gonadotropin release associated with rising estradiol levels, gonadotropin level falls to castrate level with resultant hypogonadism. This form of medical castration is very effective in inducing amenorrhea, thus breaking ongoing cycle of abnormal bleeding in many anovulatory patients. Because prolonged therapy with this form of medical castration is associated with osteoporosis and postmenopausal side-effects, its use is often limited in duration and add-back therapy in the form of low-dose hormone replacement is given. Because of the expense of these drugs, they usually are not used as a first-line approach but can be used to achieve short-term relief from a bleeding problem, particularly in patients with renal failure or blood dyscrasias.

Antifibrinolytic Therapy Using Tranexamic Acid

The Food and Drug Administration (FDA) has approved the use of tranexamic acid in oral form for heavy menstrual bleeding since 2009. The recommended dosage is 2 tablets of 500 mg for a maximum of 3 times a day for 5 days during menstrual period.[9] It is to be used with caution in women at risk for thrombogenic events and those having renal impairment.

Prostaglandin synthetase inhibitors (e.g. mefanemic acid, flufenamic acid or naproxen sodium) are particularly useful in reducing the excessive blood loss in women with DUB by striking a balance in the local prostaglandin milieu of the endometrium. It reduces the menstrual blood loss by approximately 40% in women with DUB as well as helps in counteracting dysmenorrhea.[10] It is suggested that either of the above two types of drugs be considered as first-line treatment for ovulatory DUB.

Desmopressin

On rare occasions, a young patient with anovulatory bleeding also might have a bleeding disorder. Desmopressin, a synthetic analog of arginine vasopressin, has been used as a last resort to treat abnormal uterine bleeding in patients with documented coagulation disorders. Treatment is followed by a rapid increase in Von Willebrand factor and factor VIII, which last for about 6 hours.

Surgical Care

Most cases of DUB can be treated medically. Surgical measures are reserved for situations where medical therapy has failed or is contraindicated. D and C is an appropriate diagnostic step in a patient who fails to respond to hormonal management.

Endometrial Ablation

Endometrial ablation is an alternative for those who wish to avoid hysterectomy or who are not candidates for major surgery.

Ablation techniques are varied and can employ laser, rollerball, resectoscope or thermal destructive modalities. Most of these procedures are associated with high patient satisfaction rates. The patient should be treated with an agent, such as leuprolide acetate, medroxyprogesterone acetate or danazol to thin the endometrium. The ablation procedure is more conservative than hysterectomy and has a shorter recovery time. Endometrial ablation is not a form of contraception. Some studies report up to a 5% pregnancy rate in post-ablation procedures. Some patients may have persistent bleeding and require repeat procedures or move to hysterectomy.

Rebleeding following ablation has raised concerns about the possibility of an occult endometrial cancer developing within a pocket of active endometrium.

Hysterectomy, abdominal, vaginal or laparoscopic might be necessary in patients who have failed or declined hormonal therapy, have symptomatic anemia and who experience a disruption in their quality of life from persistent, unscheduled bleeding.

Patient Education

The goal of therapy for dysfunctional uterine bleeding is to control and prevent recurrent bleeding, correct or treat any pathology present. Age, past history and amount of bleeding influence management. After initial treatment and resolution of an episode of DUB, patients need to be educated that most often chronic therapy is mandatory to prevent further episodes.

Reassure patients that most bleeding episodes stop with appropriate hormonal therapy. Explain the physiologic reason for the anovulatory bleeding pattern. This is particularly true for the adolescent patient who establishes a predictable ovulatory type of menstrual pattern over time. Perhaps, the best measure of successful treatment is a good menstrual calendar.

REFERENCES

1. Hillard P. Benign diseases of the female reproductive tract. In: Berek and Novak's Gynecology 14th ed. Philadelphia: Lippincott Williams and Wilkins. 2007:431-504.
2. Chhieng DC, Elgert PA, Cagngiarella JF, Cohen JM. Clinical significance of atypical glandular cell of undetermined significance, favor endometrial origin. Cancer. 2001;93:351-6.
3. Najeeb R, Awan AS, Bakhtiar U, Akhter S. Role of transvaginal sonography in assessment of abnormal uterine bleeding in perimenopausal age group. J Ayub Med Coll Abbottabad. 2010;22:87-90.
4. Sheth S, Sutton C. Diagnosis of DUB. In: Menorrhagia first ed. ISIS Medical Media: Informa Healthcare. 1999;23-42.
5. Conoscenti G, Meir YJ, Fischer-Tamaro L, et al. Endometrial assessment by transvaginal sonography and histological findings after D and C in women with postmenopausal bleeding. Ultrasound Obstet Gynecol. 1995;6:108-15.
6. Breitkopf D, Goldstein SR, Seeds JW; ACOG Committee on Gynecologic Practice. ACOG technology assessment in obstetrics and gynecology. Number 3, September 2003. Saline infusion sonohysterography. Obstet Gynecol. 2003;102:659-62.
7. Lindheim SR, Kavic S, Shulman SV, Sauer MV. Operative hysteroscopy in office setting. J Am Assoc Gynecol Laparosc. 2007;7:65-9.
8. Stewart A, Cummins C, Gold L, et al. The effectiveness of the levonorgestrel-releasing intrauterine system in menorrhagia: A systematic review. BJOG. 2001;108:74-86.
9. Leminen H, Hurskainen R. Tranexamic acid for the treatment of heavy menstrual bleeding: Efficacy and safety. Int J Women's Health. 2003;4:413-21.
10. Lethaby A, Augood C, Duckitt K. Nonsteroidal anti-inflammatory drugs for heavy menstrual bleeding. Cochrane Database Syst Rev. 2002:CD000400.

Chapter

34 Polycystic Ovary Syndrome

Roza Olyai, Prachi Renjhen

INTRODUCTION

Polycystic ovary syndrome (PCOS) is a heterogeneous disorder of uncertain etiology, which affects between 6% and 10% of women of the reproductive age. Stein and Leventhal (1935) were the first to report the heterogeneity of both the ovarian morphology and clinical findings in women with polycystic ovaries.

PATHOPHYSIOLOGY

The pathophysiology of the PCOS appears to be multifactorial and polygenic and involves a combination of genetic abnormalities and environmental factors, such as nutrition and body weight. There is growing consensus that the key features include insulin resistance, an alteration in cortisol metabolism, androgen excess and abnormal gonadotropin dynamics. A familial pattern (about 50% of first-degree relatives have PCOS and first-degree male relatives appear more likely to have premature baldness) in some cases suggests a genetic component but the candidate genes have not yet been identified.

Achard and Thiersin 1921 were the first to recognize the association between glucose intolerance and hyperandrogenism—the diabetes of bearded women. The state of insulin resistance noted could be due to peripheral target tissue resistance, decreased hepatic clearance, or increased pancreatic sensitivity.

- Insulin action is mediated through a protein tyrosine kinase receptor. Serine phosphorylation: The insulin receptor's inhibits tyrosine kinase activity. In at least 50% of PCOS women, potential mechanism for insulin resistance appears to be related to excessive serine phosphorylation of insulin receptor by a factor extrinsic to the insulin receptor, presumably a serine/threonine kinase and this defect in insulin action is limited to glucose metabolism. Also, serine phosphorylation of IRS-1 appears to be the mechanism of TNFα-mediated insulin resistance of obesity. Serine phosphorylation also modulate the activity of the key regulatory enzyme of androgen biosynthesis, P450c17, present in both the adrenal and ovarian steroidogenic tissue. Thus, a single defect—serine phosphorylation—

produces both the insulin resistance and the hyperandrogenism in a subgroup of PCOS women.

- Insulin leads to the inhibition of hepatic synthesis of serum sex hormone-binding globulin (SHBG), which allows free androgen and estrogen to be bioavailable. This implies that by improving insulin sensitivity and reducing circulating insulin levels, amelioration of hyperandrogenism can be achieved.
- Insulin resistance is associated with impaired glucose tolerance and type 2 diabetes mellitus, hypertension, abdominal obesity and adverse lipid profiles—all features of 'metabolic syndrome X' and these predispose the woman with PCOS to risk of cardiovascular disease. Elevated androgen levels, body fat distribution and hyperinsulinemia, also put these women at risk of dyslipidemia.
- Insulin resistance leads to elevated PAI-1 (plasminogen inhibitor activator -1) activity level which leads to increased risk of thrombotic vascular events—this is thus an independent risk factor for atherosclerosis. In PCOS, these levels decreased with improvement in insulin sensitivity mediated by weight loss or insulin-sensitizing agents.
- Elevated endothelin-1 (ET-1) levels are also seen in women with PCOS, independent of the presence of obesity. Also there is a positive correlation between plasma ET-1 levels and testosterone levels. Six months of metformin therapy reduced ET-1 concentrations in these women, suggesting that increased insulin sensitivity may offer benefit by protecting and/or restoring the endothelial barrier.
- Hyperinsulinemia increases GnRH pulse frequency, LH over FSH dominance, increased ovarian androgen production, decreased follicular maturation, and decreased SHBG binding; all these steps contribute to the development of PCOS.

HEALTH CONSEQUENCES OF PCOS

- Ischemic heart disease due metabolic syndrome
- Diabetes—as result of insulin resistance and obesity
- Endometrial cancer—unopposed exposure to estrogen predisposes to endometrial hyperplasia and can lead to endometrial cancer. Also hypertension and obesity are risk factors endometrial carcinoma
- Obesity
- Menstrual irregularity due to anovulation
- Hirsutism is manifestation of hyperandrogenism
- Infertility occurs due to chronic anovulation

DIAGNOSIS

- The syndrome is characterized by clinical, endocrine and metabolic features (Table 1). Not all women with PCOS have polycystic ovaries (PCO), nor do all women with polycystic ovaries have PCOS

Table 1: Diagnostics features of PCOS		
Clinical features	**Endocrine features**	**Metabolic aspects**
Hirsutism	Elevated androgens	Insulin resistance
Acne	Elevated luteinizing hormone	Obesity
Alopecia	Elevated estrogen	Lipid abnormalities
Anovulatory infertility	Elevated prolactin	Impaired glucose tolerance
Recurrent miscarriages		Type 2 diabetes mellitus
Menstrual abnormalities		

- The diagnosis of polycystic ovary syndrome (PCOS) is made if two out of the following three criteria are present (Rotterdam criteria):
  - Oligo and/or anovulation
  - Hyperandrogenism (clinical and/or biochemical)
  - Polycystic ovaries, with the exclusion of other etiologies such as nonclassic adrenal 21-hydroxylase deficiency, Cushing's syndrome, hyperprolactinemia and androgen-producing tumors.
- The morphology of the polycystic ovary has been redefined as an ovary with 12 or more follicles measuring 2–9 mm in diameter and/or increased ovarian volume (>10 cm). The ovaries from women with PCOS may be sonographically normal thus, the ovarian morphological changes must be distinguished from the endocrine syndrome of PCOS and be considered as a sign rather and not a disease.

INVESTIGATIONS FOR POLYCYSTIC OVARY SYNDROME

1. Pelvic ultrasound is done to assess ovarian morphology and endometrial thickness active. Transabdominal scan can be done in women who are not sexually active.
2. Testosterone (T) (normal range 0.5–3.5 nmol/L). Total testosterone is adequate for general screening. It is unnecessary to measure other androgens unless total testosterone is >5 nmol/L, in which case referral is indicated.
3. Sex hormone-binding globulin (SHBG) (normal range 16–119 nmol/L). The measurement of SHBG is not required in routine practice and will not affect management.
4. Free androgen index (FAI): <5 (T × 100/SHBG) is meant to be a predictor of free testosterone, but is a poor parameter for this and is no better than testosterone alone as a marker for PCOS.
5. Estradiol measurement is unhelpful. Estrogenization may be confirmed by endometrial assessment to diagnosis.
   Luteinising hormone (LH) (normal range 2–10 IU/L)

6. Follicle-stimulating hormone (FSH) (normal range 2–8 IU/L)
   FSH and LH are best measured during days 1–3 of a menstrual bleed. If woman is oligo or amenorrheic then random samples can be taken.
7. Serum prolactin (normal range 0.5–5 IU/L) is measured if woman is oligo- or amenorrheic.
8. Thyroid function test, thyroid-stimulating hormone (normal range <500 mU/L)
9. Fasting insulin (<30 mU/L) is not routinely measured; insulin resistance assessed by glucose tolerance test.
10. Glucose tolerance test: A 75 g oral glucose tolerance test (GTT) should be performed in women with PCOS and a body mass index (BMI) greater than 30 kg/m^2, with an assessment of the fasting and two-hour glucose concentration. For South Asian, the criteria for GTT is BMI greater than 25 kg/m^2 as they have of the greater risk of insulin resistance at a lower BMI than the white population

Investigations for Associated Conditions and Risks

Lipid profile

DIFFERENTIAL DIAGNOSIS

Other conditions causing oligo or amenorrhea and hirsutism should be considered in differential diagnosis of PCOD
- Hypothyroidism
- Congenital adrenal hyperplasia (21-hydroxylase deficiency)
- Cushing's syndrome
- Hyperprolactinemia
- Androgen-secreting neoplasms
- PCOS has been reported in other insulin-resistant situations such as acromegaly.

Management of polycystic ovarian syndrome is tailored according to the patient's need. The aim of treatment is :
- Regularization of menstruation, and prevention of endometrial hyperplasia and endometrial cancer
- Treatment of insulin resistance
- Treatment of infertility
- Treatment of hirsutism

GENERAL MEASURES

Reduction in weight helps in restoring all of the above and can be achieved by low-carbohydrate diets and sustained regular exercise. Vitamin D deficiency is known to play some role in the development of the metabolic syndrome so treatment of any such deficiency also is indicated.

SPECIFIC MEASURES

Menstrual Irregularity and Endometrial Hyperplasia

For women who desire regularization of periods, medroxyprogesterone acetate 10 mg for ten days every month can be prescribed.

Contraceptive pills can be prescribed to those who desire regular cycles and contraception .The purpose of regulating menstruation is essentially for the woman's convenience and perhaps her sense of well-being; there is no medical requirement for regular periods, so long as they occur sufficiently often. Newer contraceptive pills with combination of ethinyl estrogen and drospirenone (Yasmin/Yaz) help in regularizing the cycle and treating hirsutism as drospirenone has proven to be effective in decreasing hirsutism and testosterone levels and, more significantly, increasing sex hormone binding globulin (SHBG) levels in women who have PCOS. Drospirenone exhibits both mineralocorticoid effects and androgenic effects which makes it different from progesterones available in other combined oral contraceptive pills.

Women who do not desire regular menstrual cycle should be advised to have a menstrual bleed occur at least once in every three months. This is to prevent endometrial hyperplasia and the associated risk of cancer. This can be achieved by oral progestogen (medroxyprogesterone acetate 10 mg for ten days) taken every three months.

TREATMENT OF INSULIN RESISTANCE

Insulin sensitivity can be improved by medications such as metformin, and the newer thiazolidinedione (glitazones). National Institute for Health and Clinical Excellence recommended in 2004 that women with pcos and a body mass index above 25 be given metformin when other therapy has failed to produce results.

MANAGEMENT OF INFERTILITY IN POLYCYSTIC OVARY SYNDROME

Not all women with PCOS have difficulty in becoming pregnant. For overweight, anovulatory women with PCOS, ovulation resumes with weight loss and diet modification.

Ovulation-inducing drugs like clomiphene citrate and FSH injections are used for those who remain anovulatory after weight loss or for anovulatory lean PCOS.

For patients who do not respond to clomiphene, diet and lifestyle modification, are advised assisted reproductive technology procedures such as controlled ovarian hyperstimulation with follicle-stimulating hormone (FSH) injections followed by in vitro fertilization (IVF).

Though surgery is not commonly performed, the polycystic ovaries can be treated with a laparoscopic procedure called "ovarian drilling" (4 puncture of 4 mm with electrocautery, laser, or biopsy needles), which often results in either resumption of spontaneous ovulations or ovulations after adjuvant treatment with clomiphene or FSH. There are, however, concerns about the long-term effects of ovarian drilling on ovarian function.

MANAGEMENT OF HIRSUTISM

In women of child-bearing age who require contraception, a standard contraceptive pill containing cyproterone acetate is frequently effective in reducing hirsutism. Flutamide and spironolactone with anti-androgen effects, can also be used in treating hirsutism. Metformin can reduce hirsutism, perhaps by reducing insulin resistance, and is often used if there are other features of insulin resistance, such as diabetes or obesity. Eflornithine acts directly on the hair follicles to inhibit hair growth and can be applied locally over the skin. It is usually applied to the face.

Although these agents have shown significant efficacy in clinical trials, individuals vary in their response to different therapies. Drug treatment may be changed if one does not work. Use of hair removal creams, bleach, epilation, electrolysis or laser treatments can be offered for faster and more efficient alternative than the above mentioned medical therapies.

CONCLUSION

PCOS is a disorder of unknown etiology, characterized by menstrual disturbances, hyperandrogenism, hirsutism, obesity, infertility, insulin resistance and the presence of polycystic ovaries on ultrasound. It is associated with long-term risk of developing diabetes, endometrial hyperplasia and cardiovascular disease. The treatment is tailor-made and is directed mainly to symptom control.

SUGGESTED READING

1. Anitha P. Polycystic ovarian syndrome and hyperandrogenism. Gynaecology today Malaysia. Colour box publishing house, 2012.
2. Balen A. The current understanding of polycystic ovary syndrome. The Obstetrician and Gynaecologist. 2004;6:66-74.
3. Lucidi RS. Polycystic ovary syndrome. Available from: http://emedicine. medscape.com/article/256806-overview. Accessed June 2013.
4. Mathur R, Levin O, Azziz R. Use of ethinylestradiol/drospirenone combination in patients with the polycystic ovary syndrome. Ther Clin Risk Manag. 2008;4(2):487-92.
5. Polycystic ovary syndrome. Available from: http://en.wikipedia.org/wiki/Polycystic_ovary_syndrome. Accessed June 2013.
6. Swingler R, Awala A, Gordon U. Review Hirsutism in young Women. The Obstetrician and Gynaecologist. 2009;11:101-07.
7. Tsilchorozidou T, Overton C, Conway GS. The pathophysiology of polycystic ovary syndrome. Clinical Endocrinology. 2004;60:1-17.

Hormone Replacement Therapy

Navneet Magon, Monica Chauhan

INTRODUCTION

Hormone replacement therapy (HRT) refers to any form of hormone therapy where the patient, in the course of medical treatment, receives hormones, either to supplement a lack of naturally occurring hormones, or to substitute other hormones for naturally occurring hormones.

TYPES OF HRT

There are three main types of HRT as discussed below:

- **Estrogen-only HRT:** Estrogen-only HRT is usually recommended for women who have had their uterus and ovaries removed during a hysterectomy.
- **Cyclical HRT:** Cyclical HRT, also known as sequential HRT, is often recommended for women who have menopausal symptoms but still have their periods and uterus intact.

  There are two types of cyclical HRT:
  - **Monthly HRT:** Estrogen every day and progestogen at the end of menstrual cycle for 14 days.
  - **Three-monthly HRT:** Estrogen every day and progestogen for 14 days, every 13 weeks.

  Monthly HRT is usually recommended for women having regular periods. Three-monthly HRT is usually recommended for women experiencing irregular periods. It is useful to maintain regular periods before women progress to the last stage of the menopause.
- **Continuous combined HRT:** Continuous combined HRT is usually recommended for women who are postmenopausal.

  As the name suggests, continuous HRT involves taking estrogen and progestogen every day without a break.

NEED FOR HRT IN MENOPAUSE

HRT in menopause is based on the idea that the treatment may prevent discomfort caused by diminished circulating estrogen and progesterone hormones, or in the case of the surgical or premature menopause, that it may prolong life and may reduce incidence of dementia.[1] The main types of hormones involved are estrogens, progesterone or progestins, and sometimes testosterone.

Combination HRT is often recommended as it decreases the amount of endometrial hyperplasia and cancer associated with unopposed estrogen therapy.[1,2] Some recent therapies include the use of androgens as well.[3]

Bioidentical hormone replacement therapy refers to the use of hormones that are chemically identical to those produced in a woman's body.

HISTORY OF HRT—TIMELINE[4] (FIG. 1)

- ⊃ 1923: Natural estrogens were first isolated from the urine of pregnant mares
- ⊃ 1930: Stilboestrol, first prescribed for menopausal distress
- ⊃ 1941: First synthetic injectable estrogen developed
- ⊃ 1960s: HRT became widely available in easily deliverable oral form
- ⊃ 1966: Dr Robert Wilson published his best seller 'Feminine Forever' painting a sorry picture of physically and mentally crumbling menopausal women who could be transformed into youthful women with straight backed posture, supple breast contours, taut, smooth skin on face and neck, firm muscles and that particular vigor and grace typical of a healthy female. Promoting HRT as a 'Miracle to keep women young' through his concept—changing initiative.
- ⊃ 1975: A study from Kaiser Permanente by Dr Harry Ziel demonstrated that in the absence of progesterone, patients were at increased risk

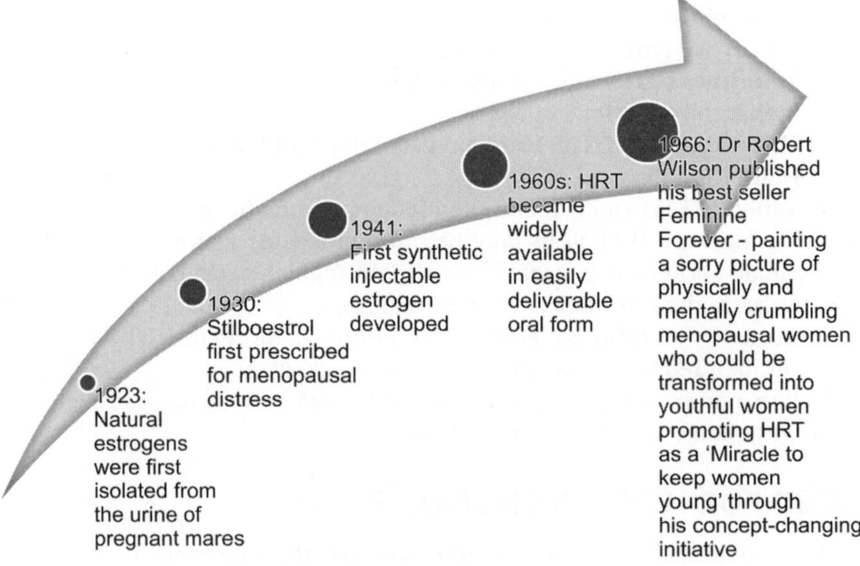

Fig. 1: History of HRT—Timeline

of endometrial cancer with unopposed estrogen therapy. After this, progestin was supplemented in women who have had not received surgical hysterectomy, to reduce the incidence of endometrial hyperplasia and cancer.

GLOBAL SCENARIO

MWS and WHI Studies

The Million Women Study (MWS) is a study of women's health analyzing data from more than one million women aged 50 and over. It is a collaborative project between Cancer Research UK and the National Health Service (NHS), with additional funding from the Medical Research Council (UK).

One key focus of the study relates to the effects of hormone replacement therapy use on women's health. The study has confirmed the findings in the Women's Health Initiative (WHI) that women currently using HRT are more likely to develop breast cancer than those who are not using HRT.[5]

WHI Studies (Table 1)

In 2002, the Women's Health Initiative (WHI) was published looking at the effects of hormonal replacement therapy in postmenopausal women.

The Women's Health Initiative (1991) consisted of clinical trials (CT) and an observational study (OS), conducted to address major health issues causing morbidity and mortality in postmenopausal women. It was designed to compare the effects of hormone replacement therapy, vitamin D and calcium and low-fat diets on more than 160,000 women. The WHI studied postmenopausal women aged 50–79 years (at time of study enrollment) over 15 years, making it the largest US prevention study of its kind. The trial was stopped 2 years early, May 31, 2002, after a mean follow up of 5.2 years.

The authors of the study concluded, "The risk-benefit profile found in this trial is not consistent with the requirements for a viable intervention for primary prevention of chronic diseases, and the results indicate that this regimen should not be initiated or continued for primary prevention of coronary heart disease."

The authors of the study recommended that women with nonsurgical menopause take the lowest feasible dose of HRT, and for the shortest possible time, to minimize risk.

These recommendations have not held up with further data analysis, however.

Later studies released by the WHI showed that all-cause mortality was not dramatically different between the groups receiving conjugated equine estrogen (CEE), those receiving estrogen and progesterone, and those not on HRT at all. Specifically, the relative risk for all-cause mortality was 1.04 (confidence interval, 0.88–1.22) in the CEE-alone trial and 1.00 (CI, 0.83–1.19) in the estrogen plus progesterone trial. Further, in analysis pooling data from both trials, postmenopausal HRT was associated with a significant reduction

Table 1: Summary of observation from WHI[6]

CT Component	Hypothesized Impact on Primary Outcome Based on previous observational, pilot, and/or laboratory studies	Supported by WHI CT Findings?	Findings of WHI
Hormone Replacement Therapy	Reduces risk of coronary heart disease (CHD)	No	Increased risk of stroke. No effect on CHD risk.
	Increases risk of breast cancer	Varies by regimen	Estrogen-progestin combination therapy increased risk. Estrogen-alone therapy showed a possible decrease in risk.
Dietary Modification	Reduces risks of CHD, stroke, and cardiovascular disease (CVD)	No	Modest, but non-significant, effects on CVD risk factors.
	Reduces risk of invasive colorectal cancer	No	Non-significant trend indicated that a longer intervention may yield more definitive results.
	Reduces risk of invasive breast cancer	No	
Calcium plus Vitamin D	Reduces risk of hip and other fractures	No	A small, but significant, improvement in bone mineral density was identified.
	Reduces risk of colorectal cancer	No	Study notes that a longer-duration study may yield more definitive results.

in mortality (Relative risk, 0.70; CI, 0.51–0.96) among women aged 50 to 59 years. This would represent five fewer deaths per 1000 women per 5 years of therapy (Table 2).

Limitations and Criticisms of WHI[7]

- Findings from the WHI are limited in that it used only one route of administration (oral) and one formulation of estrogen (conjugated estrogen) and progestogen (medroxyprogesterone acetate)
- The trial also enrolled healthy women 50 to 79 years old. As the average age of menopause is 51, this resulted in an older study population, with an average age of 63
- The WHI trial was limited by low adherence, high attrition, inadequate power to detect risks for some outcomes, and evaluation of few regimens
- To be properly double blinded, the study required that women should not be perimenopausal or have symptoms of menopause
- Most fundamentally, the WHI did not address the major indication for Menopausal Hormone Therapy (MHT) use, relief of symptoms. The study did not address the value of HRT for treatment of disruptive transitional symptoms, such as hot flashes and sleep disturbances, which can often be very serious for an individual woman
- In a more recent expert consensus statement from The Endocrine Society, evidence from the WHI trial was weighted less than that of a randomized controlled trial according to the GRADE system criteria because of the mitigating factors: Large dropout rate; lack of adequate representation of applicable group of women (i.e. those initiating therapy at the time of menopause); and modifying influences from prior hormone use[8]
- The double blinding limited validity of study results due to its effects on patient exclusion criteria
- The dominant majorities of participants were Caucasian, and tended to be slightly overweight and former smokers, with the necessary health risks for which these demographics predispose
- Furthermore, the focus of the WHI study was disease prevention. WHI was a prevention, rather than a treatment trial. Most women take hormone

Table 2: Association of breast cancer with HRT

Increased risk of breast cancer associated with hormone replacement therapy (HRT)[3,19]			
Estrogen only HRT	Up to 5 years	7 years	15 years
	No increase in risk	No increase in risk	No increase in risk
Combined estrogen/ progestogen HRT	Up to 5 years	After 5 years	
	< 1 per 1000 women per year	2 per 1000 women after 5 years	

Adapted from MacLennan AH et al 2008[19] and Sturdee DW et al 2011[3] replacement therapy to treat symptoms of menopause rather than for disease prevention, and therefore, the risks and benefits of hormone replacement therapy in the general population differ from the women included in the WHI.

Impact of WHI and MWS on HRT

- There was tremendous media attention about some of the risks and some of the benefits
- Subsequent to publication of the WHI, controversy arose regarding the applicability of its findings to women just entering menopause
- The healthcare burden of menopause and its symptoms increased significantly as the findings affected millions of American women taking hormone therapy[9]
- When the study was abruptly halted in 2002, the impact was huge, swift and charged with emotion
- Thousands of women participating in the study were instructed to stop taking the drugs and contact their doctors. For the wider population of women not in the study, the press statement advised that they should consult their physicians about stopping hormones
- For physicians, the scientific publication tried to make it clear that these findings were related to the use of hormones to prevent disease, not to the use of hormones to treat hot flashes. The findings of the research were contrary to what had been taught and thought in medical school. There was a lot of confusion about what to do and how to do it after the results were announced. There was some concern from the medical community about being caught off guard
- Since the publication of the study till date, for the last decade, there has been a disrepute and repulsion with respect to HRT among physicians and patients
- There has also been a reported increase in the use of Clonidine as alternative to estrogen for the relief of hot-flashes associated with menopause after WHI and resultant premature ovarian failure[10]
- Scientists and physicians are looking at alternative ways of administering hormones, as well as looking at alternatives to hormones. There are attempts to look at whether the skin patch is safer than taking hormones orally. Many other medications and substances are being studied or suggested as alternatives to hormone therapy for symptoms that women may experience with menopause.

Current Status—Guidelines and Recommendations

Following the need for guidance post WHI and as long-term data have become available in recent years on effects of HRT, the North American Menopause Society (NAMS) has updated its 2010 position statement in 2012 on the use of estrogen therapy (ET) and estrogen-progestogen therapy (EPT), with a seventh Advisory Panel.

Highlights of the specific recommendations of NAMS 2012 for the use of HT in menopausal women include the following[11] (Table 3):

VARIOUS APPROACHES FOR HRT

Conjugated Equine Estrogens (CEE)

Conjugated equine estrogens (CEE) are a mixture of naturally occurring estrogens and contain estrone sulfate and equilin sulfate as the main constituents. These are routinely combined with a progestational agent to prevent endometrial changes like proliferation or hyperplasia. The most popular of those regimens is CEE and medroxyprogesterone acetate (MPA). Given at varying doses from 2.5 to 10 mg per day, provides effective hormone replacement therapy (HRT) in postmenopausal women.

Table 3: Recommendations of NAMS 2012, for the use of hormone therapy in menopausal women

The most effective treatment for menopausal vasomotor symptoms and asssociated quality of life is ET or EPT.

Recommended duration of therapy differs for EPT in women with a uterus and for ET in women who have had a hysterectomy.

Heightened risk for breast cancer associated with more than 3 to 5 years of EPT use limits the duration of safe EPT use. For ET, the benefit-risk profile is more favorable. Because risk for breast cancer does not appear to increase during an average of 7 years of ET use, there is more flexibility in duration of ET treatment.

HT use is associated with a lower fracture risk, but a higher risk for ischemic stroke, venous thromboembolism (VTE), and ovarian cancer.

Compared with ET, EPT is associated with a higher risk for coronary artery disease.

The decision to use HT should still be individualized and patient-specific, based on the patient's priorities regarding health and quality of life, as well as on specific risk factors for thrombosis, cardiovascular disease, stroke and breast cancer.

NAMS recommends EPT for relief of hot flashes in women with a uterus, so that the progestogen component will protect the uterine lining from the carcinogenic effects of estrogen alone.

For women whose symptoms are limited to vaginal dryness or dyspareunia, NAMS recommends low-dose vaginal ET.

Among healthy women younger than 60 years or within 10 years of menopause, neither ET nor EPT use is associated with increased risk for cardiovascular disease. Although stroke risk may be increased, it is still a rare occurrence among women younger than 60 years.

Women with premature or early menopause and no contraindications to HT may use HT until age 51 years, which is the average age of natural menopause or longer, if needed to control symptoms.

Safety data are lacking to support HT use in breast cancer survivors.

Compared with standard doses of oral estrogen, transdermal ET and low-dose oral ET may have reduced risks for thrombosis and stroke. However, these apparent benefits need to be confirmed in randomized trials.

Future studies should investigate patient-specific effects of ET and EPT.

Estradiol Valerate (E2V)

It is a prodrug of estradiol, the principal and most biologically potent human estrogen. E2 possess the highest affinity for estrogen receptors and works by regulating transcription of target genes through binding to specific DNA target sequences. The esterification (valerate group) allows it for better absorption and avoidance of high peak estradiol levels. Given at doses of 1 or 2 mg per day, it provides effective hormone replacement therapy (HRT) in postmenopausal women.

Phytoestrogens[12]

Researches have shown that phytoestrogen containing preparations appear to demonstrate some benefits, not only for symptom relief, but also on the skeleton and cardiovascular system. Efficacy for vasomotor symptom relief is lower than the with traditional HRT (maximally, 60% symptom reduction compared to 90–100% with traditional HRT). There are as yet no hard data on major outcome measures such as coronary heart disease and fractures.

Tibolone[13]

Being a selective tissue estrogenic activity regulator (STEAR), it provides adequate relief of vasomotor symptoms of menopause, but there is evidence that tibolone results in better female sexual function, particularly with respect to desire and arousal, probably due to its combined estrogenic and androgenic properties.

The long-term Intervention on fractures with tibolone (LIFT) study showed that tibolone reduces the risk of vertebral fractures and possibly colon cancer, but increases the risk of stroke in older women with osteoporosis. Tibolone is contraindicated in known, past or suspected cases of breast cancer as shown by the LIBERATE trial.

Consensus from the Asia Pacific Tibolone Group suggests switching to tibolone from HRT will be beneficial for those who have experienced:

- An increase in breast pain, despite HRT dose adjustment
- Increased breast density that resulted in an unreadable mammogram
- Low libido
- Mood disorders and
- Persistent bleeding problems (providing no histo-pathological reasons for this exist).

Calcium and Vitamin D

Updated Recommendations from integrated medical services (IMS) 2013 conclude:

- Postmenopausal women need a dietary reference intake (DRI) of 1000–1500 mg of elemental calcium
- Excessive calcium supplementation in addition to adequate or high dietary calcium may be associated with increased cardiovascular risk

➲ The DRI for vitamin D is 800–1000 IU in the postmenopausal period
➲ Vitamin D supplementation has been shown independently to lower the risk of fracture and of falling in elderly patients.

Bisphosphonates

Updated Recommendations from IMS 2013 conclude:
➲ The bisphosphonates are potent inhibitors of bone resorption and decrease the rate of bone turnover, with proven efficacy in the prevention of vertebral and hip fractures
➲ An association has been suggested between atypical femur shaft fractures and over-suppression of bone turnover in patients exposed to bisphosphonates for longer than 3–5 years
➲ Bisphosphonates have benefits in some cancers and may prevent bone metastases from breast cancer.

Denosumab

A human monoclonal antibody to the receptor activator of nuclear factor kappa-B ligand (RANKL), at a dose of 60 mg subcutaneously, 6 monthly, significantly reduces the risk of vertebral, nonvertebral and hip fractures. As with other biological therapies, denosumab may have adverse immunological effects.

CLINICAL MANAGEMENT OF MENOPAUSAL SYMPTOMS

Osteoporosis

Osteoporosis is the disease of bones where the bone mineral density (BMD) is reduced, bone microarchitecture deteriorates, and the amount and variety of proteins in bone are altered. The underlying mechanism in all cases of osteoporosis is an imbalance between bone resorption and bone formation.

Osteoporosis is defined by the World Health Organization (WHO) as a bone mineral density of 2.5 standard deviations or more below the mean peak bone mass (average of young, healthy adults) as measured by dual-energy X-ray absorptiometry; the term established osteoporosis includes the presence of a fragility fracture.[14]

Osteoporosis may be classified as:
➲ Primary
  – Type 1
  – Type 2
➲ Secondary

The form of osteoporosis most common in women after menopause is referred to as primary type 1 or postmenopausal osteoporosis.

Primary type 2 osteoporosis or senile osteoporosis occurs after 75 years of age and is seen in both females and males at a ratio of 2:1.

Secondary osteoporosis may arise at any age and affect men and women equally. This form results from chronic predisposing medical problems or diseases or prolonged use of medications such as glucocorticoids, when the disease is called steroid- or glucocorticoid-induced osteoporosis.[15]

Hormone therapy (HT) is believed to be useful in preventing or alleviating the increased rate of bone loss that leads to osteoporosis. It is generally recommended for postmenopausal women who:

- Undergo an early menopause
- Have a low bone mass, as measured by a bone-density test and menopausal symptoms
- Have several other risk factors for osteoporosis, such as a petite, thin frame; family history of osteoporosis, or a medical problem associated with osteoporosis.

The 2010 position statement of The North American Menopause Society on the Management of osteoporosis in postmenopausal women has made the following major recommendations in its guidelines.[16]

Table 4 shows management strategies for postmenopausal osteoporosis.

Table 4: Management strategies for postmenopausal osteoporosis
NAMS recommends osteoporosis drug therapy in the following populations: ❖ All postmenopausal women who have had an osteoporotic vertebral or hip fracture ❖ All postmenopausal women who have BMD values consistent with osteoporosis (i.e. T-scores $\leq$ –2.5) at the lumbar spine, femoral neck, or total hip region ❖ All postmenopausal women who have a T-score from –1.0 to –2.5 and a 10-year risk, based on the fracture risk assessment (FRAX) calculator of major osteoporotic fracture.
It is important to encourage adherence to the treatment plan and to identify barriers to nonadherence. Providing clear information to women regarding their risk for fracture and the purpose of osteoporosis therapy may be the optimal way to improve adherence.
During therapy, it is appropriate to reevaluate the treatment goals and the choice of medication on an ongoing basis through periodic medical examination and a follow-up BMD testing. Measurement of BMD has limited use in predicting the effectiveness of antiresorptive therapies for reducing fracture risk. Also, fracture risk reductions from therapy occur much more rapidly than BMD changes. An appropriate interval for repeat BMD testing is after 1 to 2 years of treatment. There appears to be little value in repeat testing if a woman is stable (within the precision error of the original instrument).
For untreated postmenopausal women, repeat dual-energy X-ray absorptiometry (DXA) testing is not useful until 2 to 5 years have passed.
Bisphosphonates are the first-line drugs for treating postmenopausal women with osteoporosis. They have reduced the risk of vertebral fractures by 40% to 70% and reduced the incidence of nonvertebral fracture, including hip fracture, by about half this amount.
The selective estrogen-receptor modulator (SERM) raloxifene is most often considered for postmenopausal women with low bone mass or younger postmenopausal women with osteoporosis. It prevents bone loss and reduces the risk of vertebral fractures, but its effectiveness in reducing other fractures is uncertain. Extraskeletal risks and benefits are important when considering raloxifene therapy.

Contd...

Contd...

Teriparatide (parathyroid hormone [PTH] 1-34) is best offered to postmenopausal women with osteoporosis who are at high risk for fracture. Daily subcutaneous injections have been shown to stimulate bone formation and improve bone density. Therapy is indicated for no more than 24 months.

The primary indication for systemic estrogen or estrogen-progestin therapy (ET/EPT) is to treat moderate to severe menopause symptoms (e.g., vasomotor symptoms). When symptoms are controlled or cease, continued hormone therapy can still be considered for bone effects, weighing its benefits and risks against those of alternative therapies.

ET/EPT may be a treatment option for a few years of early postmenopause.

Calcitonin is not a first-line drug for postmenopausal osteoporosis treatment, as its fracture efficacy is not strong and its BMD effects are less than those of other agents. However, it is an option for women with osteoporosis who are more than 5 years beyond menopause. Calcitonin therapy may reduce vertebral fracture risk in women with osteoporosis, although the evidence documenting fracture protection is not strong. It is not recommended for treating bone pain, except bone pain from acute vertebral compression fractures.

Data are inadequate to make definitive recommendations regarding combination or serial anabolic and antiresorptive drug therapies.

The treatment of osteoporosis needs to be long term in most women.

If drug-related adverse effects occur, appropriate management strategies should be instituted. If adverse effects persist, switching to another agent may be required.

Decisions to discontinue or suspend therapy are based on the woman's risk of fracture and her response to treatment. Given the uncertainties of long-term drug safety, careful monitoring is required. Fracture risk after discontinuing therapy has not been adequately evaluated.

Vasomotor Symptoms—Hot Flashes, Night Sweats and Palpitations[17]

The NAMS recommends:
- For the relief of mild vasomotor symptoms—lifestyle changes, alone or combined with a nonprescription remedy (such as dietary isoflavones, vitamin E, or black cohosh)
- For moderate to severe menopause-related hot flashes—prescription systemic estrogen-containing products are still the therapeutic standard
- For women with concerns or contraindications to estrogen containing products, possible treatment options include prescription progestogens, venlafaxine, paroxetine, fluoxetine or gabapentin.

Estrogen Therapy and Estrogen Plus Progestogen Therapy

Many trials have shown that estrogen therapy (ET) and estrogen plus progestogen therapy (EPT) are effective in relieving menopause-related hot flashes. These therapies may take up to four weeks before the full effect is achieved.

According to the NAMS recommendations, treatment of moderate to severe menopause symptoms (including hot flashes) is the primary indication for systemic ET and EPT, NAMS recommends considering lower-than-standard doses of ET and EPT.

For all women with an intact uterus who are using ET, NAMS recommends the administration of adequate progestogen, either in a continuous-combined or continuous-sequential EPT regimen.

Medroxyprogesterone Acetate

Several studies have demonstrated that intramuscular and oral forms of this progestin effectively relieve menopause-associated hot flashes in healthy women, and in women with breast or endometrial cancer.

Megestrol Acetate

One study found a significant reduction in hot flashes in women receiving megestrol acetate. The full efficacy of this oral progestin on reducing hot flashes may not be observed until after three or four weeks of therapy. Women who are receiving concurrent tamoxifen may experience an initial increase in hot flashes before any decrease is noticed. No long-term data are available regarding the long-term safety of megestrol acetate for treatment of hot flashes in women with breast cancer. Side-effects include increased appetite, and possibly, exacerbation of preexisting diabetes and an increase in thromboembolic events.

Oral Contraceptives

NAMS supports the use of low-dose combined estrogen-progestin oral contraceptives for perimenopausal women who need hot flash relief and contraception and who do not smoke or have other contraindications.

Urogenital Problems

Vaginal Atrophy

Vaginal dryness, soreness and painful sex.

Urogenital problems are common symptoms of the menopause and as women get older, physical changes can lead to vaginal dryness, which may affect sex life and lead to relationship difficulties.

Without the production of estrogen by the ovaries, the skin and support tissues of the vulva and vagina become thin and less elastic. This is an inevitable consequence of the menopause and the majority of women will experience some form of symptoms. Vaginal dryness is commonly the first reported symptom. This is due to a reduction in the production of mucus by the glands of the vagina. Up to 40% of postmenopausal women experience vaginal dryness during the menopause. Only 20%–25% of women with these symptoms seek medical help.[18]

Alteration in the normal vaginal discharge is noticed by most women after menopause but rarely discussed. Without estrogen, the pH (acidity) of the vaginal secretions change and the normal discharge become more alkaline. This pH affects the balance of the microorganisms in the natural secretions. The discharge changes in nature, becoming watery, discolored and slightly smelly. This often leads to vaginal burning and vulval irritation.[19]

Management of Vaginal Atrophy with Local Estrogen Therapy

Vaginal dryness, soreness, burning, vulval irritation and chafing can all respond well to local estrogen treatments. This can also help greatly with discomfort, pain during sex, correcting the vaginal pH and stopping the overgrowth of abnormal vaginal flora.

Local low dose treatment with estrogen has been found to have significant effect on the postmenopausal urogenital symptoms related to atrophy.[20]

Estrogen delivered locally can be in the form of:
- Vaginal tablets or pessary: Initially taken daily, then as advised
- Creams: Taken daily initially, then as advised
- Vaginal silica ring: Inserted for a 3-month period.

Pelvic Floor Changes and Prolapse

The muscles and ligaments of the pelvic floor are also estrogen-sensitive, and changes in collagen, due to estrogen deficiency, have a profound effect on the support mechanisms of the pelvic floor. Many women who experience incontinence, link the time that it started with their final menstrual period.[19]

Many postmenopausal women become aware of ballooning or bulging of the walls inside the vagina, or even of a feeling of descent of the neck of the womb. Others simply experience a generalized pelvic dragging sensation. About half of postmenopausal women are found to have weakening of the front wall of the vagina (anterior vaginal wall prolapse), about a quarter have similar problems with the back (posterior) wall, and one-fifth with the highest part of the vagina.[21]

The role of local estrogen in the management of urinary problems is complex. Estrogen replacement therapy has been shown to alleviate urgency, urge incontinence, frequency, nocturia and dysuria.[22]

Neurological Problems

Related menopausal symptoms:
- Sleep disorders/Insomnia
- Fatigue
- Depression
- Anxiety
- Headache/Migraine
- Pain disorders
- Hot flashes

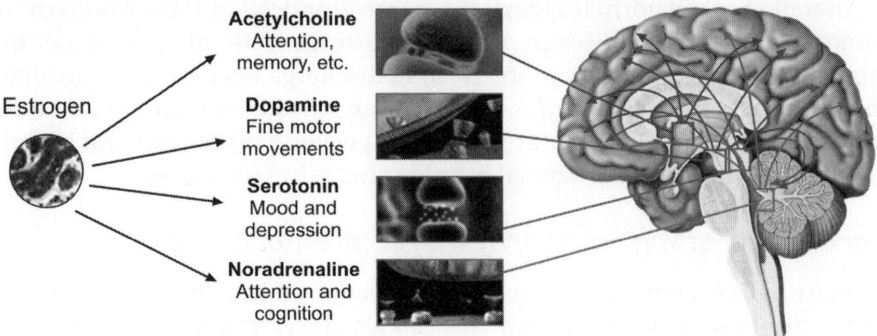

Fig. 2: Mental symptoms in postmenopausal women
(Source: http://www.34-menopause-symptoms.com/difficulty-concentrating-causes.htm)
(For color version, see Plate 3)

- Weight gain
- Memory loss
- Personality changes.

Figure 2 shows mental symptoms in postmenopausal women.

According to a 2007 presentation at the American Academy of Neurology meeting, hormone therapy taken soon after menopause may help protect against dementia, but it raises the risk of mental decline in women who do not take hormone replacement until they are older. Dementia risk was 1% in women who started HRT early, and 1.7% in women who did not (i.e. women who did not take hormone replacement seem to have had, on average, a 70% higher relative risk of dementia than women who began HRT around the time of the beginning of menopause). This suggests that there may be a critical period during which time taking HRT may have benefits, but if HRT is initiated after that period, it will not have such benefits and may cause harm. This is consistent with research that hormone therapy improves executive and attention processes in postmenopausal women.[23]

BENEFITS AND RISKS OF HRT[12]

Immediate Effects of HRT

- **Vasomotor symptoms:** One of the main indications for prescribing HRT in postmenopausal women is the relief of vasomotor symptoms. However, the optimum dose and duration should be decided according to the severity of a woman's symptoms and her response to therapy.
- **Mood:** Short-term use of HRT may improve mood and depressive symptoms during the menopausal transition and in the early menopause.
- **Sexual function:** Through its proliferative effect on the vulval and vaginal epithelium and by improving vaginal lubrication, HRT, systemic or topical, may improve sexual function in women with dyspareunia secondary to vaginal atrophy.
- **Urogenital symptoms:** Symptoms related to vaginal atrophy, such as vaginal dryness and superficial dyspareunia have been shown to gain

from estrogen therapy. It also has a proliferative effect on the bladder and urethral epithelium and may help relieve symptoms of urinary frequency, urgency and possibly reduce the risk of recurrent urinary tract infections in women with urogenital atrophy.

Long-term Effects of HRT

- **Cardiovascular:** HRT has the potential for improving the cardiovascular risk profile through its beneficial effects on vascular function, cholesterol levels and glucose metabolism in line with the 'window of opportunity' concept. Lowest effective dose should be used when prescribing HRT for the first time in women over the age of 60 years. The Kronos Early Estrogen Prevention Study, 'KEEPS' using lower doses of estradiol and progesterone in women less than three years from their last menstrual period reported neutral impact on cardiovascular risk markers such as coronary calcium scores and intima media thickness.
- **Cognition:** Based on current evidence, HRT should not be initiated for the sole purpose of improving cognitive function or reducing the risk of dementia in postmenopausal women.
- **Cancer:**
  - *Breast cancer:* A small but statistically significant decrease in breast cancer risk was detected in the WHI estrogen-alone trial. Issues were raised by the Million Women Study (MWS) over the long-term safety of HRT from the perspective of breast cancer. Recent critique of the WHI and MWS has clearly illustrated a number of key flaws which limit the ability of the trials to establish a causal association between HRT and breast cancer.
    Updated 2013 IMS recommendations conclude[24]:
    - Risk of breast cancer in women >50 years is a complex issue
    - Risk of breast cancer attributable to HRT is small and the risk decreases after treatment is stopped
    - Increased breast cancer risk is primarily related to the addition of progesterone to estrogen therapy and related to duration of use.
  - *Ovarian cancer:* Conflicting reports have been published on the incidence of ovarian cancer, with WHI suggesting no increased risk and Danish National Cancer Registry suggesting small but significant increased risk of ovarian cancer.
  - *Endometrial cancer:* Significantly lower risk of endometrial cancer has been seen in continuous combined regimens as compared to an untreated population.
  - *Colorectal cancer:* Data published over a period of years have shown a decreased risk of colorectal cancer in patients on oral HRT.
- **Venous thromboembolism (VTE):** Risk of VTE increases by almost two- to four-fold among patients taking oral HRT, with the highest risk in the first year of use. Counseling and thorough risk assessment for VTE needs to be carried out in patients requiring HRT.

Updated 2013 IMS recommendations conclude:
- Risk of VTE and ischemic stroke increases with oral HRT but the absolute risk is rare below age of 60 years
- Incidence of VTE with HRT is very low among Asian women.

➲ **Stroke:** Overall, various studies have yielded very conflicting results on stroke and HRT. As per the current evidences, HRT cannot be recommended for the primary or secondary prevention of stroke. The HERS study (the Heart and Estrogen progestogen Replacement Study) found no increased incidence of stroke with HRT.

PRECAUTIONS FOR HRT[25]

No consensus has been reached on absolute contraindications to HRT. However, patients with the following should be avoid or discontinue HRT:
➲ History of breast cancer
➲ History or known high-risk of VTE including stroke and cardiovascular disease
➲ Uncontrolled hypertension
➲ Abnormal vaginal bleeding
➲ Abnormal liver function
➲ History of endometrial or ovarian cancer
➲ High risk of gallbladder disease.

IS HRT COST EFFECTIVE?

Pure cost effectiveness of HRT is difficult to measure as HRT is principally for symptomatic treatment during menopause. However, data from the WHI study have been utilized by the modeling studies of quality of life years (QALYs), which considered fracture reduction, breast cancer, colorectal cancer, coronary heart disease, stroke, and venous thromboembolic events over five years of HRT use.

The result showed HRT was more cost effective in all women compared with no treatment but that the cost effectiveness was greater in those with more severe vasomotor symptoms.

PATIENT COUNSELING

➲ Menopause occurs when the ovaries stop forming eggs and releasing female hormones *viz* estrogen and progesterone, as a result, the period ceases
➲ Menopause can lead to a series of symptoms which might adversely affect the quality of life in certain situations
➲ Hormone replacement therapy (or HRT) contains 2 natural hormones of the body: Estrogen and progestogen
➲ HRT is a safe and effective treatment for relief from menopausal symptoms like hot flushes and night sweats at menopause

➲ It may also improve sleep, joint aches and pains, and vaginal dryness and protects against fractures resulting from osteoporosis

➲ Benefit-risk profile of HRT varies from patient to patient and thorough assessment should be carried out to customize the treatment plan.

SUMMARY

➲ The woman should be encouraged to make a decision whether to use HRT by giving sufficient information, so as to make a fully informed choice

➲ HRT should to be customized as per the signs and symptoms with regular assessment/monitoring of patient's condition

➲ If women start HRT around the time of menopause, the risk is very small, it is not usually appropriate for women over 60 years of age to start HRT

➲ Women suffering with premature ovarian insufficiency should be encouraged to use HRT at least until the average age of the menopause

➲ Always start the therapy with a lower dose and if the symptoms persist, higher dose can be administered

➲ HRT can play a vital role in optimizing quality of life and facilitating the primary prevention of long-term conditions which might create a personal, social and economic burden.

REFERENCES

1. Shuster, Lynne T, Rhodes, Deborah J, Gostout, Bobbie S, et al. "Premature menopause or early menopause: Long-term health consequences". Maturitas. 2010;65(2):161-6. doi:10.1016/j.maturitas.2009.08.003

2. Eden KJ, Wylie KR. Quality of sexual life and menopause. Women's Health. 2009;5(4):385-96. doi:10.2217/whe.09.24.

3. Ziaei S, Moghasemi M, Faghihzadeh S. Comparative effects of conventional hormone replacement therapy and tibolone on climacteric symptoms and sexual dysfunction in postmenopausal women. Climateric. 2010;13:147-56. doi:10.1016/j.maturitas.2006.04.014.

4. Wright J. Hormone replacement therapy: An example of McKinlay's theory on the seven stages of medical innovation. Journal of Clinical Nursing. 2005;14:1090-7.

5. Million Women Study C, Reeves G, Bull D. "Breast cancer and hormone-replacement therapy in the Million Women Study". Lancet. 2003;362(9382):419–27.

6. Hays J, Hunt JR, Hubbell FA, Anderson GL, Limacher M, Allen C, et al. "The Women's Health Initiative recruitment methods and results." Annals of epidemiology. 2003 Oct;13(9 Suppl):S18-77.

7. Nelson HD, Walker M, Zakher B, Mitchell J. "Menopausal hormone therapy for the primary prevention of chronic conditions: A systematic review to update the US Preventive Services Task Force recommendations". Annals of internal medicine. 2012;157(2):104-13.

8. Santen RJ, Utian WH. "Executive Summary: Postmenopausal Hormone Therapy: An Endocrine Society Scientific Statement". J Clin Endocrinol Metab. 2010;95:S1-66 (Supplement 1). Retrieved Feb 7, 2013.

9. Lagro-Janssen T, Rossner WW, Van Weel C. Breast cancer and hormone-replacement therapy: Up to general practice to pick up the pices. Lancet. 2003;362(9392):414-5.

10. Austin P, Mamdani M, Tu K. The impact of the Women's Health Initiative study on incident Clonidine use in Ontario, Canada. Can J Clin Pharmacol. 11:e191-4.

11. The 2012 Hormone Therapy Position Statement of The North American Menopause Society. Menopause. 2012 March;19(3):257-71. doi:10.1097/gme.0b013e31824b970a.

12. Nick Panay, Haitham Hamoda et al. The 2013 British Menopause Society and Women's Health Concern recommendations on hormone replacement therapy. Menopause Int OnlineFirst, 2013 doi:10.1177/1754045313489645.

13. Huang KE, Baber R, et al. Updated clinical recommendations for the use of tibolone in Asian women. CLIMACTERIC. 2010;13:317-27.

14. WHO. "Assessment of fracture risk and its application to screening for postmenopausal osteoporosis. Report of a WHO Study Group". World Health Organization technical report series. 1994;843:1-129.

15. Alldredge BK; Kimble K, Anne M, Lloyd Y, Kradjan WA, Guglielmo BJ. Applied therapeutics: The clinical use of drugs. Philadelphia: Wolters Kluwer Health/Lippincott Williams and Wilkins. 2009;p. 101-3.

16. Management of osteoporosis in postmenopausal women: 2010 position statement of The North American Menopause Society. Menopause. 2010;17(1):25-54.

17. Neff MJ. Practice Guidelines: NAMS Releases Position Statement on the Treatment of Vasomotor Symptoms Associated with Menopause. Am Fam Physician. 2004;70(2):393-9.

18. Bachmann GA, Nevadunsky NS. Diagnosis and treatment of atrophic vaginitis. Am Fam Physician. 2000;61:3090-6.

19. Iosif C, Bekassy Z. Prevalence of genitourinary symptoms in the late menopause. Acta Obstet Gynecol Scand. 1984;63:257-60.

20. Eriksen PS, Rasmussen H. Low dose 17 beta-estradiol vaginal tablets in the treatment of atrophic vaginitis: A double-blind placebo controlled study. Eur J Obstet Gynecol Reprod Biol. 1992;44(2):137-44.

21. Versi E, et al. Urogenital prolapse and atrophy at menopause: A prevalence study. Int. Urogynecol J Pelvic Floor Dysfunct. 2001;12:107-10.

22. Milson I, Molander U. Urogenital ageing. J Br Menopause Soc. 1998;151-6.

23. Schmidt R, Fazekas F, Reinhart B, Kapeller P, Fazekas G, Offenbacher H, et al. "Estrogen replacement therapy in older women: A neuropsychological and brain MRI study". J Am Geriatr Soc. 1996;44(11):1307-13.

24. de Villiers TJ, Pines A, Panay N, et al. Updated 2013 International Menopause Society recommendations on menopausal hormone therapy and preventive strategies for midlife health. CLIMACTERIC. 2013;16:316-37.

25. Hickey M, et al. Hormone replacement therapy BMJ. 2012;344:e763. doi: 10.1136/bmj.e763.

Chapter

36

Adenomyosis

Meena Samant

INTRODUCTION

Adenomyosis is presence of endometrial gland and stroma within the myometrium with secondary myometrial hyperplasia and is situated at least 2.5 mm below the endometrial-myometrial junction. Adenomyosis has often been referred to as endometriosis interna. This term is misleading because endometriosis and adenomyosis are clinically different diseases. The only common feature is the presence of ectopic endometrial glands and stroma. Adenomyosis is derived from aberrant glands of the basalis layer of the endometrium. Therefore, these glands do not usually undergo the traditional proliferative and secretory changes that are associated with cyclic ovarian hormone production.

CLINICAL FEATURES

Over 50% of women with adenomyosis are asymptomatic or have minor symptoms that do not annoy them enough to seek medical care. Symptomatic adenomyosis usually presents in women between the ages of 35 and 50. The severity of pelvic symptoms increases proportionally to the depth of penetration and the total volume of disease in the myometrium. The classic symptoms of adenomyosis are secondary dysmenorrhea and menorrhagia. The acquired dysmenorrhea becomes increasingly more severe as the disease progresses. There may be abdominal pressure and bloating. Occasionally, the patient complains of dyspareunia, which is midline in location and deep in the pelvis.

On pelvic examination, the uterus is diffusely enlarged, usually two to three times normal size. It is most unusual for the uterine enlargement associated with adenomyosis to be greater than a 14-week-size gestation unless the patient also has uterine myomas. The uterus is globular and tender immediately before and during menstruation.

Adenomyosis is a common condition. It is found in 15–27% of hysterectomy specimens. It is most often diagnosed in middle-aged women and women who have had children. Some studies also suggest that women, who have had prior uterine surgery, may be at risk for adenomyosis. Though, the cause of adenomyosis is not known, studies have suggested that various hormones, including estrogen, progesterone, prolactin, and follicle-stimulating hormone, may trigger the condition.

ADENOMYOSIS AND FERTILITY

Adenomyosis co-exists with endometriosis in 20% cases. Because of the coexistence, it is difficult to tell precisely what role adenomyosis may play in fertility problems. In theory, adenomyosis is a condition that can affect a woman's fertility if it develops during her childbearing years, but research is still preliminary. As more and more women are planning their pregnancy in later years, which corresponds to the age of adenomyosis and also of diminishing ovarian reserve, the problem may be compounded.

Women who become pregnant with adenomyosis are at increased risks of pregnancy complications. Juang et al. noted an increase in premature labor and delivery, low birth weight, and preterm premature rupture of membranes in a large case-control series of women with adenomyosis.

INVESTIGATIONS—IMAGING AND NEWER INSIGHTS

Until recently, the only definitive way to diagnose adenomyosis was to perform histopathological examination after a hysterectomy. However, imaging technology has made it possible to recognize adenomyosis without surgery. Using MRI or transvaginal ultrasound, characteristics of the disease in the uterus can be identified to a great extent.

Transvaginal ultrasonography (TVS) and magnetic resonance imaging (MRI) are able to evaluate the inner myometrial layers underlying the endometrium and has been termed JZ or the junctional zone. This portion of myometrium is Mullerian in origin and measures 5 mm in thickness. Uterine peristaltic wave originates in JZ and has a role in sperm transfer and nidation. Heterotopic endometrial tissue on JZ in adenomyosis induces neoangiogenesis and exaggerated myometrial peristalsis.[1]

Ultrasound

Though ultrasound cannot definitively diagnose adenomyosis, it can help to rule out other conditions with similar symptoms. Pitfalls in diagnosis of uterine adenomyosis include leiomyomas, endometrial carcinomas, myometrial contractions and muscular hypertrophy. Imaging features that favor adenomyosis instead of leiomyoma are poorly defined borders, minimal mass effect, an elliptical instead of globular shape, and absence of large vessels at the margin of the lesion. At endovaginal US, the presence of echogenic nodules or linear striations favor the diagnosis of adenomyosis along with absence of calcification, edge shadowing, and a whorled appearance. The presence of adenomyosis alters and distorts the USG appearance of the three uterine zones.[2] Adenomyosis most commonly appears as areas of decreased echogenecity of the myometrium, a sign found in approximately 75% of patients. The presence of dilated cystic glands or hemorrhagic foci within the heterotopic endometrial tissue results in presence of small myometrial cysts (usually < 5 mm in diameter) in approximately 50% of patients. When large or confluent, the areas of heterotopic endometrial tissue result in discrete echogenic nodules (> 5 mm in diameter). The sensitivity of endovaginal USG is 80–86%, the specificity 50–96% and the overall accuracy is 68–86%.

Magnetic Resonance Imaging (MRI)

It can be used to confirm a diagnosis of adenomyosis in women with abnormal uterine bleeding. MRI is currently regarded as the best imaging tool for differential diagnosis.[3] Thin-section high-resolution MRI acquired with a pelvic multicoil array are optimal for diagnosis of adenomyosis. Abnormal widening of the junctional zone is one of the MRI features associated with adenomyosis. When maximal junctional zone is 12 mm or greater, adenomyosis is diagnosed with a high degree of accuracy. With a maximal junctional zone thickness of 8–12 mm, secondary findings, such as relative thickening of the junctional zone in a localized area; poor definition of borders or high signal in intensity foci on T1 or T2 weighted images can be used to diagnose adenomyosis.[4,5]

With the advent of high-resolution imaging techniques, adenomyosis can be diagnosed with a high degree of accuracy. The imaging signs demonstrated with endovaginal US and MR imaging correspond closely to the varied appearances of this disease at histopathologic analysis. Endovaginal US can be used as the initial imaging modality in patients suspected of having adenomyosis, but US must be performed meticulously and in real time. MR imaging can be reserved for cases that are indeterminate at endovaginal US and for patients who will undergo uterus-sparing surgery.

HISTOPATHOLOGICAL DIAGNOSIS

Adenomyosis is a histopathological diagnosis. Histological examination will note benign endometrial glands, and stroma within the myometrium. These glands rarely undergo the same cyclic changes as the normal uterine endometrium. Studies have demonstrated both estrogen and progesterone receptors in tissue samples from adenomyosis. Histologically the glands exhibit an inactive or proliferative pattern. Rarely, one sees cystic hyperplasia or a pseudodecidual pattern. In general, there is a lack of inflammatory cells surrounding the foci of adenomyosis. Although, the areas do not undergo full menstrual-type changes, bleeding may occur in these ectopic areas, as evidenced by both gross and microscopic findings. Some foci of adenomyosis undergo decidual changes either during pregnancy or during estrogen-progestin therapy for endometriosis. The reaction of the myometrium to the ectopic endometrium is hyperplasia and hypertrophy of individual muscle fibers. Surrounding most foci of glands and stroma are localized areas of hyperplasia of the smooth muscle of the uterus. This change in the myometrium produces the globular enlargement of the uterus.

Adenomyosis can be diffuse or focal. Diffuse adenomyosis is found in two-thirds of cases. In the diffuse type, uterus is uniformly enlarged, usually two to three times normal size. The second presentation is a focal area or adenomyoma. This results in an asymmetrical uterus, and this special area of adenomyosis may have a pseudo capsule. It is often difficult to distinguish on physical examination from uterine leiomyomas. On visual inspection, the two entities are quite different. When a knife transects the myometrium, the cut surface protrudes convexly and has a spongy appearance and is whorled in myoma. The cut surface of a uterus with adenomyosis is darker than the white surface of a myoma. Sometimes, there are discrete area of adenomyosis that are not densely encapsulated and contain small, dark cystic spaces. There is no distinct cleavage plane around focal adenomyoma as there is with uterine myomas.

TREATMENT

Most women have some adenomyosis as they near menopause but few women have symptoms, and most women do not require any treatment. In symptomatic patients, treatment can be an enigma.

Medical Approach

For symptoms of dysmenorrhea and menorrhagia, simple pain relievers and nonsteroidal anti-inflammatory drugs (NSAIDs) may be useful. NSAIDs are usually started one or two days before beginning of menstruation and continued through the first few days of period.

Hormone Therapy

Symptoms such as heavy or painful periods can be controlled with hormonal therapies to relax the uterus, such as a levonorgestrel-releasing IUD (which is inserted into the uterus), aromatase inhibitors and oral contraceptive pill. In 2002, Imaoka et al, investigated a possible role of gonadotropin-releasing hormone analogs for the treatment of diffuse adenomyosis, as evidenced by MRI. They administered the analog over a 6-month period to 31 patients with MRI features suggestive of diffuse adenomyosis and concluded that use of gonadotropin-releasing hormone analogs is associated with a decrease in myometrium JZ width. Furthermore, asymmetric adenomyosis with high-signal intensity foci appears to be the most sensitive to hormonal therapy.

Inhibitors of Angiogenesis

New knowledge of a modified angiogenesis in heterotopic uterine mucosa in case of adenomyosis is opening the way for a new treatment line. Starting from the observation that dopamine and its agonists, such as cabergoline (Cb2), promote endocytosis of VEGF receptor (VEGFR)-2 in endothelial cells, thereby preventing VEGF–VEGFR-2 binding and reducing neoangiogenesis.[6]

Another approach aimed at inhibiting angiogenesis has been studied by the group of Creatsas using pentoxifylline, a phosphodiesterase inhibitor.[7]

Surgical Approach

Uterine Artery Embolization

In this minimally invasive procedure, tiny particles are used to block the blood vessels that provide blood flow to the adenomyosis. The particles are guided through a tiny tube inserted into the vagina through the cervix. With blood supply cut off, the adenomyosis shrinks.[8]

Endometrial Ablation

This minimally invasive procedure destroys the lining of the uterus. Endometrial ablation has been found to be effective in relieving symptoms in some patients when adenomyosis has not penetrated deeply into the muscle wall of the uterus.

MRI Focused Ultrasound

Thermal ablative effect of MRIgFUS[9] on adenomyosis in improving clinical parameters has been documented in recent trials. Most adenomyotic lesions could be satisfactorily ablated close to the serosal surface or the endometrium and, at 6 months, the mean uterine volume decreased by 12.7%. Symptom severity score improved significantly during the 6 months of follow-up and no serious complications were observed. Therefore, it seems that MRIgFUS represents a new, safe and effective method for the ablation of adenomyotic tissue.

Hysterectomy

Unfortunately, the disorder tends to progress and not uncommonly ultimately results in hysterectomy where the diagnosis is finally formally made. Hysterectomy is the definitive treatment if this therapy is appropriate for the woman's age, parity, and plans for future reproduction. Size of the uterus, degree of prolapse, and presence of associated pelvic pathology determine the choice of surgical approach. For the woman in her late 40s, the ovaries are often removed as a risk-reducing measure against ovarian carcinoma.

PROGNOSIS

Symptoms usually go away after menopause. Hysterectomy completely relieves symptoms. Medical, hormonal treatment and conservative surgeries have a role in alleviating symptoms where hysterectomy is not desirable and fertility conservation is a priority.

REFERENCES

1. Fusi L, Cloke B, Brosens JJ. The uterine junctional zone. Best Pract Res Clin Obstet Gynaecol. 2006;20:479-81.
2. Reinhold C, Tafajoli F, Wang L. Imaging features of adenomyosis. Hum Reprod update. 1998;4:337-49.
3. Reinhold C, McCarthy S, Bret PM, et al. Diffuse adenomyosis: comparison of endovaginal US and MR imaging with histopathologic correlation. Radiology. 1996;199:151-8.
4. Togashi K, Ozasa H, Konishi I, et al. Enlarged uterus: differentiation between adenomyosis and leiomyomas with MR imaging. Radiology. 1989;171:531-4.
5. Polina, et al. Indian J Radiol imaging. 2012;22(2):93-7.
6. Novella-Maestre E, Carda C, Noguera I, et al. Dopamine agonist administration causes a reduction in endometrial implants through modulation of angiogenesis in experimentally induced endometriosis. Hum. Reprod. DOI: 10.1093/humrep/den499 (2009).
7. Vlahos NF, Gregoriou O, Deliveliotou A, et al. Effect of pentoxiphylline on vascular endothelial growth factor C and flk-1 expression on endometrial implants in the rat endometriosis model. Fertil. Steril. DOI: 10.1016/j.fertnstert.2008.10.056 (2009).
8. Kim MD Won JW, Lee DY, Ahn CS: Uterine artery embolisation for adenomyosis without fibroids. Clin. Radiol. 2004;59(6):520-6.
9. Fukunishi H, Funaki K, Sawada K, et al. Early results of magnetic resonance-guided focused ultrasound surgery of adenomyosis: analysis of 20 cases. J Min Inv Gynecol. 2008;15:571-9.

Uterine Polyps

Pankaj Desai, Purvi Patel

INTRODUCTION

A polyp is defined as an abnormal growth of tissue projecting from a mucous membrane. If it is attached to the surface by a narrow elongated stalk, it is said to be pedunculated. If no stalk is present, it is said to be sessile polyp. Uterine polyps, also known as endometrial polyps are a common cause of abnormal uterine bleeding in premenopausal and postmenopausal women. Many uterine polyps, however, can be asymptomatic and can be found accidentally on a USG scan of the subject for some other pathology.

Endometrial polyps are obviously localized endometrial intrauterine overgrowth that may be single or multiple, may measure from a few millimeters to centimeters, and may be sessile or pedunculated.[1] Pedunculated polyps are more common than sessile ones. It is estimated that 10% of women have endometrial polyps.[2] In 20% cases, they are multiple. Most polyps arise from the fundal region of the uterus and extend towards the internal os of the cervix. Occasionally, they project through the external cervical os and can be seen in the vagina. Endometrial polyps consist of endometrial glands, stroma, and blood vessels.[3] These polyps are usually benign, although some can be malignant or can eventually turn malignant (precancerous polyps).

ETIOLOGY

The exact cause of polyps is unknown, and their heterogeneity makes identification of a single causative factor unlikely. However, there is a broad consensus to the fact that there is some strong endocrinal basis for development of polyps in the uterus. Estrogens have been thought to play a major role in formation of polyps. Their response seems to follow the endometrial response to estrogen—growing with estrogens.

Genetic factors may be contributory to the development of endometrial polyps, with reports identifying clusters of anomalies in chromosomes 6 and 12, which may alter the proliferative process, resulting in endometrial overgrowth and polyp formation.[4] The preponderance of polyps in the postmenopausal group may be partly explained by an increase in a proliferation—regulating protein, p63, in this group. This protein is also a marker of reserve cells of the basalis layer, from which polyps are believed to arise.[5]

Risk factors for the development of endometrial polyps include age, hypertension, obesity, and tamoxifen use.[6,7] Increasing age appears to be the best-documented risk indicator for endometrial polyps. The prevalence of endometrial polyps appears to increase by age during the reproductive years, but it is not clear whether it continues to rise or decrease after menopause.[8,9] An increased level of estrone is the likely mechanism in obese women, although the link with hypertension may be a confounder of obesity, rather than a direct correlation to the causation of polyps.

Tamoxifen is a weak estrogen agonist in postmenopausal endometrial tissue, and a spectrum of endometrial abnormalities is associated with its use, including polyps. Women using tamoxifen are at specific risk for development of polyps, with studies reporting up to 30% to 60% prevalence.[10-12] In another study, the incidence of endometrial polyps reported in women treated with tamoxifen than in untreated women was 8–36% versus 0–10%.[13] Tamoxifen-related polyps are different.

Whether hormone replacement therapy leads to development of endometrial polyps is not clear as some studies report higher prevalence of endometrial polyps in women using hormone therapy[8,14] whereas others do not.[15,16] A progestogen with high antiestrogenic activity, as well as use of oral contraceptive pills may have a protective effect on the development of endometrial polyps.[8]

Endometrial polyps have found to be associated with other benign diseases like myomas, cervical polyps, and endometriosis.

The reported prevalence of endometrial polyps varies widely and ranges from 7.8% to 34.9%, depending on the definition of a polyp, diagnostic method used, and the population studied.[8,9]

PATHOLOGY

The central core of the polyp consists of basal type of endometrium covered by functional endometrium, which may vary from inactive to secretory type. The stroma is typically fibrous but may contain endometrial stroma or occasionally smooth muscles. The glands are irregularly outlined and may be out of phase with endometrium. A cluster of thick walled vessels is found in the base of the stalk, which tend to send a solitary vessel in the stalk, identified on color Doppler.

Those in the lower uterine segment may contain endocervical glands.

Histologically, the polyps can be classified as hyperplastic (resemble diffuse nonpolypoid endometrial hyperplasia), atrophic (low columnar or cuboidal cells lining cystically dilated glands, typically in postmenopausal patients) or functional (resemble normal cycling endometrium, rare). Typical histopathological appearance of a polyp is shown in Figure 1.

The tamoxifen-associated polyps are large (mean diameter, 5 cm) sessile with a honeycomb appearance containing bizarre stellate shape of glands and frequent epithelial and stromal metaplasias with periglandular

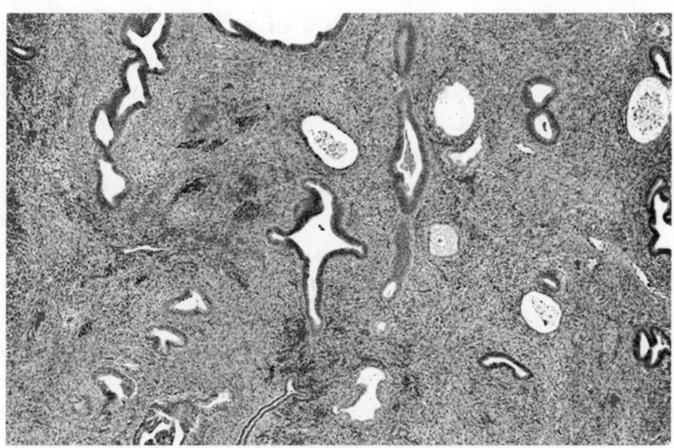

Fig. 1: Histological section of endometrial polyp
(For color version, see Plate 4)

stromal condensation. They result in malignant transformation in up to 3% cases. They are microscopically differentiated from usual polyps by their mixture of proliferative activity (cystic glandular dilatation), unusual epithelial differentiation (metaplasia), and focal periglandular stromal condensation.[17,18]

CLINICAL PRESENTATION

Although abnormal uterine bleeding is a common presentation, women with a polyp may be asymptomatic and may be diagnosed incidentally on imaging for other indications. Most women with symptomatic endometrial polyps present with abnormal uterine bleeding which has been recently classified abnormal uterine bleeding (AUB) associated with polyps (AUB-P) for premenopausal women, which has been approved by the FIGO Executive Board as a FIGO Classification system.[19] Overall, 64% to 88% of premenopausal women with endometrial polyps have symptoms,[20] most commonly presenting with menorrhagia, irregular menses, postcoital bleeding, or intermenstrual bleeding. Endometrial polyps account for 39% of all abnormal vaginal bleeding in premenopausal women,[21] and this bleeding is believed to be due to stromal congestion within the polyp leading to venous stasis and apical necrosis.[22] It is important to note that symptoms do not correlate with polyp number, diameter, and site.[23]

Increasing age appears to be the best-documented risk indicator for endometrial polyps. The prevalence of endometrial polyps appears to increase by age during the reproductive years, but it is not clear whether it continues to rise or decreases after menopause. For both premenopausal and postmenopausal women with an endometrial polyp, abnormal vaginal bleeding occurs in approximately 64% of cases and is the most common presenting symptom for women with this disease.[20]

In the postmenopausal period, 56% of women with an endometrial polyp present with symptoms such as postmenopausal bleeding.[20,23] In premenopausal women, endometrial polyps are associated with infertility, although the causal relationship remains uncertain. Hypotheses include mechanical obstruction hindering ostium function and affecting sperm migration,[24] or biochemical effects of polyps on implantation or embryo development. The latter reflects the finding of increased levels of metalloproteinases and cytokines such as interferon-gamma found in polyps when compared with normal uterine tissue.[25] Endometrial polyps can distort the endometrial cavity, may have a detrimental effect on endometrial receptivity and increase the risk of implantation failure.[26] Women treated with gonadotropins for infertility are exposed to a higher level of estrogen, which can predispose them to development of endometrial polyps. The incidence of polyps occurring in infertile women is widely variable, ranging between 3.8% to 38.5% of women with primary infertility, 1.8% to 17% of women with secondary infertility, and 1.9% to 24% of infertile women when combined.[27]

There is a significantly increased association of endometrial polyps with endometriotic infertility and hysteroscopy is recommended if endometriosis is detected in a woman undergoing evaluation for infertility, even if hysterosalpingography and transvaginal ultrasonography does not suggest endometrial polyps.[28,29]

Most endometrial polyps are benign; however, they may become hyperplastic, with malignant transformation developing in 0% to 12.9% of polyps in various case series reported to date. Although the risk of malignancy is low in premenopausal women, it has been significantly correlated with increasing age and menopausal status; polyps with a size greater than 1.5 cm; and hypertension and tamoxifen use.

A study found a 27% spontaneous regression rate in incidentally detected endometrial polyps at 1 year.[30] Smaller polyps <1 cm are more likely to regress spontaneously, whereas those >1 cm are more likely to persist and cause abnormal uterine bleeding. Polyp regression may be associated with isolated episodes of menorrhagia associated with cramping possibly due to the passage of endometrial polyps followed by resumption of normal menstruation.

DIAGNOSIS

Imaging Modalities

Transvaginal Ultrasonography

On transvaginal ultrasonography (TVS), an endometrial polyp typically appears as a hyperechoic lesion with regular contours within the uterine lumen, outlining the endometrial walls on which it rests, surrounded by a thin hyperechoic halo. Cystic spaces corresponding to dilated glands filled with proteinaceous fluid may be seen within the polyp or the polyp may appear as a nonspecific endometrial thickening or focal mass within the endometrial cavity. Similar findings may be visualized in endometrial hyperplasia or submucosal fibroid. To aid in the diagnosis of an endometrial polyp, TVS is best performed in premenopausal women before day 10 of the cycle when the endometrium is at its thinnest to minimize the risk of false-positive and false-negative findings. In a single large prospective study evaluating the causes of menorrhagia, the reported sensitivity, specificity, positive and negative predictive values (PPV and NPV) of TVS for the diagnosis of endometrial polyps were 86%, 94%, 91% and 90%, respectively.[31]

Color flow Doppler or power Doppler may help to identify vascular network and the feeding vessel of polyp and may improve the diagnostic capability of TVS. However, Doppler examination is not a substitute for surgical removal of polyps followed by pathologic evaluation when malignancy is suspected.

Saline Infusion Sonography

The use of saline infusion sonography (SIS) or sonohysterography (SHG) increases sonographic contrast of the endometrial cavity, enabling delineation of the size, location and other features of an endometrial polyp (Fig. 2). With SIS, polyps appear as echogenic, smooth, intracavitary masses with either broad bases or thin stalks outlined by fluid. This technique may outline small endometrial polyps missed on gray-scale TVS and is likely to improve the diagnostic accuracy.

Differentiating endometrial polyps from submucosal fibroids can still be difficult, but examination of lesion echotexture and identification of overlying echogenic endometrium are useful features to distinguish the two.

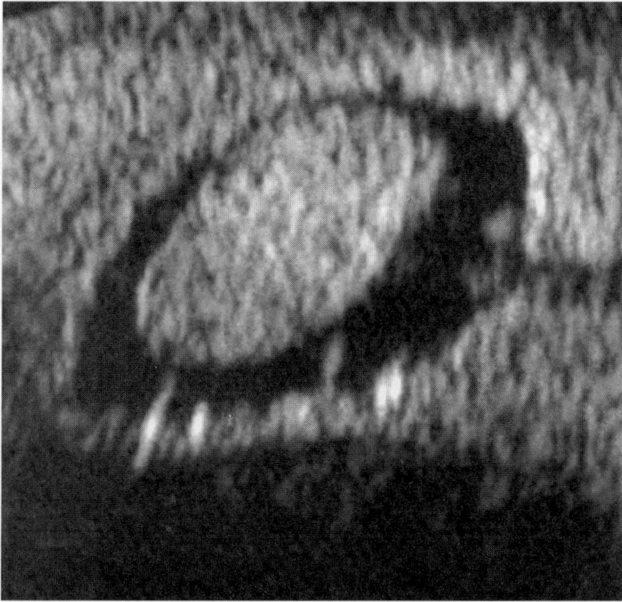

Fig. 2: Endometrial polyp on saline infusion sonography
(For color version, see Plate 4)

SIS has the advantage of assessing both the uterine cavity and other uterine and pelvic structures and the potential to assess tubal patency in patients with infertility. Disadvantages of SIS include an inability to determine final endometrial disease, a longer learning curve compared with non-contrast TVS, and patient discomfort caused by fluid leakage or pain with the use of a balloon catheter.

Studies with noncontrast 3-dimensional (3D) TVS show limited improvement to diagnosis when compared with 2D TVS. Adding saline solution contrast into the endometrial cavity to perform 3D SIS is slightly superior for the diagnosis of endometrial polyps. Considering the greater expense of 3D sonography and its less-frequent availability, 2D US with intrauterine contrast should be preferred as an effective and reliable noninvasive method to diagnose polyps.

Histological Diagnosis

Blind Dilation and Curettage

Blind dilation and curettage is inaccurate in diagnosing endometrial polyps and should not be used as a diagnostic method. A curette can miss pedunculated polyps and fragmentation of sessile polyps may make histological diagnosis difficult.

Hysteroscopic-guided Biopsy

Hysteroscopy with guided biopsy is the gold standard in the diagnosis of endometrial polyps. The main advantage of hysteroscopy is the ability to visualize and remove polyps concurrently. Typical appearance of the endometrial cavity, endometrium and polyp on hysteroscopy has been shown in Figure 3. Hysteroscopic appearance of multiple polyps is shown in Figure 4.

With continuing technological improvements producing narrow diameter hysteroscopes, operative hysteroscopy can be readily performed in an outpatient setting. However, polyps larger than the diameter of the internal cervical os may be best removed with the patient under general anesthesia given the increased patient discomfort and longer operating time.

Other Modalities

The use of ionizing radiation, iodinated contrast materials and patient discomfort, limit the usefulness of hysterosalpingography (HSG) for this indication. Endometrial polyps can be identified on magnetic resonance imaging (MRI) as low signal intensity intracavitary masses surrounded by high signal intensity fluid and endometrium by T2-weighted magnetic resonance imaging. Very high cost and limited availability with limited advantages over sonography preclude this technique from routine use. Computed tomography scanning has limited role because of its low sensitivity compared to TVS, even with contrast enhancement.

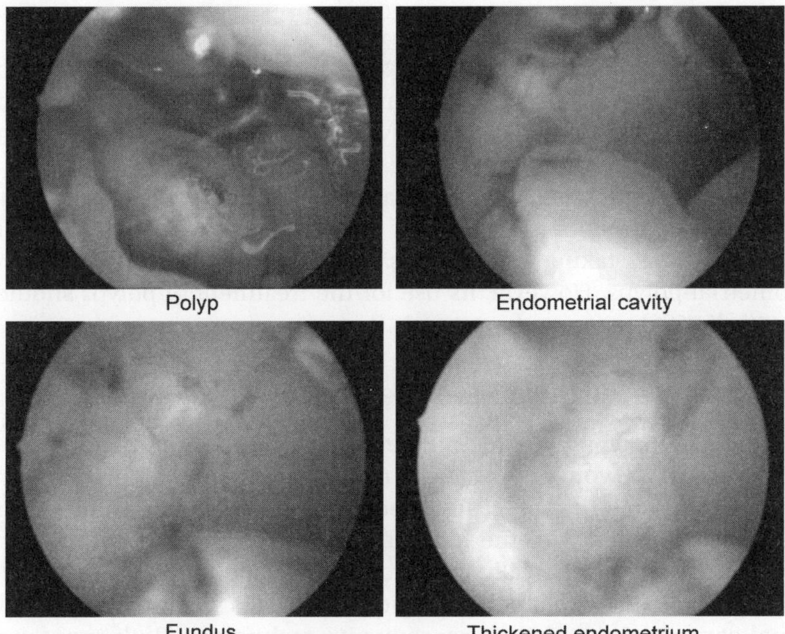

Fig. 3: Endometrial polyp on hysteroscopy
(For color version, see Plate 4)

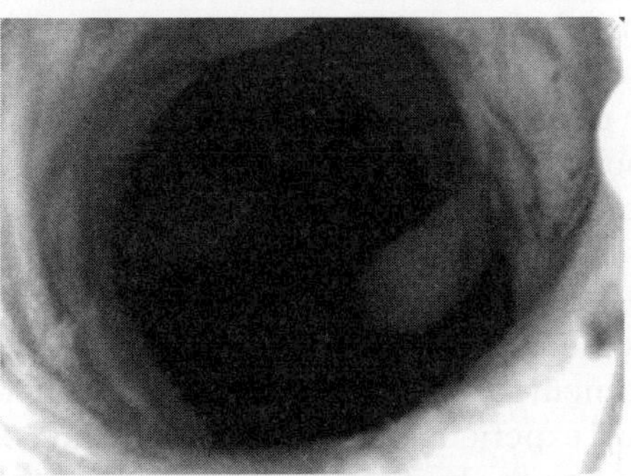

Fig. 4: Multiple polyps on hysteroscopy
(For color version, see Plate 5)

MANAGEMENT

Conservative Management

Since most polyps are benign, there is a place for expectant management; especially for asymptomatic small polyps less than 1 cm, which are likely to regress. Asymptomatic postmenopausal polyps are unlikely to be malignant and observation is an option after discussion with the patient.

Medical Management

Medical management has a limited role for endometrial polyps. GnRH agonists are reported to give short-term symptomatic relief for endometrial polyps, but cost, side effects and symptom recurrence after treatment cessation preclude its use for this indication.

The use of some types of hormonal therapies may have a preventative role for polyp formation.[32] The use of levonorgestrel releasing intrauterine system in women taking tamoxifen is reported to reduce the incidence of endometrial polyps. However, its use for the treatment of polyps should be currently limited to research protocols.[33]

Conservative Surgical Management

Symptomatic polyps should be removed in the premenopausal or postmenopausal woman because evidence reports improvement in symptoms in majority of cases. Because postmenopausal bleeding in women is associated with the highest risk of premalignant and malignant tissue changes, it is especially important to exclude this histologically. For the infertile patient with a polyp, surgical removal is recommended to allow natural conception or assisted reproductive technology. Both spontaneous pregnancy rates and those associated with assisted reproductive technology are reportedly increased after polypectomy.

Studies indicate that removal of endometrial polyps by blind curettage is successful less than 50% of the time, and in many cases removal is incomplete.[34,35] When hysteroscopic treatment is available, blind curettage should not be used as a diagnostic or therapeutic intervention. If hysteroscopy is not available, the patient should be referred for appropriate treatment.

Hysteroscopic polypectomy is effective and safe as both a diagnostic and therapeutic intervention. It is the gold standard treatment for endometrial polyps. There are a variety of methods practiced to remove polyps at hysteroscopy; however, there are no differences in clinical outcomes with different hysteroscopic polypectomy techniques.

The type of instruments used for polyp removal is dependent on availability, expense, and surgical experience, as well as the size and location of the lesion. Large and sessile polyps are best removed with a hysteroscope fitted with an electrosurgical loop (resectoscope), whereas small and pedunculated polyps may be removed with either scissors or small polyp grasping forceps in an operating hysteroscope under direct vision. While there is no recurrence of polyps in the resectoscopic group, the use of grasping forceps may be associated with a small recurrence rate.

Other instruments include bipolar systems and the hysteroscopic morcellator, although these techniques may be limited by availability and the cost of disposable and specialized equipment.

Radical Surgical Options

Hysterectomy is the definitive treatment for endometrial polyps. Although this guarantees no recurrence and no potential for malignancy, its invasive nature, risk of surgical morbidity, cost, and implication for future fertility are factors that require careful consideration.

REFERENCES

1. Kim KR, Peng R, Ro JY, Robboy SJ. A diagnostically useful histopathologic feature of endometrial polyp: the long axis of endometrial glands arranged parallel to surface epithelium. Am J Surg Pathol. 2004;28:1057-62.
2. Jane B. Practical gynaecological ultrasound. Cambridge University Press. 2007.p.65. ISBN 1-900151-51-0.
3. Peterson WF, Novak ER. Endometrial polyps. Obstet Gynecol. 1956;8:40-9.
4. Vanni R, Dal Cin P, Marras S, et al. Endometrial polyp: Another benign tumor characterized by 12q13-q15 changes. Cancer Genet Cytogenet. 1993;68:32-3.
5. Nogueira AA, Sant'Ana de Almeida EC, Poli Neto OB, Zambelli Ramalho LN, Rosa e Silva JC, Candido dos Reis FJ. Immunohisto-chemical expression of p63 in endometrial polyps: evidence that a basal cell immunophenotype is maintained. Menopause. 2006;13:826-30.
6. Cohen I. Endometrial pathologies associated with postmenopausal tamoxifen treatment. Gynecol Oncol. 2004;94:256-66.
7. Onalan R, Onalan G, Tonguc E, Ozdener T, Dogan M, Mollamahmutoglu L. Body mass index is an independent risk factor for the development of endometrial polyps in patients undergoing in vitro fertilization. Fertil Steril. 2009;91:1056-60.
8. Dreisler E, Stampe Sorensen S, Ibsen PH, Lose G. Prevalence of endometrial polyps and abnormal uterine bleeding in a Danish population aged 20-74 years. Ultrasound Obstet Gynecol. 2009;33:102-08.
9. Anastasiadis PG, Koutlaki NG, Skaphida PG, Galazios GC, Tsikouras PN, Liberis VA. Endometrial polyps: prevalence, detection, and malignant potential in women with abnormal uterine bleeding. Eur J Gynaecol Oncol. 2000;21:180-3.
10. Hann LE, Gretz EM, Bach AM, Francis SM. Sonohysterography for evaluation of the endometrium in women treated with tamoxifen. AJR Am J Roentgenol. 2001;177:337-42.
11. Exacoustos C, Zupi E, Cangi B, Chiaretti M, Arduini D, Romanini C. Endometrial evaluation in postmenopausal breast cancer patients receiving tamoxifen: an ultrasound, color flow Doppler, hysteroscopic and histological study. Ultrasound Obstet Gynecol. 1995;6:435-42.
12. Reslova T, Tosner J, Resl M, Kugler R, Vavrova I. Endometrial polyps: a clinical study of 245 cases. Arch Gynecol Obstet. 1999;262:133-9.
13. Schlesinger C, Seiryu K, Ascher SM, Kendell M, Lage JM, Silverberg SG. Endometrial polyps: a comparison study of patients receiving tamoxifen with two control groups. Int J Gynecol Pathol. 1998;17:302-11.
14. Maia H Jr, Barbosa IC, Marques D, Calmon LC, Ladipo OA, Coutinho EM. Hysteroscopy and transvaginal sonography in menopausal women receiving hormone replacement therapy. J Am Assoc Gynecol Laparosc. 1996;4:13-8.

15. Elliott J, Connor M, Lashen H. The value of outpatient hysteroscopy in diagnosing endometrial pathology in postmenopausal women with and without hormone replacement therapy. Acta Obstet Gynecol Scand. 2003;82:1112-9.
16. Perrone G, DeAngelis C, Critelli C, et al. Hysteroscopic findings in postmenopausal abnormal uterine bleeding: a comparison between HRT users and non-users. Maturitas. 2002;43:251-5.
17. Ismail SM. Pathology of endometrium treated with tamoxifen. J Clin Pathol. 1994;47:827-33.
18. Cohen CJ. Tamoxifen and endometrial cancer: tamoxifen effects on the human female genital tract. Semin Oncol. 1997;24(suppl 1):S1-55-S1-64.
19. Munro M, Critchley HO, Broder MS, Fraser IS. FIGO Working Group on Menstrual Disorders. FIGO classification system (PALM-COEIN) for causes of abnormal uterine bleeding in nongravid women of reproductive age. Int J Gynecol Obstet. 2011;113:3-11.
20. Golan A, Sagiv R, Berar M, Ginath S, Glezerman M. Bipolar electrical energy in physiologic solutionda revolution in operative hysteroscopy. J Am Assoc Gynecol Laparosc. 2001;8:252-8.
21. Valle RF. Hysteroscopy for gynecologic diagnosis. Clin Obstet Gynecol. 1983;26:253-76.
22. Jakab A, Ovari L, Juhasz B, Birinyi L, Bacsko G, Toth Z. Detection of feeding artery improves the ultrasound diagnosis of endometrial polyps in asymptomatic patients. Eur J Obstet Gynecol Reproduct Biol. 2005;119:103-7.
23. Hassa H, Tekin B, Senses T, Kaya M, Karatas A. Are the site, diameter, and number of endometrial polyps related with symptomatology? Am J Obstet Gynecol. 2006;194:718-21.
24. Shokeir TA, Shalan HM, El-Shafei MM. Significance of endometrial polyps detected hysteroscopically in eumenorrheic infertile women. J Obstet Gynaecol Res. 2004;30:84-9.
25. Inagaki N, Ung L, Otani T, Wilkinson D, Lopata A. Uterine cavity matrix metalloproteinases and cytokines in patients with leiomyoma, adenomyosis or endometrial polyp. Eur J Obstet Gynecol Reproduct Biol. 2003;111:197-203.
26. Alansari LM, Wardie P. Endometrial polyps and subfertility. Hum fertile (camb). 2012;15(3):129-33.
27. Preutthipan S, Linasmita V. A prospective comparative study between hysterosalpingography and hysteroscopy in the detection of intrauterine pathology in patients with infertility. J Obstet Gynaecol Res. 2003;29:33-7.
28. Shen L, Wang Q, Huang W, Wang Q, Yuan Q, Huang Y, et al. High prevalence of endometrial polyps in endometriosis-associated infertility. Fertil Steril. 2011;95(8):2722-4.
29. Kim MR, Kim YA, Jo MY, Hwang Kj, Ryu HS. High frequency of endometrial polyps in endometriosis. J Am Assoc Gynecol Laparosc. 2003;10(1):46-8.
30. Lieng M, Istre O, Sandvik L, Qvigstad E. Prevalence, 1-Year regression rate, and clinical significance of asymptomatic endometrial polyps: Cross-sectional study. J Minim Invasive Gynecol. 2009;16:465-71.
31. Vercellini P, Cortesi I, Oldani S, Moschetta M, De Giorgi O, Crosignani PG. The role of transvaginal ultrasonography and outpatient diagnostic hysteroscopy in the evaluation of patients with menorrhagia. Hum Reprod. 1997;12:1768-71.

32. Oguz S, Sargin A, Kelekci S, Aytan H, Tapisiz OL, Mollamahmutoglu L. The role of hormone replacement therapy in endometrial polyp formation. Maturitas. 2005;50:231-6.
33. Gardner FJ, Konje JC, Bell SC, et al. Prevention of tamoxifen induced endometrial polyps using a levonorgestrel releasing intrauterine system long-term follow-up of a randomised control trial. Gynecol Oncol. 2009;114:452-6.
34. Bettocchi S, Ceci O, Vicino M, Marello F, Impedovo L, Selvaggi L. Diagnostic inadequacy of dilatation and curettage. Fertil Steril. 2001;75:803-5.
35. Svirsky R, Smorgick N, Rozowski U, et al. Can we rely on blind endometrial biopsy for detection of focal intrauterine pathology? Am J Obstet Gynecol. 2008;199:115.e1-115.e3.

Chapter 38

Pelvic Organs Prolapse

Navneet Magon, Reeti Mehra

Pelvic organ prolapse is the downward displacement of structures that are normally situated adjacent to the vaginal vault i.e. urethra, bladder, uterus, rectum and pouch of Douglas through the pelvic floor. They may be considered as hernias as each one of them is associated with defect in the supporting structures of the uterus and vagina.

CLINICAL TYPES

Genital prolapse is broadly classified into:
- Vaginal
- Uterine prolapse

Vaginal

Vaginal prolapse may occur without uterine prolapse.
- Cystocele: Herniation of the bladder through the lax anterior vaginal wall. It is seen as descent of the upper 2/3rd of the vagina.
- Urethrocele: Herniation of urethra through the lower 1/3rd of vagina.
- Cystourethrocele: Both may coexist.
- Rectocele: Laxity of lower 2/3rd of the posterior vaginal wall, associated with herniation of the rectum.
- Relaxed perineum: Torn perineal body produces a gaping introitus and deficient perineum.
- Enterocele: Herniation of upper 1/3rd of posterior vaginal wall, may contain omentum or small bowel loop.

Vault Prolapse

Prolapse of the vault of vagina following an abdominal or vaginal hysterectomy.

Nulliparous prolapse/Uterovaginal prolapse: Uterus prolapse occurs first, followed by the vagina due to congenital weakness of the ligaments as in spina bifida occulta or other connective tissue disorders. So cystocele and rectocele may not be associated and cervical elongation may be absent.

ETIOLOGY

Vaginal delivery with consequent injury to the supporting system is the single most important predisposing factor.

- Premature bearing down efforts
- Instrumental delivery
- Prolonged second stage of labor
- Fundal pressure
- Precipitate labor
- Ill nourished mothers
- Early resumption of activities
- Repeated pregnancy and childbirth

All the above factors predispose the female to prolapse.

Vaginal delivery in such predisposing factors leads to:

- Overstretching of Mackenrodt and uterosacral ligaments
- Breaks in the endopelvic fascia
- Loss of levator function
- Neuromuscular damage of levator muscles.

Besides childbirth, other aggravating factors may be:

- Postmenopausal atrophy due to hypoestrogenism
- Increased abdominal pressure as in bronchitis, asthma and constipation
- Under nutrition
- Obesity
- Myohyperplasia or fibroids
- Neuropathy of diabetes
- Smoking also has antiestrogenic activity
- Corticosteroid use in certain medical disorders. They weaken the connective tissue
- Connective tissue disorders like Ehlers Danlos syndrome.

SUPPORTS OF THE UTERUS

The uterus is normally anteflexed and anteverted, the external os is at the level of ischial spines. Pelvic support structures include:

- The muscles and connective tissue of the pelvic floor
- The fibromuscular tissue of the vaginal wall
- The endopelvic connective tissue
- Bony element

Also there is described a three tier system of uterine support where-in:

- **The upper tier:** Supports the uterus and keeps it in anteverted position. It includes:
    - Endopelvic fascia covering the uterus
    - Round ligaments
    - Broad ligaments with intervening pelvic cellular tissues
- **The middle tier:** They are the strongest support system. They are composed of:

- Pericervical ring: It is in the shape of a collar encircling the supravaginal cervix and consists of fibroelastic connective tissue.
  - Function: Cervical stabilization within the inter ischial diameter.
  - Connections:
    a. The pericervical ring connects with pubocervical ligaments at 11 o'clock and 1 o'clock position and proximal pubocervical ligament centrally
    b. Cardinal ligaments at 3 and 9 o'clock position
    c. Uterosacral ligaments at 5 o'clock and 7 o'clock position and proximal rectovaginal septum centrally

These ligaments are condensations of the deep endopelvic connective tissue and are the primary proximal suspensory elements of the urogenital complex.

- Pelvic cellular tissue
  Consists of: - Connective tissue
  - Smooth muscles

Blood vessels and nerves pass through the pelvic cellular tissue.

The connective tissue of the pelvis is also called endopelvic fascia.

The endopelvic fascia may be divided into:

⊃ Parietal fascia
⊃ Visceral fascia
⊃ Deep endopelvic connective tissue

Parietal fascia: They are dense membranes around the pelvic surface of skeletal muscles including:

⊃ Obturator fascia
⊃ Levator ani fascia
⊃ Coccygeus fascia
⊃ Piriformis fascia

The visceral fascia is the fascia around the vagina, uterus, bladder and rectum. The tubes and ovaries are not invested by a visceral fascia.

THE DEEP ENDOPELVIC CONNECTIVE TISSUE

This deep endopelvic tissue gets condensed at places to form ligaments which are the primary proximal supports of the uterovaginal complex and are attached to the cervical ring as mentioned before.

⊃ Mackenrodt—also called cardinal ligaments
⊃ Uterosacral ligaments
⊃ Pubocervical ligament/fascia.

Inferior Tier

The support is given by:

⊃ Pelvic floor muscles—mainly levator ani
⊃ Endopelvic fascia
⊃ Perineal body
⊃ Urogenital diaphragm.

The pelvic diaphragm or levator ani forms a basin covering the pelvic outlet. The defect in the diaphragm is the urogenital hiatus through which the prolapse occurs.

The puborectalis, pubococcygeus and iliococcygeus cover the posterior and lateral position of the pelvic outlet. The superior insertion of iliococcygeus extends as arcus tendineus, levator ani from the ischial spine posteriorly to the pubic tubercle anteriorly. Immediately inferior to the muscular arch is the thickening of the parietal fascia of the iliococcygeus which is called the "white line" or arcus tendineus pelvic fascia. This white line serves the function of midvaginal lateral support.

The levator ani is like a hammock supporting the urethra, vagina and the canal and guards the urogenital hiatus.

The levator plate: Thick band of connective formed by medial fibers of the two levator ani. It extends from the anorectal junction and the coccyx and some fibers encircle the anorectal junction and insert into the perineal body. It forms a horizontal shelf over which the rectum, upper vagina and uterus rests. The horizontal posterior of the plate is maintained by pubococcygeus and iliococcygeus.

Perineal Body

Solid pyramidal structures at the center of the perineum, which receive the muscles, like the hub of a wheel. Superficially passing in the perineal body are the external anal sphincter muscles, bulbospongiosis and superficial transverse perinei muscles. Deeper is a fascial layer and then the deep transverse perinei muscles and the levator ani. Clinically, holding the perineum between two fingers inside the introitus and the thumb outside assesses it.

DE LANCY'S BIOMECHANICAL ANALYSIS

He has divided the weakening of vaginal support in three levels:

Proximal Level I

Suspension by ligaments of the paracolpium results in:
- Uterovaginal prolapse
- Post hysterectomy vaginal vault prolapse
- Enterocele
  The cause of problems is at or above the level of ischial spines.

Mid Vaginal Level II Support

It is due to lateral attachment of fascial septa to the pelvic sidewall. The septa attached to the white line and its muscle and weakening leads to:
- Paravaginal defect
- Pararectal defect

Level III Support

It is due to fusion of urogenital diaphragm anteriorly and perineal body posteriorly. Damage leads to:

- Stress urinary continence
- Perineal body deficits

Cystocele and rectocele are central defects within the pubocervical and rectovaginal septum.

SYMPTOMS OF PROLAPSE

There are variable symptoms, from minor to profound.

- Feeling of something coming down per vaginum
- Discomfort during walking
- Backache
- Dragging pain in lower abdomen
- Urinary symptoms (more in cystocele)
  - Difficulty in passing urine
  - Incomplete evacuation
  - Urgency
  - Frequency
  - Repeated UTIs
  - Retention of urine
  - Stress urinary incontinence (SUI) in urethrocele
  - May have to reduce cystocele to be able to pass urine
- Bowel symptoms
  - Incomplete evacuation
  - May have to reduce mass to evacuate
- Decubitus ulcer may cause white discharge or blood stained discharge

CLINICAL EVALUATION

- POP (pelvic organ prolapse) is evaluated by pelvic examination in both dorsal and standing position.
- The patient is asked to strain or cough or perform valsalva maneuver and sometimes even asked to squat/strain to show the degree of prolapse to retract the posterior vaginal wall.
- A Sims speculum may be used to retract the posterior vaginal wall to demonstrate the cystourethrocele.
- The same speculum or an anterior vaginal wall retractor may be used to demonstrate the enterocele which is in the upper posterior vagina close to the cervix and the rectocele which is in the mid and lower posterior vagina.
- A rectovaginal examination may be done and then patient asked to strain. A bulge appearing above the rectal finger is the enterocele.

- SUI is demonstrated by examining the patient in full bladder and the cystocele must be reduced before asking the patient to cough to look for SUI.
- Note is made of degree of uterine prolapse, any decubitus ulcer, any depigmentation.
- For procidentia, the entire uterus and its fundus should be palpable and so a thumb placed anterior to the uterus would oppose a finger placed posterior to the uterus.
- Pap smear should be taken and if suspicious, biopsy from decubitus ulcer may be taken as rarely cancer may develop.
- Huge cystocele may lead to obstructive uropathy leading to bladder hypertrophy, UTI, hydronephrosis.
- Rarely a prolapse may be incarcerated and irreducible. It will require ice packs and magnesium sulphate dressings to reduce the edema.

EXTENT OF PROLAPSE/QUANTIFICATION METHODS

- Degrees of prolapse—I, II, IIIrd degree and procidentia
- Baden Walker Halfway system
- POP-Q, pelvic organ quantification system.

Clinical Degrees of Uterine Prolapse

- First degree: Uterus descends from its normal position (ischial spine) but external os still in the vagina
- Second degree : External os protrudes up to the hymen
- Third degree: The external os protrudes outside the hymen, but part of uterus body still inside the vagina
- Fourth degree/Procidentia: Uterine body lies outside the introitus with eversion of the vagina.

Baden Walker Halfway System

Extent of prolapse is recorded using a number 0 to 4 at each of the six defined sites in the vagina, i.e.

1. Urethral
2. Vesical
3. Uterine
4. Cul de sac
5. Rectal
6. Perineal

0 = Normal anatomic position

4 = Maximal prolapse

- When grade in doubt—use the greater grade
- If grade still in doubt—examine while patient standing

➲ Strength of levator contraction on performing Kegel's exercises may be mentioned as 0–4.

Example

13/44/33

1 = Small urethrocele

3 = Cystocele significant coming halfway past hymen

4 = Complete out uterus

4 = Complete out enterocele (cul de sac)

3 = Rectocele coming halfway past hymen

3 = Perineal attenuation

    2/4 Levator tone

Pelvic Organ Prolapse-Quantification System (POP-Q)

This was developed more objectively. Measurements are used in centimeters instead of grades. Nine specific sites are used.

1. Aa = (Point A on anterior wall—corresponds to urethrocele)
   3 cm proximal to the external urethral meatus on the ant vaginal wall
2. Ba = Point B on ant wall—corresponds to cystocele
   Points of maximal prolapse on the anterior wall
3. C = Cervix or Cuff (corresponds to the Point 3, i.e. uterine in the Baden Walker system)
4. Ap = Point A on posterior wall
   3 cm proximal to the hymen on the posterior vaginal wall
5. Bp = Point B on posterior wall
   Point of maximal execution on the posterior vaginal wall
6. D = Posterior fornix (corresponds to point 4, i.e. cul de sac of Baden Walker)
7. gh = Genital hiatus (from external urethral meatus to mid posterior point on introitus)
8. pb = Perineal body (mid posterior point on introitus to mid anterior point on external anal sphincter)
9. tvl = Total vaginal length (taken with prolapsed completely reduced)

On a sagittal diagram (Fig. 1), the sites are clearly depicted.

The stage of prolapse is then assigned as stage 0 (no prolapse) to stage V (complete prolapse) according to POP Quantitative Scoring (International Continence Society Terminology, American Urogynecological Society, Society of Gynae Surgeons; 1996).

Stage	Description
0	No descent
I	Leading edge not below 1 cm above the hymen
II	Leading edge between 1 cm above to 1 cm below the hymen
III	1 cm beyond the hymen ring but not complete vaginal eversion
IV	Complete vaginal eversion

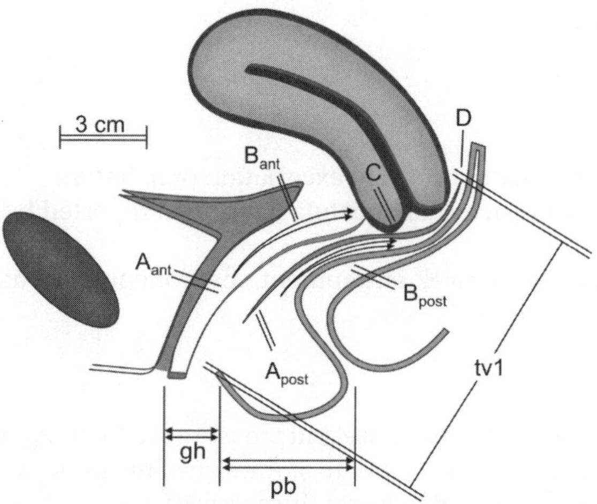

Fig. 1: Measurements used in POP-Q system

TREATMENT

It can be surgical or nonsurgical.

Nonsurgical

In mild-to-moderate prolapse:
- Where women desire future childbearing
- Who do not desire surgical option
- Patient is unfit for anesthesia/surgery or very advanced age of patient with comorbidities
- Currently pregnant patient.

1. Pelvic floor muscle training and Kegel's exercises
   In mild cases:
   - It may prevent worsening of prolapse
   - It may decrease severity of symptoms
   - May delay surgery
   - Increases the strength of pelvic floor muscle
2. Other life style modifications suggested to alleviate symptoms are:
   - Weight reduction if patient is obese
   - Reduce heavy weight lifting or squatting or reduction of activities that increase the intra abdominal pressure

Pessaries—Two Types

1. Ring pessary which are support providing
2. Space filling: Like Gel horn pessary
   Space filling are more useful in advanced, stage 3 and 4 prolapse as ring pessary may not be retained.

Complications

- Vaginal discharge
- Foul odor
- Failure to retain
- Too large a pessary may lead to excoriation or irritation
- Rarely cases of vesicovaginal fistula have been reported by forgotten ring pessary
- Rarely urosepsis, bowel entrapment, hydronephrosis have also been reported.

Insertion

With 2 fingers, reduce the prolapse and measure the total vaginal length up to the subpubic arch to get an estimate of the size of the pessary required.

- A lubricant may be used to insert the pessary
- Fold the ring pessary and it is inserted in the postvaginal fornix as high up as possible and anteriorly behind the symphysis avoiding the urethra
- After inserting, ask the patient to perform Valsalva in standing position to see if it is retained.

Follow-up

- 1st visit in 1–2 weeks
- 2nd visit in 4–6 weeks
- Patient can be taught to remove, clean and wash the pessary and reinsert. If she can not then she can be called at 4–12 weekly intervals for the same.
- Always check for irritation, pressure sores, ulceration, if required estrogen cream for short duration may be prescribed to improve the quality of vaginal tissue at initial visit or prior to fitting.

Surgical Management

Approaches to Surgery — Vaginal
                         — Abdominal
                         — Combined

- Route depends on extent and location of prolapse and the surgeons training and experience
- Surgery for urinary and fecal incontinence may be required at the same sitting
- Sexual function must be considered in choosing the appropriate procedure and in certain cases obliterative procedures may be used to close or partially close the vagina (colpocleisis).

Historically, the treatment for uterine prolapse is vaginal hysterectomy in combination with vaginal apical suspension along with repair of co-existent defects.

Vaginal Hysterectomy with Pelvic Floor Repair (PFR) for Prolapse

This would include:

- Vaginal hysterectomy to remove the uterus from the vaginal route and apical suspension.
- Correction of enterocele by McCall's culdoplasty incorporating both the uterosacrals.
- Approximation of pedicles in the midline to form a buttress.
- Fixation of uterosacrals to the vault to prevent vault prolapse.
- Anterior colporrhaphy to correct cystocele. Correct any SUI with appropriate surgery.
- Posterior colpoperineorrhaphy to treat the rectocele and the perineal defect.

Transvaginal apical suspension is important to prevent future vault prolapse and the procedures include:

- Uterosacral ligament suspension—intraperitoneal
- Iliococcygeal suspension—extraperitoneal
- Sacrospinous suspension—extraperitoneal
- McCall culdoplasty—intraperitoneal

Accepted practice is that the vaginal apex should be suspended in a posterior cephalad direction. Anterior apical suspension changes the direction of the vaginal apex and gives rise to higher incidence of posterior compartment defect like rectocele, enterocele and sigmoidocele. Postapical suspension may bring forth a stress urinary incontinence.

Uterosacral Ligament Suspension

- This procedure is one of the most commonly used, prophylactically and therapeutically during abdominal hysterectomy as well as vaginal hysterectomy.
- Excellent success rates have been reported.
- The ligaments can be approximated in the midline to prevent and treat enterocele as well as to close the pouch of Douglas.

Most surgeons suspend the left and right vaginal apex to the ipsilateral uterosacral.

Success rate and side effects: 2–5%. Recurrent apical prolapse is reported.

Ureteral kinking has been reported in as many as 11% cases.

Sacrospinous Ligament Fixation

The procedure was first described in 1958 and subsequently modified. The rectovaginal space is dissected to approach the ischial spine. The ligament that runs between the ischial spine and coccyx is exposed and the vault sutured to the ligament, 2 cm medial to the ischial spine taking care to avoid the sciatic nerve and pudendal vessels and nerves. This procedure is also used for treatment of vault prolapse.

Disadvantages of the procedure
- Difficulty in exposing the ligament
- Unilateral lateral vaginal deflection

Iliococcygeal Vaginal Suspension

Attachment of the vaginal apex to the iliococcygeus. This is the least commonly used procedure. No. I, polydioxanone suture is passed like a pulley stitch bilaterally.

Anterior Compartment—Cystocele Repair

- Anterior vaginal colporrhaphy is performed
- Steps:
    - Vesicovaginal space is dissected
    - Excess vaginal mucosa is excised
    - Midline plication of the fibromuscular tissue is done
    - The apical support sutures should be passed before but tied only after the anterior colporrhaphy has been done
- SUI if present needs to be repaired simultaneously

Paravaginal Repair of Cystocele

It is to be done in the presence of lateral defects.
- The anterior lateral vaginal sulcus is attached to the obturator internus fascia or muscle.
- Repair of a central defect, where the redundant vaginal tissue is excised, makes it difficult to suspend the vagina laterally to the obturator internus. In such cases repairing the central defect and suspending the apical defect may be a better option.
- Graft placement to augment the paravaginal tissue strength is another option in such cases.

Enterocele Repair

- Transvaginal McCall's suture may be used in a purse string maneuver. A suture (delayed absorbable) is passed from one uterosacral to the highest possible posterior peritoneum after and if required removing the redundant peritoneum and then from the opposite uterosacral. This is the more effective way of preventing future enterocele rather than just purse string suture at the neck of the sac and is recommended in the RCOG guidelines as well.
- During abdominal hysterectomy, procedures used are:
    - Moschowitz procedure: Obliterating the pouch of Douglas (POD) by purse string concentric sutures incorporating the uterosacral and peritoneum over the rectosigmoid. One may have to take 3 or 4 concentric sutures depending on the depth of POD.

– Halban's procedure: POD is obliterated by 3–4 sutures passed from anterior to posterior rather than concentric.

Site Specific Posterior Repair

They are used to correct posterior defects. The inverted T incision in the vagina beginning from the posterior mucocutaneous junction is extended as high as the defect which may be as high as the vault. The vagina is separated from the underlying rectum and fibromuscular tissue. The fibromuscular pararectal tissue is approximated in a manner similar to correction of cystocele at the level of the defect, so that the rectum is positioned at the pelvic floor. The perineal body is reinforced after the site specific posterior repair.

Repair of Rectocele

- Skin at the mucocutaneous junction at perineum is excised
- Dissection is done in an inverted T manner to separate the vagina from the rectum
- The prerectal fascia is plicated in the midline with delayed absorbable suture
- The levator and the superficial muscles of the perineum and bulbospongiosus are plicated in the midline.

Complications
- Defecatory dysfunction
- Dyspareunia due to vaginal stricture
- Over tight introitus
- Scarring
- Levator spasm
- Neuralgia

Colpocleisis

It is used for very elderly patients with comorbidities, with moderate anesthesia risk to shorten the duration of surgery.

Most surgeons prefer partial colpocleisis where some vaginal tissue is left which forms two passages by the sides for drainage to occur. In total colpocleisis, the complete vagina from the posterior mucocutaneous junction is removed up to 0.5–2 cm of the urethral opening.

Vault Prolapse

Incidence is 3–6 per 1000. It is a delayed complication of abdominal or vaginal hysterectomy. It may occur because of:
- Technical error in previous surgery
- Age and estrogen deficiency
- Failure to identify and repair enterocele at first surgery
- Chronic cough, obesity, chronic constipation
- Pessary treatment may be offered to patients with poor anesthesia risk.

Prevention

- McCall culdoplasty at the time of vaginal hysterectomy is a recommended measure to prevent enterocele formation.
- Suturing the cardinal and uterosacral ligaments to the vaginal cuff at the time of hysterectomy is a recommended measure to avoid vault prolapse.
- Sacrospinous fixation at the time of vaginal hysterectomy is recommended when the vault descends to the introitus during closure.

Surgical treatment of vault prolapse

Sacrospinous colpopexy

- It was 1st described by Richter in 1968
    - Bilateral is rarely required and only right sided may be performed
    - Success rate of 90% has been claimed
    - Cystocele may develop at a later date
- Transabdominal sacral colpopexy
    - Using Mersilene tape or mesh
    - Mesh erosion: 3% incidence
    - Recurrence reported: 10%
- Colpocleisis
- Le Fort's partial obliteration of vagina
- Lately laparoscopic colpopexy has been used
- Caution is advised with vaginal uterosacral ligament suspension, although it is effective for post hysterectomy vaginal vault prolapse, there is a risk of ureteric injury.

Abdominal Sacrocolpopexy

Graft material, usually synthetic prolene mesh is attached to the vault and vagina anteriorly after reflecting the bladder and posteriorly as low down as possible if rectocele is present. The other end of the mesh is then attached to the anterior longitudinal ligament of the sacrum at the level of S_1–S_2.

- Cervical sacral suspension may also be done if uterine conservation is desired
- Most surgeons use no. 0 to 3, 0 polypropylene, prolene, and monofilament or nylon sutures
- Variations are seen in choice of mesh, choice of suture, extent to which the mesh is attached to the vagina both anteriorly and posteriorly
- The mesh must be covered by peritoneum to avoid gut complications
- Enterocele may be corrected by simultaneously performing Halban's or Moschowitz repair.

Complications

- Erosion of mesh
- Mesh infection
- Intraoperative hemorrhage especially in presacral space
- Postoperative ileus

- Small bowel obstruction
- Adhesions
- Wound complications
- Postoperative sacral osteomyelitis has also been described
- Chronic backache
- SUI and cystocele dye to posterior cephalad suspension

Sacrospinous Ligament Fixation

The ligament that runs between the ischial spine and coccyx is exposed and the vault sutured to the ligament, 2 cm medial to the ischial spine taking care to avoid the sciatic nerve and pudendal vessels and nerves (described earlier in the text).

Side effects were noted as 2% for each and 7% and 4% in one study with the two procedures respectively.

Use of Mesh and Prosthetics

10–30% of women suffer recurrent prolapse and may need repeat surgical intervention.

The second surgery will depend on the route and method used in first surgery.

Prosthetics are increasingly being used for treatment of recurrence and also in primary surgery to reduce recurrence in high risk cases.

The recurrence rates may be lower but there are other more frequent complications like:

- Erosions and infections
- Severe dyspareunia and sexual dysfunction due to excessive scarring
- Bothersome discharge

A systematic review in 2008 (114) reported that there is insufficient evidence to evaluate their use in prolapse. The US FDA has also released a warning stating that:

- Physicians should obtain specialized training for placement.
- They should be aware of its risks.
- Be vigilant for adverse effects like erosion and infection.
- To watch out for complications like bowel, bladder, blood vessel perforation associated with placement techniques.
- Inform patient about the side effects and the fact that it is permanent.

1. Synthetic material
   - Macroporous, nonabsorbable synthetic mesh: Most preferred. Pore size more than 75 mm to allow infiltration by macrophages, fibroblasts, new vessels and collagen fibers.
   - Absorbable polygalactin (Vicryl):
     Long term results need evaluation
2. – Biological material
     Autologous — Rectus fascia
                  — Fascia lata
   - Xenografts of porcine

3. New systems
   - Polypropylene tape
   - Apogee/Perigee

Mesh may be sutured over fascial defects as inlay or whole vagina can be surrounded by mesh (Total mesh). Theoretically it is suitable for any degree of anterior or posterior vaginal prolapse. In anterior defects, objective failure rates of about 9% have been described with use of nonabsorbable synthetic mesh, 23% with synthetic absorbable mesh, 18% with absorbable biologic mesh as against 30% without mesh . The subjective failure reports are however comparable.

Subjective failure rates however are 2% with mesh and around 11% without mesh.

For posterior repairs, 9 RCTs did not show any significant difference in the failure rate or quality of life after 6 months. The side effects with use of mesh are however serious and can be distressing in the form of erosions and infections around 6–10% depending on type of mesh used and may need reoperation 16–36% have reported dyspareunia due to excessive scarring. Besides, there are reports of bladder injury, rectal perforations and hematomas especially with use of trocar introducer systems for mesh.

Laparoscopic and Robotic Techniques

As with most surgeries, both laparoscopy and Da Vinci have been used in lieu of laparotomies to offer benefit of minimally invasive techniques, but they are limited by need for high level of technical skill.

CONCLUSION AND RECOMMENDATIONS

Awareness of a vaginal bulge or protrusion is the only symptom specific to prolapse. Pessaries can be fitted in most women with prolapse, regardless of stage of prolapse or site of predominant prolapse, in case they are unwilling to undergo surgery. Alternative operations for uterine preservation in women with prolapse include uterosacral or sacrospinous ligament fixation vaginally, or abdominal sacral hysteropexy. Compared with vaginal sacrospinous ligament fixation, abdominal sacral colpopexy has less apical failure and less postoperative dyspareunia and SUI. A recent Cochrane database review has also concluded that sacral colpopexy has superior outcomes to a variety of vaginal procedures including sacrospinous colpopexy, uterosacral colpopexy and transvaginal mesh.

Stress-continent women with positive stress test results (prolapse reduced) are at higher risk for developing postoperative SUI after prolapse repair alone compared with women with negative stress test results. For stress-continent women planning abdominal sacral colpopexy, regardless of the results of preoperative stress testing, the addition of the Burch procedure substantially reduces the likelihood of postoperative SUI. For subset of these women who are planning vaginal route of prolapse repair, midurethral sling offers prevention from postoperative SUI.

The use of synthetic mesh for anterior vaginal wall repair reduces the risk of recurrent prolapse, however, it comes at a cost of increased operating time, blood loss, rate of apical or posterior compartment prolapse, de novo stress urinary incontinence, and reoperation rate for mesh exposures associated with the use of polypropylene mesh. Presently, evidence does not support use of any meshes or grafts for posterior vaginal repair.

SUGGESTED READING

1. Deffleux X, Letouzey V, Savary D, et al (CNGOF): Prevention of Complications related to the use of prosthetic meshes in prolapse in surgery. Eur J Obstet Gynecol Reprod Biol. 2012;165(2):170-80.
2. Maher C, Feiner B, Baessler K, Schmid C. Surgical management of pelvic organ Prolapse in Women. Cochrane Database. Syst Rev. 2013;4.
3. National Guideline Clearinghouse: Pelvic Organ Prolapse. Based on ACOG Practice Bulletin No. 85.September 2007.
4. Surgical Repair of Vaginal Wall prolapse using mesh (IPG267) NICE Guidance, June 2012.
5. Zimmerman CW. Pelvic Organ Prolapse. In: Rock JA Jr, Jones III HW (Ed). Te Linde's Operative Gynecology, 9th Edition. Lippincott, Williams and Wilkins.

Vault Prolapse After Hysterectomy

Suchitra N Pandit, Rakhee R Sahu

Vaginal vault prolapse after hysterectomy is not uncommon, but the precise frequency is unknown. Vaginal prolapse has negative impact on women's quality of life due to associated urinary, anorectal and sexual dysfunction.

Vaginal vault prolapse has been defined by the International Continence Society as descent of the vaginal cuff below a point that is 2 cm less than that the total vaginal length above the plane of the hymen and it occurs when the upper vagina bulges into or outside the vagina.[1]

Eversion of the vaginal vault can be seen with or without coincident enterocele, cystocele and rectocele, almost 75% of the time they coexists.[2]

Being of separate etiology, each must be recognized and repaired independently during surgical reconstruction. A retrospective follow-up study showed the incidence of vault prolapse was 11.6% in surgery done for genital prolapse and 1.8% of those performed for other indications.

Preexisting pelvic floor defect prior to hysterectomy is the most important risk factor for vault prolapse.[3,4]

Surgeons who would subject a patient with uterine prolapse to a routine hysterectomy without special attention to supporting the vaginal vault do not appreciate the fact that a dropped uterus is the result of a genital prolapse and not the cause.

The upper vaginal axis is almost horizontal because the vagina lies on an intact and more or less horizontal levator plate formed by the fused posterior portion of the pubococcygeus extending from the posterior surface of the rectum to the sacrum. As the levator plate relaxes and tips downwards, the genital hiatus becomes larger, through which the vagina can prolapse.

The risk factors of vault prolapse include aging and menopausal loss of estrogenic support, multiparity, chronic intra-abdominal pressure, as with heavy weight lifting, chronic cough in asthmatics, smokers, and obesity.

Vault prolapse after hysterectomy may occur if there was partial degrees of cystocele or rectocele or enterocele which was undiagnosed or otherwise unattended, which will generally progress. A poorly supported vault during hysterectomy may be pushed down later. During hysterectomy, the vaginal angles are suspended to uterosacral ligaments for vault support. But if in case of procidentia, the uterosacral ligaments may become flimsy with poor tone providing no support to the vault.

Vault prolapse and enterocele are often associated with complains of backache, pelvic heaviness and pressure exacerbated with prolonged standing. There may be vaginal discomfort and dyspareunia due to dryness of exteriorized vagina. When rectocele coexists, the patient may experience difficulty in bowel evacuation. There may be need to digitally reduce the bulge to void or defecate. Urinary complaints are uncommon unless displacement cystocele coexists and there is an inability to empty bladder, resulting in stagnation of urine with overflow incontinence.

Bonney described two general systems that maintain pelvic integrity: the upper suspensory system and the lower supportive system. After the prolapsed organs have been gently replaced, even in a patient with total eversion of the vagina, the patient is asked to bear down, as in valsalva maneuver. The site of primary damage appears first at the vulva, followed by the sites of secondary damage. When damage to the upper suspensory system is primary, the cervix or the vaginal vault appears first, followed by any cystocele and rectocele. With primary damage to the lower supportive system, a cystocele and rectocele will appear first, followed by the cervix or vaginal vault. While planning the patient's surgery, the surgeon should remember Bonney's rule: the primary site of damage should be identified and over-repaired to lessen the chance of recurrence.

An effective way of distinguishing between enterocele, rectocele and vault prolapse is in standing position. The patient is asked to stand, and the vaginal examination is repeated, first with the patient at rest, then holding, and finally straining. The vault is replaced to its highest position within the pelvis, and the patient is asked to bear down. The result of this maneuver is observed, and the presence or absence of incontinence is redetermined. If, in this situation, a peritoneal sac containing omentum or a palpable loop of bowel comes down between the thumb (placed in vagina) and the index finger (place in rectum), the patient has enterocele.

Pelvic organ prolapse quantification (POP-Q) is an objective and standardized system of prolapse classification introduced in 1996, by the International continence society. It is a useful tool in assessing the extent of prolapse. It has the added advantage of its use in evaluating surgical and non-surgical treatment outcomes and for clinical research purposes. The vaginal cuff scar corresponds to point C on the POP-Q grid.

At the time of initial hysterectomy, steps should be taken to prevent postoperative enterocele and vault prolapse like culdoplasty and vault suspension to uterosacral ligaments.

The cardinal and uterosacral ligaments form a complex of visceral supporting tissues to the upper vagina and cervix and, after hysterectomy, to the vaginal vault. They pull the upper vagina horizontally back towards the sacrum and thus, suspend it over the muscular levator plate.

Careful preoperative examination should be done to rule out mild enterocele and rectocele. During hysterectomy, after the uterus has been removed, before the peritoneum is closed, one should hook a finger in the cul-de-sac to see if there is an extraperitoneum that should be excised. If the uterosacral ligaments are strong, they should be used to support the vaginal vault. After vaginal hysterectomy, a high purse string closure of the peritoneal cavity is advised. The suture used in peritoneal closure should penetrate both the uterosacral and round ligaments. The surgeon should be mindful of the course of ureter to avoid kinking them when the suture is tied.

Royal College of Obstetricians and Gynecologists (RCOG) green-top guidelines no. 46 recommends McCall culdoplasty at the time of vaginal hysterectomy to prevent enterocele formation.

Preserving vaginal depth and axis is an important prophylactic feature of all genital prolapse surgery. Ventral fixation of the prolapsed uterus or vaginal vault to the anterior abdominal wall was once popular. Although the uterine fundus remains fixed, the uterus and cervix elongate until ultimately the vagina and those organs to which it is attached come down again. By changing the axis of the vagina, ventral fixation leaves a vulnerable cul-de-sac exposed to increases in abdominal pressure. When Burch presented his excellent results in treating urinary incontinence by fixation of the vagina to the Cooper ligament, it was pointed out that the incidence of subsequent enterocele was between 11–15%, which was most likely caused by the change in vaginal axis.

When the vagina is completely everted, its lateral attachments to the arcus tendineus may have been severely compromised or avulsed. Support of the vault by colpopexy and colporrhaphy may restore vaginal support.

MANAGEMENT OF VAULT PROLAPSE

Conservative management will include pelvic floor exercise and pessaries, commonly ring and shelf pessaries. Their role in vault prolapse is unclear and there is no evidence to suggest that pelvic floor exercise is helpful.[5]

However, pessaries may have a limited role in the very frail and elderly, in whom surgery is not an option.

The surgical management of vault prolapse should consider all the aspects of prolapse pathology, patient's lifestyle, age, sexual function and presence of comorbidities must be taken into consideration.

Abdominal sacrocolpopexy and transvaginal sacrospinous fixation are the surgeries recommended by the RCOG Green-top Guideline no. 46.

Surgical Technique of Transvaginal Sacrocolpopexy

The procedure was first described by Miyazaki in 1987[6] and later popularized by Sharp et al. and Lang et al.[7]

It was originally described as a bilateral procedure but subsequently studies showed, unilateral procedure equally effective.

Transvaginal sacrocolpopexy is done in women uterine prolapse but without strong uterosacral ligaments for vault support. After the uterus is removed, any enterocele is identified and excision of peritoneum with high ligation of the sac and closure of the peritoneal cavity is done. The technique comprises of incision on the perineal skin and posterior vaginal mucosa to open the rectovaginal space. The right ischial spine is identified and the right rectal pillar is penetrated with either with artery forceps or blunt dissection with fingers. Through the window created in the rectal pillar, the sacrospinous ligament-coccygeus muscle complex is palpated which courses from the ischial spine to the sacrum. The sacrospinous ligament-coccygeus muscle complex is held by Allis forceps and penetrated with Deschamps ligature carrier or simple needle holder under direct visualization or Miya hook ligature.[8] Two nonabsorbable sutures are placed through the ligament, not too deep as it could endanger the sciatic nerve and pudendal nerves and vessels. The free end of suture is attached to the under surface of posterior vaginal wall. If a tug is applied to the sutures placed through the sacrospinous ligament, one can actually move the patient on table, and this also indicates the proper placement of sutures.

Anterior colporrhaphy is completed and when the posterior colporrhaphy reaches the mid-portion of the vagina, the sacrospinous sutures are tied with no intervening bridge of suture material.

Although infrequent, hemorrhage is the most common complication but is rarely life-threatening. There could be injury to the pudendal vessels, nerve or the hypogastric venous plexus.

Other complications include injury to the rectum, urinary bladder or sciatic nerve. Immediate and severe postoperative gluteal pain radiating to the posterior surface of leg suggests sciatic nerve injury. The recommended treatment is immediate operation for release of the offending suture and repositioning it to a more medial position.[9]

Abdominal Sacrocolpopexy

Abdominal sacrocolpopexy involves the attachment of the vaginal vault to the sacral promontory by interposition of a suspensory synthetic prothesis. This procedure was first described by Lane in 1962.[10]

This method has been proven to be superior to the other surgical techniques in terms of restoration of normal vaginal axis and maintains vaginal depth and function.

A vertical incision is usually performed as it allows optimal exposure and access to the deep pelvis and sacrum. The bladder and rectum is dissected away from the vaginal vault. Any weakness in the integrity of the vaginal vault is repaired with nonabsorbable sutures for good vault support and post-operative mesh erosion. Around 8–10 permanent sutures (prolene No 1) is placed around the vaginal vault and kept long. Mersilene mesh is secured to the vaginal vault by bringing out the vaginal vault sutures through it and tied. The rectosigmoid is retracted to the patient's left and the peritoneum over the sacral promontory is opened extended in midline inferiorly till the sacral hollow. Then permanent sutures are placed into the periosteum of the anterior surface of sacrum from the promontory to the hollow of sacrum till S3-4 level and kept long. When the peritoneum is reflected to expose the anterior surface of sacrum and sutures are placed, care is taken to avoid injury to the presacral vessels. Any injury to these vessels can result in severe hemorrhage, which is difficult to control as the vessels retract into the bone. The standard methods of controlling bleeding from these vessels are often unsuccessful and insertion of steel thumbtacks or bone glue at the site of hemorrhage can be dramatically effective. Next it is important to do culdoplasty which is an essential component of this surgery. The pouch of Douglas is obliterated either with Halban's anteroposterior sutures or Moschowitz sutures. The culdoplasty sutures are brought out through the suspensory mesh to prevent herniation of small bowel between the mesh and superior surface of culdoplasty. The free end of mersilene mesh is pulled towards the sacrum till there is appropriate tension on the mesh fixed to vaginal vault. The sacral fixation sutures are then brought out through the mesh and tied at points that maintain this support. The posterior peritoneum is closed, and the bladder flap and vesical peritoneum is used to cover the remaining exposed mesh. Mesh erosion was reported in 2–2.7% of cases which necessitated removal or revision of the mesh.[11]

Laparoscopic Approach

Laparoscopic Sacral Colpopexy

The operative steps remain the same as abdominal sacrocolpopexy, with laparoscopy being the mode of surgical access. In a study by Hsiao et al. in 2004, comparing laparoscopic sacrocolpopexy (25 patients) and abdominal sacrocolpopexy (22 patients), it showed that blood loss and hospital stay was significantly less in the laparoscopic group (P = 0.002), though operation time was longer (P < 0.001). However, there was no difference in efficacy of both methods. Success rates of 95% for abdominal and 100% for laparoscopic techniques has been reported.[12]

Other Procedures for Vault Prolapse

Iliococcygeal Fixation

This technique was described by Sze and Karram in1997 and comprises the fixation of the everted vaginal apex to the iliococcygeal fascia just below the ischial spine.[13] The iliococcygeal muscle can be approached through either an anterior or posterior vaginal wall incision. It is usually done as a bilateral procedure as it causes less tension on the vaginal wall than sacrospinous fixation. This procedure is relatively easier than sacrospinous fixation. In a small series Carey reported 14% recurrence following iliococcygeal fixation as compared to 11% following sacrospinous fixation.

The RCOG guidelines no. 46 states iliococcygeal fixation does not reduced the incidence of anterior vaginal wall prolapse associated with sacrospinous fixation and should not be routinely recommended.[14]

Uterosacral Suspension

The aim of the procedure is to place sutures through the uterosacral ligament at the level of the ischial spine, with one arm brought out through the lateral aspect of rectovaginal fascia and the other through the pubocervical fascia on each side. These are tied anchoring the vaginal cuff to the uterosacrals. This has been described as bilateral procedure carried out vaginally; it can also be performed via an abdominal or laparoscopic approach.[15]

There is a high-risk of ureteric injury, so cystoscopy is advised after suture placement.

Infracoccygeal Sling Sacropexy

The principle of this technique is to create artificial uterosacral ligaments by inserting woven nylon tapes along their anatomical path.

The technique comprises a transverse incision on the posterior vaginal wall 1.5–2 cm below the hysterectomy scar line and opened anteroposteriorly. The enterocele sac is placed backwards and allowed access to the laterally displaced uterosacral ligaments. At this point, the enterocele sac is reduced with a purse string suture. The next step is making bilateral incisions 0.5 cm long in the perianal skin at 4 and 8 o'clock, halfway between the coccyx and external anal sphincter. Having slid the conical head of the tunneller subdermally to the level of 3 and 9 o'clock, the handle is lifted upward 90 degrees so that the head is parallel to the floor. The shaft of the tunneller is then thrust forward into the ischiorectal fossa. This action penetrates the levator plate and brings the conical head into a position behind the uterosacral ligament. Under direct vision, with finger placed in the rectum to locate the position of the rectal wall, the conical tip of the tunneller is gently inclined medially towards the vaginal vault. The tip is then penetrating the fascia adjoining the vagina and rectum. A 6 mm woven nylon tape was threaded into the eye of the plastic insert and brought into the transverse incision. The procedure is repeated on the contralateral side, leaving the tape as a U entirely unfixed at the sacral end. The tape is then sutured to the vault at each corner at the estimated insertion site of the uterosacral ligament. The tape is then gently stretched by pulling on each perineal end, and left entirely free and unfixed.

In his series of 75 patients, Petros reported 5% recurrence of vault prolapse at a follow up between 1–4 years, 16% de novo anterior wall prolapse, and 4% partial rectocele.[16]

Colpocleisis

Colpocleisis involves surgical obliteration of the lumen of the vagina. Basically the vaginal epithelium is mobilized anteriorly and posteriorly leaving about 2 cm from the vault above and also from the urethral meatus below. The prolapse is reduced by placing progressive sutures anteroposteriorly, till the prolapsed tissues are above the level of the levator plate. It can also be carried out as a partial or total procedure. The partial procedure is usually reserved for women with an intact prolapsed uterus with the aim of giving access to any discharge or bleeding from the uterus via a small opening.

It is suitable for the frail elderly woman who is not sexually active and for whom conservative methods like the pessary is not ideal. It has the advantage that it can also be carried out under local anesthesia and involves a shorter operation time. Essentially, it is about improving the quality of life. De novo urinary stress incontinence of up to 27% in previously continent women has been reported,[17] though no intraoperative complication has been reported in the literature.[18]

ROLE OF MESH IN VAULT PROLAPSE

Synthetic mesh has been commonly used to manage pelvic organ and prolapse, even though the more traditional suture repair technique is still the primary choice, with the mesh mainly reserved for repeat procedures and large defects.

A multicenter retrospective study[19] involving 110 patients, of whom 59 had total mesh repair, (transvaginal) using the prolift (Gynecare) system, showed a recurrence rate of 4.75% at 3 months follow-up. In spite of the short follow-up in this study, the total mesh may possibly address the issue of high rate of recurrence commoner with the more traditional methods. Other types of mesh like the Apogee (posterior vaginal wall) and Perigee (anterior vaginal wall) have been used for management of recurrent cystocele and rectocele with or without vault prolapse. Success rate of 93% has been reported.[20] However, there are no randomized controlled studies to compare this procedure with abdominal sacrocolpopexy or uterosacral suspension for now.

CONCLUSION

There is no consensus on the mechanism and management of vault prolapse, but what is accepted by all is the need to properly assess these patients, involve them in the management and to agree on the type of surgery that will be suitable for their own peculiar circumstance. The mesh is gaining in popularity, but there are no studies yet on its long term efficacy though initial results are very encouraging. Vaginal sacrospinous fixation and abdominal sacrocolpopexy have the most commonly performed and successful surgeries for vault prolapse.

REFERENCES

1. Abrams P, Cardozo L, Fall M, et al. The standardization of terminology of lower urinary tract function: report from the standardization sub-committee of the international continence society. Neurology and Urodynamics. 200;21(2):167-78.
2. Sederl J. Zur operation des prolapses der blind endigenden sheiden. Geburtshilfe Frauenheilkd. 1958;18:824-8.
3. Marchionni M, Bracco GL, Checcucci V, et al. True incidence of vaginal vault prolapse: thirteen years of experience. Journal of Reproductive Medicine for the Obstetrician and Gynecologist. 1999;44(8):679-84.
4. Baden WF, Walker TA, Lindsey JH. The vaginal profile. Tex Med. 1968;64:56-8.
5. Hagen S, Stark D, Maher C, Adams E. Conservative management of pelvic organ prolapse in women. Cochrane Database of Systematic Reviews. 2006;(4) Article ID CD003882.

6. Miyazaki FS. Miya Hook ligature carrier for sacrospinous ligament suspension. Obstetrics and Gynecology. 1987;70(2):286-8.

7. Sharp TR. Sacrospinous suspension made easy. Obstetrics and Gynecology. 1993;82(5):873-5.

8. Pollak J, Takacs P, Medina C. Complications of three sacrospinous ligament fixation techniques. International Journal of Gynecology and Obstetrics. 2007;99(1):18-22.

9. Shull BL, Capen CV, Riggs MW, Kuehl TJ. Bilateral attachment of the vaginal cuff to iliococcygeus fascia: an effective method of cuff suspension. Am J of Obs and Gyne. 1993;168(6):1669-77.

10. Lane FE. Repair of posthysterectomy vaginal vault prolapse. Obstetrics and Gynecology. 1962;20:72-7.

11. Iglesia CB, Fenner DE, Brubaker L. The use of mesh in gynecologic surgery. Int Urogynecol J Pelvic Floor Dysfunct. 1997;8(2):105-15.

12. Hsiao KC, Latchamsetty K, Govier FE, Kozlowski P, Kobashi KC. Comparison of laparoscopic and abdominal sacrocolpopexy for the treatment of vaginal vault prolapse. Journal of Endourol. 2007;21(8):926-30.

13. Sze EHM, Karram MM. Transvaginal repair of vault prolapse: a review. Obstetrics and Gynecology. 1997;89(3):466-75.

14. RCOG Green-top Guideline no 46; 2007.

15. Barber MD, Visco AG, Weidner AC, Amundsen CL, Bump RC. Bilateral uterosacral ligament vaginal vault suspension with site-specific endopelvic fascia defect repair for treatment of pelvic organ prolapse. Am J Obs Gynecol. 2000;183(6):1402-11.

16. Petros PEP. Vault prolapse II: restoration of dynamic vaginal supports by infracoccygeal sacropexy, an axial day-case vaginal procedure. Int Urogynecol J Pelvic Floor Dysfunct. 2001;12(5):296-303.

17. FitzGerald MP, Brubaker L. Colpocleisis and urinary incontinence. Am J Obs Gynecol. 2003;189(5):1241-4.

18. Latthe PM, Kamakshi K, Arunkalaivanan AS. Colpocleisis revisited. The Obstetrician and Gynaecologist. 2008;10:133-8.

19. Fatton B, Amblard J, Debodinance P, Cosson M, Jacquetin B. Transvaginal repair of genital prolapse: preliminary results of a new tension-free vaginal mesh (ProliftTM technique)—a case series multicentric study. Int Urogynecol J Pelvic Floor Dysfunct. 2007;18(7):743-52.

20. Gauruder-Burmester A, Koutouzidou P, Rohne J, Gronewold M, Tunn R. Follow-up after polypropylene mesh repair of anterior and posterior compartments in patients with recurrent prolapse. Int Urogynecol J Pelvic Floor Dysfunct. 2007;18(9):1059-64.

Chapter 40

Stress Urinary Incontinence

JB Sharma, Manisha Yadav

DEFINITION OF STRESS URINARY INCONTINENCE

Stress urinary incontinence (SUI) is a symptom that refers to leakage of urine during events that result in increased abdominal pressure, such as sneezing, coughing, physical exercise, lifting, bending and even changing positions. There are two principal causes of this urine leakage—stress urinary incontinence and, more rarely, stress-induced detrusor overactivity, which involves involuntary detrusor contractions that are caused by sudden increase in abdominal pressure.

SYMPTOMS

- Mild incontinence is light leakage with vigorous activity, such as exercise or from sneezing, laughing, coughing or lifting
- Moderate/more severe incontinence is leakage with any movement such as standing up, walking, or bending over.

RISK FACTORS

Risk factors for SUI include:
- Age
- Caucasian or Hispanic race
- Obesity
- Smoking
- Chronic cough
- Pregnancy and childbirth
- Nerve injuries to the lower back
- Pelvic surgery.

PREVALENCE

The involuntary loss of urine is a common medical condition occurring in about one, out of every three women at some time in their lives. Among these women, about six in ten have both SUI and overactive bladder. Prevalence of urinary incontinence is approximately 30% in women aged 30 to 60 years, with about half of the cases attributed to SUI.

NATURE OF URETHRAL SUPPORT

The important components are the levator ani muscles, which run from the pubic bone to the anal sphincter and behind the rectum in a position where they can support the pelvic organs. These muscles lie lateral to the arcus tendineus fasciae pelvis, a band of endopelvic fascia that stretches between the pubic bone and the ischial spine. Endopelvic fascia ties the anterior vaginal wall to the arcus tendineus. The layer formed by the anterior vaginal wall and its connection to the arcus tendineus fasciae pelvis by the endopelvic fascia forms a hammock-like layer in which the bladder and vesical neck rest. Although, this fascial support is usually thought to be a passive rather than an active mechanism, the connection between the fascia and the levator ani muscle is an important element of this system. This connection permits active contraction of the pelvic muscles to elevate the vesical neck and their relaxation to allow it to descend. In addition, the normal constant activity of the levator ani muscle supports the vesical neck during normal activities.

PATHOPHYSIOLOGY OF STRESS URINARY INCONTINENCE

Urine storage and release involve numerous reflexes. Stress urinary incontinence (SUI) is mainly caused by pelvic floor muscle (PFM) weakness. It is characterized by the loss of small amounts of urine accompanying coughing, laughing, sneezing, exercising or other movements that increase intra-abdominal pressure, and thus, increase pressure on the bladder. Physical changes resulting from pregnancy, childbirth and the menopause often cause SUI. Loss of urethral support lead to urethral hypermobility and proximal urethra is displaced downwards with sudden increase in intra-abdominal pressure. SUI may also result from intrinsic sphincter deficiency, in which the urethra is unable to generate enough outlet resistance to keep it closed at rest or with minimal physical activity.

HOW IS SUI DETERMINED?

Initial Evaluation

The initial evaluation should include:

Focused History

The healthcare provider should ask the patient about duration of incontinence, frequency and intensity of the incontinence, use of protective pads, impact of symptoms on lifestyle, degree of bother experienced by the patient, and patient's expectations of treatment.

Validated questionnaire: One or more validated questionnaires that ask about lifestyle and medical history (Donovan, 2005), such as the incontinence quality of life (I-QOL) questionnaire (Patrick, 1997), should be completed.

Physical Examination

The examination includes a pelvic examination and assessment of the strength of the pelvic floor muscles and to determine the presence and degree of pelvic organ prolapse. Prolapse includes cystocele and uterine prolapse.

Pad test: The patient wears an absorbent pad while exercising, and the weight of the pad is measured.

Stress test: Demonstration of leakage with increasing abdominal pressure.

Sphincter function: Diagnosed by examination, Valsalva leak point pressure, urethral pressure profile.

Degree of urethral mobility: Diagnosed by estimation at time of physical examination, cotton-swab test, or imaging.

Urodynamics

This is a function test of the lower urinary tract that assesses the storage and emptying ability of the bladder. The basic study involves evaluation of bladder capacity, filling pressures, urethral function, bladder outlet resistance, and bladder emptying ability (post-void residual). Additional parameters that might add to the basic study to provide further information include pressure-flow analysis, electromyelogram, and fluoroscopic/visual imaging of the bladder.

The healthcare provider may perform further testing if there are indications such as concomitant overactive bladder symptoms, prior lower urinary tract surgery, including failed anti-incontinence procedures, known or suspected neurogenic bladder, a negative stress test, abnormal urinalysis, such as unexplained hematuria or pyuria, excessive residual urine volume, grade III or greater pelvic organ prolapse, or any evidence of dysfunctional voiding.

Nonsurgical Management of SUI

Pelvic Floor Muscle Exercises

Vaginal palpation can be used to assist patients in isolating the correct muscles to use in daily exercise. In addition, biofeedback can be helpful for patients. These special computerized devices teach patients how to strengthen the pelvic floor muscles.

Pelvic Floor Stimulation

Through the controlled delivery of stimulation to the nerves and muscles of the pelvic floor and bladder, this treatment can help patients strengthen their pelvic floor.

Lifestyle Changes

Patients should be counseled about lifestyle changes that can positively impact their stress urinary incontinence. Maintaining a healthy weight and good overall health can improve urinary incontinence. Additionally, smoking cessation is critical in reducing chronic cough, which results in pressure on the pelvic floor muscles.

Urinary Devices or Inserts

Occlusive devices include urethral inserts and patches, inserted into the urethra, which exert pressure inside the pelvis; these may be used during significant activity in order to minimize the risk of urethral irritation and urinary tract infections. A pessary is a small silicone ring inserted into the vagina and held in place by pelvic floor muscles and the pelvic bone. It provides pressure to the urethra which results in better closure at the bladder neck; these can be used as a long-term alternative with few complications.

Medications

There are currently no FDA-approved medications for SUI.

Topical Estrogen

This treatment aids postmenopausal women by addressing thinning of the vaginal lining. However, it is not a curative therapy; once the treatment is discontinued, SUI will recur.

Surgical Management of SUI

Commonly recommended surgical options include:

Periurethral Bulking Agents

In this procedure, biologic or synthetic bulking materials are injected into the layers of the urethra to "bulk" it up and help tighten up the valve muscle. A cystoscope and local anesthesia are used for this office procedure.

Injectable agents have a role after other procedures have failed; for example, when a diagnosis of intrinsic sphincter deficiency is made, the short-term continence rate is 48%, with an improvement rate of 76%. The effect decreases over time and repeat injections may be needed. The bulking agents (e.g. collagen, carbon coated beads, and fat) are injected in a retrograde (more common) or antegrade fashion in the periurethral tissue at the bladder neck and proximal urethra.

Retropubic Colposuspension

A retropubic suspension suspends the neck of the bladder behind the pubic bone. Bladder neck suspension is traditionally carried out for SUI secondary to urethral hypermobility and several procedures have been described.

The most extensively studied include the Marshall-Marchetti-Krantz (MMK) procedure and Burch colposuspension. The principle of open retropubic colposuspension is fixation of the bladder neck and proximal urethra to a retropubic position in order to reduce urethral hypermobility.

MMK procedure: It was initially described in late 1940's. Paravesical endopelvic fascia is attached to periosteum of back of pubic symphysis. Complications of the MMK procedure include wound infection, urinary tract infection (UTI), injury to urinary tract, postoperative voiding problems, pelvic organ prolapse and detrusor overactivity. In the MMK procedure, sutures are placed through the pubic symphysis and this carries the risk of osteitis pubis.

Burch colposuspension: It was introduced in the early 1960s. The sutures are passed through the ipsilateral Cooper's ligament and tied with gentle tension, leaving a suture bridge so as not to over-elevate and distort the bladder neck. The subjective and objective of early continence rates following the Burch procedure are described as 89.6% and 84.3%, respectively. Furthermore, a recent Cochrane review of surgery for SUI concludes that Burch colposuspension should be regarded as the standard procedure for open retropubic colposuspension due to its improved and more durable cure rates.

This is a more invasive surgical procedure that has become less popular with the advent of the less invasive sling procedures.

Midurethral Sling Procedures

Since its introduction, this minimally invasive midurethral procedure used to treat stress incontinence has been aggressively marketed.

Tension-free vaginal tape (TVT) procedure: The TVT procedure developed by Ulmsten et al. in the early 1990s, a midurethral sling, has been shown to have long-term effectiveness and equivalent efficacy of TVT to Burch. Studies have shown TVT to be a safe and effective surgical procedure for managing female stress urinary incontinence. TVT is a minimally invasive midurethral sling that is passed through the retropubic space and that was designed to replace functionally deficient pubourethral ligaments.

The TVT kit consists of two curved stainless steel needles attached to a prolene mesh sling sheathed in plastic, a detachable handle to facilitate retropubic passage of the needles, and a guide to make a Foley catheter rigid. Three small incisions are made—two suprapubic and one on the anterior vaginal wall at the midurethra. The TVT needles are then passed from the vagina through retropubic space, exiting through the suprapubic incisions. Cystoscopy is performed to ensure there have been no bladder perforations. The tape is adjusted to an appropriate snugness. Excess sling is then trimmed and the incisions closed with sutures.

Complications with retropubic slings include bleeding, hematoma, erosion of the mesh into the urethra or vagina, bladder perforation, de novo urge symptoms, voiding dysfunction, and infection.

Transobturator tape (TOT) procedure: The transobturator approach to midurethral slings was developed in 2001, with the following proposed advantages:

- It avoids the retropubic area, thus decreasing the risk of bowel perforation and vascular injury.
- It requires less operating room time.
- It is believed to mimic the natural support system in the pelvic floor better than the TVT.

In 2006, a surgical device requiring only one suburethral incision was introduced. Its purported advantages over existing midurethral procedures were the following:

- Complications associated with suprapubic and groin incisions will be eliminated.
- Cystoscopy will not be necessary.
- Operating room time will be shorter than with other midurethral sling techniques.

There is insufficient evidence to permit an evaluation of the advantages of outside-in versus inside-out transobturator routes, as long-term studies with significant results have yet to be published.

Alternative midurethral sling kits: TVT SECUR (Gynecare) is a new short midurethral sling tape with a novel securing mechanism. It is a modification of the TVT and TVT-O, with the ends of the tape held in place initially by friction between the tissue and a PDS/Vicryl pledget. It can be placed in a "U" (like the TVT) or hammock (like the TOT) orientation. Initial results suggest a steep learning curve and lower success rates than the traditional TVT.

Artificial Urinary Sphincter

In 1972, the artificial urethral sphincter (AUS) was introduced for the treatment of severe intrinsic sphincter deficiency. These devices can be successfully used after a previous failed continence surgery, but AUSs have a high morbidity rate and can result in a need for further surgery. As a primary procedure for SUI, the AUS has a cure rate of 80% and an improvement rate of 90%. The risks associated with this device are malfunction of the AUS or cuff erosion.

Complications from surgery for stress urinary incontinence may include:

- Urinary retention
- Gastrointestinal complications
- Infectious complications
- Perioperative genitourinary complications.
- Vascular complications
- General medical complications
- Neurological complications.

Overactive Bladder

JB Sharma, Manisha Yadav

Overactive bladder (OAB) is a clinical diagnosis characterized by presence of bothersome urinary symptoms. The International Continence Society (ICS) defines OAB as presence of "urinary urgency, usually accompanied by frequency and nocturia, with or without urge incontinence, in the absence of UTI or other obvious pathology".

OAB symptoms consist of four components:

1. *Urgency:* It is defined by ICS as the "complaint of sudden, compelling desire to pass urine which is difficult to defer." Urgency is considered as the hallmark symptom of OAB, but it has proven difficult to precisely define or to characterize for research or clinical purpose.
2. *Urinary frequency:* It can be reliably measured with a voiding diary. Traditionally, up to seven micturition episodes during waking hours has been considered normal, but his number is highly variable based upon hours of sleep, fluid intake, comorbid medical conditions and other factors.
3. *Nocturia:* It is the complaint of interruption of sleep one or more time because of need to void. Three or more episode of nocturia constitutes moderate or major bother.
4. *Urgency urinary incontinence:* It is defined as involuntary leakage of urine, associated with a sudden compelling desire to void. Incontinence episodes can be measured with pad tests. However, in patients with mixed urinary incontinence (both stress and urgency incontinence), it can be difficult to distinguish between incontinence subtypes.

OAB, because it is a symptom complex, is primarily a diagnosis of exclusion.

EPIDEMIOLOGY

OAB prevalence rate ranges from 7% to 27% in men, and 9% to 43% in women. Higher prevalence is reported in females then males. OAB symptom prevalence and severity tend to increase with age.

Negative impact of OAB symptoms on psychological functioning and quality of life has been well documented. Carrying out the activities of daily life and engaging in social and occupational activities can be profoundly affected by lack of bladder control and incontinence. The negative impact is evident among older adults (> 65 years), resulting in significant impairment in quality of life (QOL), including high rate of anxiety and depression.

Successful treatment of OAB symptoms with behavioral approach, antimuscarinic medications, neuromodulation therapies and botulinum toxins, all have been reported to improve patient QOL.

PATIENT PRESENTATION

Symptoms

When symptoms of urinary frequency (both daytime and night) and urgency with or without urgency incontinence may be diagnosed with OAB.

Differential Diagnosis

1. *Nocturnal polyuria:* In nocturnal polyuria, nocturnal voids are frequently normal or large volume as opposed to small volume voids commonly observed in nocturia associated with OAB. Sleep disturbances, vascular and/or cardiac disease and other medical conditions are often associated with nocturnal polyuria.
2. *Polydipsia:* Frequency that is result of polydipsia and resulting polyuria may mimic OAB; the two can only be distinguished with use of frequency-volume charts.
3. *Diabetes insipidus:* It is also associated with frequent large volume voids and should be distinguished from OAB.
4. *Interstitial cystitis:* It shares the symptoms of urinary frequency and urgency, with or without urgency incontinence; however, bladder and/or pelvic pain, including dyspareunia, is a crucial component of its presentation in contradistinction to OAB.

DIAGNOSTIC APPROACH

History

Clinician should carefully elicit the patient's bladder symptoms to document duration of symptoms and baseline symptom levels, to ensure that symptoms are not the consequence of some other condition and to determine whether the patient constitutes a complex OAB presentation.

Questions should assess bladder storage symptoms associate with OAB (urgency, frequency and nocturia), other bladder storage problems (e.g. stress urinary incontinence) and bladder emptying (e.g. hesitancy, straining to void, prior history of retention and force of stream).

Excessive fluid intake can produce voiding pattern that mimic OAB symptoms. For this reason, an enquiry into fluid intake habits should be performed, including asking patients how much fluid and of what type (e.g. with or without caffeine) they drink each day. Patients who do not appear able to provide accurate intake and voiding information should fill out a fluid diary.

Current medication use also should be reviewed to ensure that voiding symptoms are not a consequence of a prescribed medication, particularly diuretics.

Comorbid conditions should be completely elicited as these conditions may directly impact bladder function. Patients with comorbid conditions and OAB symptoms would be considered complicated OAB patients. These comorbid conditions include neurologic diseases (i.e. stroke, multiple sclerosis, spinal cord injury), mobility deficits, medically complicated/uncontrolled diabetes, fecal motility disorders (fecal incontinence/constipation), chronic pelvic pain, history of recurrent urinary tract infections (UTIs), gross hematuria, prior pelvic/vaginal surgeries (incontinence/prolapse).

Physical Examination

A careful, directed physical examination should be performed. An abdominal examination should be performed to assess for scars, masses, hernias and areas of tenderness as well as for suprapubic distension that may indicate urinary retention. Examination of lower extremities for edema should be done to give the clinician an assessment of the potential for fluid shifts during periods of postural changes. A rectal/genitourinary examination to rule out pelvic floor disorders (e.g. pelvic floor muscle spasticity, pain, pelvic organ prolapse) in females and prostatic pathology in males should be performed. In menopausal females, atrophic vaginitis should be assessed as a possible contributing factor to incontinence symptoms. The examiner should assess for perineal skin for rash or breakdown. The examiner also should assess perineal sensation, rectal sphincter tone and ability to contract the anal sphincter in order to evaluate pelvic floor tone and potential ability to perform pelvic floor exercises (e.g. the ability to contract the levator ani muscles) as well as to rule out impaction and constipation.

Neurological Examination

Cognitive impairment is related to symptom severity and has therapeutic implications regarding goals and options. The mini-mental state examination (MMSE) is a standardized, quick and useful assessment of cognitive function. An MMSE should be conducted on all patients who may be at risk for cognitive impairment to determine whether symptoms are aggravated by cognitive problems, to ensure that they will be able to follow directions for behavioral therapy and/or to determine the degree of risk for cognitive decline with anti-muscarinic therapy.

Urinalysis

A urinalysis to rule out UTI and hematuria should be performed. A urine culture is not necessary unless indication of infection (i.e. nitrites/leukocyte esterase on dipstick, pyuria/bacteriuria on microscopic examination) is found and may be done at the discretion of the clinician. If evidence of infection is detected, then a culture should be performed, the infection should be treated appropriately and the patient should be queried regarding symptoms once the infection has cleared. If evidence of hematuria not associated with infection, then the patient should be referred for urologic evaluation.

Urine Culture

Urinalysis is unreliable for identification of bacterial counts below 100,000 cfu/mL. In some patients with irritative voiding symptoms but without overt signs of infection, a urine culture may be appropriate to completely exclude the presence of clinically significant bacteriuria.

Post-void Residual (PVR)

Measurement of the post-void residual (PVR) is not necessary for patients who are receiving first-line behavioral interventions or for uncomplicated patients (i.e. patients without a history of or risk factors for urinary retention) receiving antimuscarinic medications. Because antimuscarinic medications can induce urinary retention, particularly in complicated patients with retention risk factors. PVR should be assessed in patients with obstructive symptoms, history of incontinence or prostatic surgery, neurologic diagnoses and in other patients at clinician discretion when PVR assessment is deemed necessary to optimize care and minimize potential risks.

PVR should be measured with an ultrasound bladder scanner immediately after the patient voids. If an ultrasound scanner is not available, then urethral catheterization may be used to assess PVR. For any patient on anti-muscarinic therapy, the clinician should be prepared to monitor PVR during the course of treatment should obstructive voiding symptoms appear. As there is considerable overlap between storage and emptying voiding symptoms, baseline PVRs should be performed for men with symptoms prior to initiation of anti-muscarinic therapy.

Bladder Diaries

Diaries that document intake and voiding behavior may be useful in some patients, particularly the patient who cannot describe or who is not familiar with intake and voiding patterns. Diaries also are useful to document baseline symptom levels so that treatment efficacy may be assessed.

In particular, self-monitoring with a bladder diary for three to seven days is a useful first step in initiating behavioral treatments for OAB.

Urodynamics, cystoscopy and diagnostic renal and bladder ultrasound should not be used in the initial workup of the uncomplicated patient.

TREATMENT

Issues to Consider

It is important to recognize that OAB is a symptom complex that may compromise quality of life (QoL) but generally does not affect survival. Given this context, in pursuing a treatment plan, the clinician should carefully weigh the potential benefit to the patient of a particular treatment against that treatment's risk for adverse events, the severity of adverse events and the reversibility of adverse events. Clinician should counsel patients and should develop an individualized treatment plan that optimizes quality of life. In developing the treatment plan, the balance between benefits and risks/burdens (i.e. adverse events) should be considered.

First-line Treatment: Behavioral Therapies

Behavioral treatments are a group of therapies that improve OAB symptoms by changing patient behavior or changing the patient's environment. Most effective behavioral treatment programs include multiple components and are individualized to the unique needs of the patient and his/her unique living situation. There are two fundamental approaches to behavioral treatment for OAB. One approach focuses on modifying bladder function by changing voiding habits, such as with bladder training and delayed voiding. The other approach, behavioral training, focuses on the bladder outlet and includes pelvic floor muscle training to improve strength and control and techniques for urge suppression. Specific components of behavioral treatment can include self-monitoring (bladder diary), scheduled voiding, delayed voiding, double voiding, pelvic floor muscle training and exercise (including pelvic floor relaxation), active use of pelvic floor muscles for urethral occlusion and urge suppression (urge strategies), urge control techniques (distraction, self-assertions), normal voiding techniques as biofeedback, electrical stimulation, fluid management, caffeine reduction, dietary changes (avoiding bladder irritants), weight loss and other lifestyle changes. In addition, behavioral therapies have the advantage that they can be combined with all other therapeutic techniques. Behavioral therapies are most often implemented by advance practice nurses (e.g. continence nurses) or physical therapists with training in pelvic floor therapy.

Clinicians should offer behavioral therapies (e.g. bladder training, bladder control strategies, pelvic floor muscle training, and fluid management) as first line therapy to all patients with OAB.

Second-line Treatment: Antimuscarinics

Clinicians should offer oral antimuscarinics, including darifenacin, fesoterodine, oxybutynin, solifenacin, tolterodine or trospium as second-line therapy.

The choice of oral antimuscarinics as second-line therapy reflects the fact that these medications reduce symptoms but also can commonly have non-life-threatening side effects, such as dry mouth, constipation, dry or itchy eyes, blurred vision, dyspepsia, UTI, urinary retention and impaired cognitive function. Rarely, life-threatening side effects, such as arrhythmias have been reported.

If an immediate release (IR) and an extended release (ER) formulation are available, then ER formulations should preferentially be prescribed over IR formulations because of lower rates of dry mouth.

ER formulations of oxybutynin and tolterodine resulted in statistically significantly fewer patient reports of dry mouth than the IR formulations of both medications.

Transdermal preparations of oxybutynin may be offered instead of oral anti-muscarinics to patients who are at risk of or who have experienced dry mouth with oral agents.

Clinicians should not use antimuscarinics in patients with narrow angle glaucoma unless approved by the treating ophthalmologist and should use anti-muscarinics with extreme caution in patients with impaired gastric emptying or a history of urinary retention.

Third-line Treatment: Neuromodulation Therapies (FDA Approved)

Clinicians may offer sacral neuromodulation (SNS) as third-line treatment in a carefully selected patient population characterized by severe refractory OAB symptoms or patients who are not candidates for second-line therapy and are willing to undergo a surgical procedure.

Sacral neuromodulation (SNS) is FDA-approved for the treatment of urinary frequency and urgency incontinence.

SNS is an appropriate therapy that can have durable treatment effects but in the context of frequent and moderately severe adverse events, including the need for additional surgeries. Patients should be counseled that the device requires periodic replacement in a planned surgical procedure and that the length of time between replacements depends on device settings. Patients also must be willing to comply with the treatment protocol because treatment effects typically are only maintained as long as the therapy is maintained and they should have the cognitive capacity to use the remote control to optimize device function. In addition, patients must accept that the use of diagnostic MRIs is contraindicated in individuals with the device implanted.

Peripheral tibial nerve stimulation (PTNS) is FDA-approved for the treatment of urinary urgency, frequency and urgency incontinence.

Non-FDA-approved: Intradetrusor Injection of Onabotulinum Toxin A

Clinicians may offer intradetrusor onabotulinum toxin A as third-line treatment in the carefully-selected and thoroughly-counseled patient who has been refractory to first- and second-line OAB treatments. The patient must be able and willing to return for frequent post-void residual evaluation, and able and willing to perform self-catheterization if necessary.

SURGERY

In rare cases, augmentation cystoplasty or urinary diversion for severe, refractory, complicated OAB patients may be considered.

In general, surgery is not recommended for OAB patients except in extremely rare cases. The vast majority of case series that document the effects of augmentation cystoplasty and diversion focus on neurogenic patients. Little is known regarding the impact of these procedures on non-neurogenic OAB patients and, particularly, on their quality of life. There are substantial risks to these procedures, however, including the likely need for long-term intermittent self-catheterization and the risk of malignancy.

Genitourinary Fistulas

Reeti Mehra, Navneet Magon

INTRODUCTION

Genitourinary fistulas are among the most distressing complications of gynecological and obstetrical procedures. A fistula is defined as an abnormal communication between two or more epithelial surfaces and as an abnormal communication between the urinary and genital tract. It may be acquired or congenital and presents as involuntary escape of urine into the vagina. The incidence is estimated to be as high as 0.5–3% of gynecological admission in referral hospitals. It may be of different types depending on the communication.

Bladder : Vesicovaginal
          Vesicouterine
          Vesicocervical
          Vesicourethra vaginal
Urethra : Urethrovaginal
Ureter   : Ureterovaginal
          Ureterouterine
          Ureterocervical

The most common is the vesicovaginal fistula (VVF).

ETIOPATHOGENESIS

It may be classified as:

- Congenital
- Acquired
  - Obstetric following childbirth
  - Gynecologic
    - After gynecologic surgery
    - Malignancy
    - After radiation therapy
- Traumatic
- Rarely after infections like tuberculosis, syphilis, lymphogranuloma venereum (LGV)
- After forgotten vaginal pessaries.

Vesicovaginal fistulae (VVF) in childhood usually occurs following penetrating trauma, foreign bodies and genitourinary surgery. Congenital cases are extremely rare. Prolonged obstetric labor remains a common cause in underprivileged countries, whereas elective vaginal and urogynecological surgeries are the leading cause in the developed states. Kelly from England[1] found that 95% of fistulas were from nonobstetric cause. In contradiction, in a study of 1443 cases from Nigeria, [2] which is one of the largest series, obstructed labor was the cause in 98%. Only 1% was associated with antecedent surgery. Similar results were seen in one of the largest studies on 14928 cases in Ethiopian women,[3] where VVF was more common in primipatients.

In developing countries, obstetric trauma remains the leading cause of vesicovaginal fistula and is largely unreported. Prolonged, neglected and obstructed labor, results in pressure necrosis and sloughing of tissue. Obstetric fistulas are usually large, trigonal and may also involve urethra and cervix.

Other contributing causes may be:
- Introital stenosis secondary to female circumcision
- Cephalopelvic disproportion
- Hydrocephalus may contribute
- Android pelvis
- Malnutrition
- Orthopedic disorders including rickets
- Misuse of forceps
- Destructive instruments used to deliver stillborn infants
- As complication of surgical abortions
- Rarely, symphysiotomy in shoulder dystocia
- Traditional harmful practices like Gishiri (anterior vaginal incision) and use of intravaginal caustic agents to cauterize vaginal lesions or postpartum, used to restore the vagina to its pre-pregnant state have also been reported to cause VVF.

The underlying mechanism in posthysterectomy fistulas is multifactorial:
- Avascular necrosis secondary to crush injury
- Thermal injury from cautery use
- Unrecognized bladder lacerations or partial bladder tear
- Wrong plane of dissection especially with previous surgeries, as in previous cesareans
- Suture placement in the bladder theoretically may cause erosion and a resultant fistula. However, in a study by Meeks et al[4], in a rabbit model, suture material intentionally placed through vaginal cuff and bladder was not associated with VVF.

Tancer in a group of 151 females[5] with VVF reported that gynecological surgery was responsible in 125 cases. Abdominal hysterectomy was the most common procedure in 73% or 110 cases. Factors thought to contribute were:
- Prior cesarean sections
- Pelvic inflammatory disease (PID)

- Endometriosis
- Cervical fibroids
- Prior radiation or ablative therapy for malignancy
- Diabetes
- Atherosclerosis
- Postoperative cuff abscess

Tancer also found that the most common association was prior surgery, particularly previous cesarean sections which were seen in 29% of his cases. However, 67% of VVF had none of the above risk factors. In the Cochrane review of 2009,[6] laparoscopic hysterectomies though offer many advantages, but at the cost of more operative injuries to the bladder and ureter. In general, most studies report 1–1.5% incidence of bladder injury in abdominal hysterectomy and 2–2.6% in laparoscopic hysterectomy. These surgical fistulas are smaller, usually supratrigonal and may be associated with ureteral fistulas. Malinowski et al[7] also reported an incidence of 1.26% ureterovaginal fistulas, occurring 2–3 weeks after laparoscopic hysterectomy due to thermal injury.

Bladder injury and urogenital fistulae are also known after anti-incontinence surgery. Urethrovaginal fistulae are also seen in such surgeries. Other types of urologic and gastrointestinal surgeries also contribute to the incidence of VVFs like surgical repair of urethral diverticulum, electrocautery of bladder papilloma, and surgery for pelvic carcinoma. Two case reports of fistula have also been linked with relatively innocuous periurethral collagen placement.[8] Also, there are a couple of cases reported after a forgotten vaginal pessary.[9]

PREVENTION OF OBSTETRICAL FISTULA

- Adequate antenatal care to screen high-risk women
- Early detection by using partograph
- Drainage by catheter for 7–10 days in obstructed labor.

PREVENTION OF FISTULA AT THE TIME OF GYNECOLOGICAL SURGERY

- Adequate exposure: It avoids inadvertent injury and also prompt identification
- Identify the high-risk cases and carefully delineate the anatomy during surgery
- In high-risk cases, preoperative ureteric stenting may not prevent injury but will help in delineating and identifying the course of the ureters intra-operatively
- Minimize bleeding and hematoma formation
- Wide mobilization of the bladder and correct dissection of the pubo-cervicovaginal plane. Both these measures serve to prevent an inadvertent clamping or suturing of the bladder

- Intraoperative retrograde filling of the bladder helps to delineate bladder limits and also to detect injury, if any
- Postoperatively, cystourethroscopy may be done to see bladder integrity and ureteral openings
- Knowledge and care about energy sources, especially when working close to bladder and ureters, especially in laparoscopic surgery. Bipolar cautery has less lateral spread of heat as compared to monopolar source.

CLINICAL PRESENTATION

Most common presenting feature is continuous leakage of urine from the vagina, most commonly in the first 10 days after surgery and less commonly between 10th and 20th postoperative day. The size and location of the fistula, determines the degree of leakage.

Patients with small fistula may void normally and notice only small position dependant drainage. Alternatively, there may be leakage only at maximal bladder capacity. They may be recurrent cystitis, pyelonephritis, unexplained fever, hematuria, flank, vaginal or suprapubic pain and abnormal urinary stream.

Irritation of vagina and vulval mucosa and perineum will be present and women complain of foul ammoniacal odor. The constant leakage makes the patient a social recluse, disrupts sexual relations, and leads to depression, low self-esteem and insomnia. Urethrovaginal fistulas may present as spraying of urine, altered stream, stress urinary incontinence (SUI) or even be asymptomatic.

PREOPERATIVE ASSESSMENT

A thorough assessment is mandatory. In series by Goodwin et al,[10] 12% of patients were found to have coexistent ureterovaginal fistulas. In a report by Lee et al,[11] 19% of urethrovaginal fistulas were associated with VVF also. In a recent study by Rangnekar et al[12] also, almost 37% patients have multiple fistulae.

Assessment would include:
- Detailed history
- Physical examination with a speculum in adequate light and position
- Leakage from the vagina is noted
- Vaginal fluid may be sent for—Urea, C/S, Urine R/E
- Renal function tests
- Intravenous urography to aid the location of the fistula and ureteric involvement
- Retrograde pyelography may be done, if IV urography does not reveal a ureteric fistula and clinical suspicion is high
- Dye test has been traditionally used as 3 swab test.

In this test with the patient in position for pelvic examination, a 16 FR Foley's catheter is placed and the vagina is inspected by a Sims speculum.

The fistula, if large will be visualized and urine is seen coming through it. If not visualized, dilute methylene blue dye is instilled in the bladder with the Foley's catheter and observed. If the dye appears immediately, VVF is diagnosed and the site is seen carefully. If the dye does not appear, a tampon or 3 swabs in upper, mid and lower vagina are inserted in the vagina and the patient is asked to move about for 10–15 minutes.

In a ureterovaginal fistula, the tampon will be wet but not blue. Blue staining of the tampon at the apex indicates a small VVF. If the distal end of tampon is wet, urethral incontinence is suspected.

- An IV urogram or retrograde pyelogram is indicated to see ureteric injury. Retrograde pyelography is one of the investigations of highest diagnostic accuracy for diagnosing the site and presence of a coexisting ureteral fistula
- Cystourethroscopy is a crucial adjunct and should be done in all patients to see the size, location, number and margins of the fistula and to note the ureteral openings. Large fistulas may prevent bladder distension and make cystoscopy difficult. In such conditions, the vagina may have to be packed with gauge
- Other radiological investigations mentioned are CT scan with IV contrast and colored Doppler USG with contrast media. They have only limited value
- Preoperative urodynamic testing is defended by some authors by the fact that it may prepare patients for a less than perfect outcome and protect the surgeon medicolegally.[13] However, for the typical posthysterectomy VVF, de novo detrusor instability is rare. However, voiding difficulties even after successful repair has been described by Agarwal M et al.[14]

ANATOMIC CONSIDERATIONS

Post total abdominal hysterectomy (TAH) fistulae are usually supratrigonal and medial to both ureteral openings. Vaginally, it corresponds to the vaginal cuff. Fistulae from obstetric cause may be larger, more distal and associated with urethral injury.

PREOPERATIVE CARE

- Cystitis, vaginitis and perineal dermatitis should be treated with appropriate agents
- Zinc oxide ointments or creams containing lanolin are needed for skin dermatitis
- Appropriate antibiotics may be used for the cystitis
- Estrogen cream may be used for patient with poor quality vaginal tissue.

CONSERVATIVE MANAGEMENT

A trial of conservative treatment that uses continuous bladder drainage, supplemented by anticholinergics may be used in some cases of very small fistula. There are reports of spontaneous closure in small fistulas, less than 1 cm in size and diagnosed with 7 days of index surgery. Continuous bladder drainage for 3–4 weeks through a urethral or suprapubic catheter is recommended. If it has failed to close spontaneously after 30 days of continuous catheterization, it is unlikely to do so without definitive surgery. Also this technique is unlikely to be successful, if the fistula tract has matured (after 6 weeks), or if it is associated with irradiation or malignancy.

Timing of Repair

Fistula is an anguishing experience for both the patient and the surgeon. The timing of repair depends on the overall medical condition of the patient and very importantly the tissue quality surrounding the fistula. While the emotional status of the patient should not be underestimated, it also should not play a dominant role in the decision process of when to repair a VVF. Many authors simply recommend delaying surgery until tissue inflammation and infection has settled. Use of estrogen cream and indwelling catheter in the waiting period may expedite tissue recovery. It usually takes 6–8 weeks for the same in most cases. Surgeons no longer advocate 3–6 months wait, as was done earlier.

In the guidelines used at teaching hospitals, University of Rome Campus Biomedico and University of Miami School of Medicine,[15] a minimum of a 4–6 week's wait from the onset of the fistula is recommended. In a study by Raasen TJ et al also on 888 women with fistulae, patients operated within 3 months had a better surgical outcome and is also expected to restore the social status of the patients.[16] Fresh injuries, if detected within 24–48 hours post-operative must be operated immediately. Longer intervals are universally accepted as the standard of care only in infected or irradiated tissue. As long as 1 year interval for radiation-induced fistulas, may be required to insure full resolution of tissue necrosis.

Surgical Treatment

Sims in 1852,[17] published his first famous successful surgical repair of VVF in a maid using a silver wire. Since then, there have been many changes and developments. Most authors agree that the best chance at closure of the fistula is at first attempt. Factors that affect the success of a fistula repair include:
- Duration of fistula
- Etiology
- Presence of necrotic tissue
- Surgical technique and experience of the surgeon.

The best chance for a surgeon to achieve successful repair is by using the type of surgery with which he or she is most familiar and comfortable with. Techniques of repair include:
- The vaginal approach
- The abdominal approach
- Electrocautery
- Fibrin glue

- Endoscopic closure using fibrin glue with or without adding bovine collagen
- The laparoscopic approach
- Using interposition flaps or grafts.

The several surgical principles proposed to improve success rates are:
- Wide mobilization of bladder and adequate exposure
- Excision of scar tissue at the risk of increasing the fistula size, in an attempt to create a fresh bladder injury
- Tension free and water tight layered closure of bladder and vagina
- Non-traumatizing technique
- Good hemostasis
- Complete drainage of the bladder postoperatively.

Most literature on fistula repairs is by retrospective studies and these are individual series published by individual surgeons or individual fistula centers. However, management of these fistulas has been better defined and standardized over the last decade. In the guidelines used at teaching hospitals, University of Rome Campus Biomedico and University of Miami School of Medicine, their preferred approach is a transvaginal repair.[15]

The vaginal repair techniques can be categorized as to those that are modifications of the Latzko procedure or a layered closure with or without a martius flap. The most frequently used abdominal approaches are the bivalve technique or the fistula excision. Radiated fistulas usually require a more individualized management and complex surgical procedures. The rate of successful fistula repair reported in the literature varies between 70 and 100% in nonradiated patients, with similar results when a vaginal or abdominal approach is performed, the mean success rates being 91 and 97%, respectively. Fistulas in radiated patients are less frequently repaired and the success rate varies between 40 and 100%. In this setting, many institutions prefer to perform a urinary diversion. They recommend waiting at least 4–6 months or even a year in certain cases, prior to attempting repair of a vesicovaginal fistula in irradiated fistulas.

Vaginal Approach

It has many advantages and is the preferred route in most cases, as elucidated:
- It avoids the potential morbidity associated with abdominal surgery
- Quicker recovery
- More cosmetic and comfortable to the patients
- Success rate of 98% to 100% have been reported in most series.

Abdominal Approach

It is favored in:
- Larger fistulas
- If located high on posterior wall
- If located close to ureters
- If concomitant abdominal pathology or associated ureteric involvement

⊃ If bowel is required for augmentation cystoplasty.

If the fistula repair is attempted vaginally in a case where it is high in an immobile vaginal vault, result may not be satisfactory.

Surgical Technique

Vaginal repair

Two techniques commonly used are:

⊃ Flap splitting technique

⊃ Latzko procedure.

Flap splitting technique

It involves:

⊃ Wide mobilization of vaginal mucosa from the edge of fistula

⊃ Bladder is closed in two layers, a submucosal line of interrupted Lembert sutures, and a second layer to close the muscularis to reduce tension on the previous line

⊃ Trigonal defects are repaired in a transverse direction as vertical closure will draw the ureters close to the midline and may cause ureteric obstruction

⊃ There is no vaginal shortening in this method.

Latzko procedure

It is an excellent procedure for correcting small post hysterectomy fistulae at the vaginal apex, but cannot be performed if cervix is in situ. In this procedure, there is partial colpocleisis of upper 2–3 cm of vagina surrounding the fistula. In a recent publication by Dorairajan LN et al,[18] they have recommended that this technique is simple and is an excellent age-old technique that has stood the test of time. They recommend that it deserves wider adoption by the urological community.

It involves:

⊃ An elliptical portion of vaginal epithelium is stripped from anterior and post-vaginal walls around the fistula, at least 2.5 cm in all direction.

⊃ The vesical edges of the fistula are not denuded

⊃ Vaginal epithelium is mobilized

⊃ Delayed absorbable interrupted sutures are placed, so that the post-vaginal wall becomes the posterior bladder wall and it epithelizes with the urothelium

⊃ The vagina which has been mobilized around 2 cm is now closed over it with interrupted delayed absorbable suture.

Advantage: Theoretically, there is no suture in the bladder wall and so bladder can fill without tension.

Interposition grafts:

May be used in – Large fistulae
– Recurrent fistulae
– Urethral fistulae
– Bladder neck fistula.

- In 1928, Martuis[19] first described the use of lateral fat pad
- Bir Khoff and colleagues[20] reported a 100% success rate using the Martius technique. Etkins and colleagues[21] reported a success rate of 96%
- Fugiwara and associates[22] have described gracilis myocutaneous flap in radiation induced VVF and rectovaginal fistulae
- Pedicled flap of vagina has also been described by Hurley and Previte in a case report[23]
- Peritoneal flap has been used successfully by Razs et al[24] and is also recommended by Lentz SS et al.[25]

Note: Regardless of the route of repair, the closure should be water tight which should be checked with methylene blue or indigo carmine. Most authors leave a suprapubic catheter for 3 weeks and a vaginal pack for 24 hours. The patient is on antibiotics till the catheter is in situ.

Abdominal repair

O'Connor's technique:
- Can be done extraperitoneally or intraperitoneally
- Bladder is bisected with wide mobilization of bladder and vagina
- Fistula is excised
- Bladder and vagina finally closed in 2 layers.

Results

Mondet and coworkers[26] in their review gave an 85% success rate, and 33% patients required ureteral reimplantation.

Cetin and colleagues[27] have described a modification of the Connor's technique where extraperitoneal repair is done through a small vertical anterior cystostomy. Success rates are comparable.

Tissue grafts in abdominal route: The following flaps have been used:
- Omental flaps
- Rectus muscle flaps.

In a recent review by Evans,[28] all repairs with grafts were successful, whereas success rate without grafts was 64%.

Minimally Invasive Management

This has been used in very small fistulas in some case reports. Fibrin glue (thrombin and fibrinogen combination) to occlude small VVF was first reported in 1979 by Petterson et al.[29] Occlusion therapy using fibrin glue is considered useful and safe for intractable fistulas. Fibrin glue facilitates healing by recruiting macrophages and providing a semisolid support structure rich in growth and angiogenic factors. This system continues to support the fibroblast to connective tissue transition.

Fulguration of small VVF that are just pinhole size followed by continuous drainage has been described by Storsky et al.[30] Recently Dogra and Nabi,[31] used the term laser welding where they used endoscopic neodymium-doped yttrium aluminum garnet (Nd:YAG) laser to fulgurate a small 2–3 mm VVF.

Denuding the tract probably led to spontaneous closure of the fistula after 3 weeks continuous drainage.

Laparoscopic repair was first reported in 1994 by Nezhat et al[32] and has also been described by Putambekar et al[33] and others, but it is limited by its steep learning curve.

Repairs using the Da Vinci have also been reported but are only of academic interest as of now.

POSTOPERATIVE CARE

Bladder Drainage

Continuous bladder drainage postoperatively is vital for successful urogenital fistula (UGF) repair. A large caliber catheter minimizes the potential for catheter blockage by blood clots, mucus, and calcaneus deposits. For fistulas involving the lower portion of the bladder trigone, bladder neck, or urethra, transurethral bladder, catheters should not be used. In post hysterectomy VVF repairs, both transurethral and suprapubic catheters may be placed. The urethral catheter may be discontinued on the fifth to seventh day. Most surgeons remove the suprapubic catheter after 2–3 weeks. Surgeries to repair pelvic radiotherapy-associated VVFs require longer periods of drainage.

Acidification of urine to diminish risks of cystitis, mucus production, and formation of bladder calculi is a consideration for patients with an indwelling catheter. Vitamin C, methenamine mandelate and sodium acid phosphate can also be administered to achieve urine acidification.

Control of Postoperative Bladder Spasms

Urised is effective for control of postoperative bladder spasms. It is a combination of antiseptics (methenamine, methylene blue, phenyl salicylate, and benzoic acid) and parasympatholytics (atropine sulfate and hyoscyamine sulfate).

Antibiotic Therapy

Many physicians administer oral antibiotic prophylaxis to patients with VVF postoperatively until the Foley catheter is discontinued. Others administer antibiotic therapy only when urine cultures are positive for bacterial growth. Close follow up and prompt evaluation for any urinary tract infections and antibiotic therapy are mandatory.

Minimizing Valsalva Maneuvers

Stool softeners and a high fiber diet are given postoperatively.

Examination: Avoid pelvic and speculum vaginal examinations during the first 4–6 weeks postoperatively because the tissue is delicate.

Pelvic rest: Prohibit coitus and tampon use for a minimum of 4–6 weeks.

Complicated Fistulas

They can be defined as:
- ⊃ Fistulas of large size ≥ 3 cm in diameters
- ⊃ Fistulas occurring after prior closure
- ⊃ Those associated with radiation therapy
- ⊃ Fistulas associated with malignancy
- ⊃ Fistulas in compromised operative fields due to poor healing or host characteristics
- ⊃ Fistulas involving trigone, bladder neck and/or urethra.

These are operative challenges and need individualized treatment.

URINARY DIVERSION AND RECONSTRUCTION

In irreparable or recurrent VVF following radiation therapy, these are used as last resorts to achieve a socially acceptable solution. Ureteral implantation into an isolated ileal loop or into a continent colon or ileal pouch is now the preferred method.

FISTULA: A DEVASTATING PUBLIC HEALTH PROBLEM

An obstetric fistula is classically regarded as an "accident of childbirth". Obstetric fistula is highly stigmatizing and afflicted women often become social outcasts. Although obstetric fistula has been eliminated from advanced industrialized nations, it remains a widespread and incompletely documented public health problem in the world's poorest countries. Several million cases of obstetric fistula are currently thought to exist in Sub-Saharan Africa and South Asia. Estimates suggest that at least 3 million women in poor countries have unrepaired vesicovaginal fistulas, and that 30,000–1,30000[34] new cases develop each year in Africa alone. Such a high occurrence is largely because of the complex interactions among medical, social, economic and environmental factors present in these third world countries. Mostly, the women are in labor for days being helped by untrained *dais* and unskilled family members. They deliver a stillborn child and then develop a urogenital or rectal fistula and become divorced and outcasts. An article by Wall LL et al uses the Haddon matrix,[35] a standard tool for injury analysis, to examine the factors influencing obstetric fistula formation in low-resource countries. Construction of a Haddon matrix provides that fistula prevention, will involve enhanced surveillance of labor, competent medical care for women both during and after obstructed labor, and the development of specialist fistula centers to treat injured women where fistula prevalence is high.[35] Time interval from obstructed labor to delivery is critical and this time delay can be reduced by improving transportation, better healthcare infrastructure at rural areas. Competent obstetric care delivered promptly and at low cost is the key. The long-term strategies to eradicate obstetric fistula must include universal access to emergency obstetric care, improved access to family planning services, increased education for women, and community economic development. Successful eradication of the obstetric fistula will require the mobilization of sufficient political will at both the international and individual country levels to insure that adequate resources are devoted to this problem and that maternal health becomes a high priority.

REFERENCES

1. Kelly J. Vesicovaginal and rectovaginal fistulae. J R Soc Med. 1992;85:257.
2. Hilton P, Ward A. Epidemiological and surgical aspects of urogenital fistulae: A review of 25 years experience in South-East Nigeria. Int Urogynecol J Pelvic Floor Dysfunct. 1998;9:189-94.
3. Muleta M, Rasmussen S, Kiserud T. Obstetric fistula in 14, 928 Ethiopian women. Acta Obstet Gynecol Scand. 2010;89(7):945-51.
4. Meeks GR, Sams JO, Field K, et al. Formation of vescicovaginal fistula: The role of suture placement into the bladder during closure of the vaginal cuff after transabdominal hysterectomy. Am J Obstet Gynecol. 1997;177:1298.
5. Tancer ML. Observation or prevention and management of VVF after total hysterectomy. Surg Gynecol Obstet. 1992;175:501-6.
6. Nieboer TE, Johnson N, Lethaby A, Tavender E, Curr E, Garry R, et al. Surgical approach to hysterectomy for benign gynecological disease. Cochrane Database Syst Rev. 2009;8(3).
7. Malinowski A, Makowska J, Antosiak B. Total laparoscopic hysterectomy—indications and complications of 158 patients. Ginekol Pol. 2013;84(4):252-7.
8. Pruthi R, Petrus C, Bundrick WJ. New onset vesicovaginal fistula after transurethral collagen injection in women who underwent cystectomy and orthotopic neobladder creation: Presentation and definitive treatment. J Urol. 2000;164:1638-9.
9. Penrose KJ, Ma Yin J, Tsokos N. Delayed vesicovaginal fistula after ring pessary usage. Int Urogynecol J. 2013 Jun 26[ahead of print].
10. Goodwin WE, Scardino PT. Vesicovaginal and ureterovaginal fistulae: A summary of 25 years experience. J Urol. 1980;123:370.
11. Lee RA, Symmonds RE, Williams TJ. Current status of genitourinary fistula. Obstet Gynecol. 1988;72:313.
12. Rangnekar NP, Imdad Ali N, Kaul SA, Pathak HR. Role of the martius procedure in the management of urinary-vaginal fistulas. J Am Coll Surg. 2000;191(3):259-63.
13. Hinton P. Urodynamic findings in patients with urogenital fistualae. Br J Urol. 1998;81:539.
14. Agarwal MM, Raamya SM, Mavuduru R, Mandal AK, Singh SK. Voiding dysfunction after repair of giant trigonal vesicovaginal or urethrovesicovaginal fistulae: A need for long term follow-up. Indian J Urol. 2012;28(4):405-8.
15. Angioli R, Penalver Muzii L, Mendez L, Mirhashemi R, Bellati F, et al. Guidelines of how to manage vesicovaginal fistula. Crit Rev Oncol Hematol. 2003;48(3):295-304.
16. Raassen TJ, Verdaasdonk EG, Vierhout ME, et al. Prospective results after first-time surgery for obstetric fistulas in East African women. Int Urogynecol J Pelvic Floor Dysfunct. 2008;19(1):73-9.
17. Sims JM. On the treatment of vesico-vaginal fistula (classic articles in Urogynecology). Urogynecol J Pelvic Floor Dysfunct. 1998;9:236-48.
18. Dorairajan LN, Khattar N, Kumar S, Pal BC. Latzko repair for vesicovaginal fistula revisited in the era of minimal-access surgery. Int Urol Nephrol. 2008;40(2):317-20.
19. Martius H. Die operative Wiederherstellung der vollkommen feblenden, Harnrohre und des Schiessmuskels derselben. Zentralbl Gynakol. 1928;52:480.

20. Birkhoff JD, Wechsler M, Romas NA. Urinary fistulae: Vaginal repair using a labial fat pad. J Urol. 1977;117:595.
21. Elkins TE, DeLancey JOL, McGuire EJ. The use of modified martius graft as an adjunctive technique in vesicovaginal and ractovaginal fistula repair. Obstet Gynecol. 1990;75:727.
22. Fugiwara K, Koshima I, Tanaka K. Radiation-induced vsicovaginal fistula successfully repaired using a gracilis myocutaneous flap. Int J Clin Oncol. 2000; 5:338-44.
23. Hurley LJ, Previte SR. Vaginal pedicled flap for closure of vesicovaginal fistula. Urology. 2000;56:856.
24. Raz S, Bregg KJ, Nitti VW. Transvaginal repair of vesicovaginal fistula using a peritoneal flap. J Urol. 1993;156:56.
25. Lentz SS. Transvaginal repair of the posthysterectomy vasicovaginal fistula using a peritoneal flap: The gold standard. J Reprod Med. 2005;50(1):41-4.
26. Mondet F, Chartier-Kastler EJ, Conort P. Anatomic and functional results of transperitoneal-transvesical vsicovaginal fistula repair. Urology. 2001;58:882-6.
27. Cetin S, Yazicioglu A, Ozgur S. Vescovaginal fistula repair: A simple uprapubic transvesical approach. Int Urol Nephrol. 1988;20:265-8.
28. Evans DH, Madjar S, Politano VA. Interposition flaps in transabdominal vasicovaginal fistula repairs: Are they really necessary? Urology. 2001;57:670.
29. Pettersson S, Hedelin H, Jansson I. Fibrin occlusion of a vesicovaginal fistula. Lancet. Apr 1979;28:933.
30. Stovsky MD, Ignatoff JM, Blum MD. Use of electrocoagulation in the treatment of vesicovaginal fistulae. J Urol. 1994;152:1443.
31. Dogra PN, Nabi G. Laser welding of vasicovaginal fistula. Int Urogynecol J Pelvic Floor Dys. 2001;12:69.
32. Nezhat CH, Nezhat F, Nezhat C. Laparoscopic repair of a vesicovaginal fistula: A case report. Obstet Gynecol. May 1994;83:899-901.
33. Puntambekar SR, Desai R, Galagali A, Joshi S, Kenawadehar R, Pandit A, et al. Laparoscopic transvesical approach for vesicovaginal fistula repair. Minim Invasive Gynecol. 2013;20(3):334.
34. Wall LL. Obstetric vesicovaginal fistula as an international public-health problem. Lancet. Sept 30 2006;368(9542):1201-9.
35. Wall LL. Preventing Obstetric fistulas in low-resource countries: Insights from a Haddon matrix. Obstet Gynecol Surv. 2012 Feb;67(2):111-21.

Chapter
43

Vulval Pruritis

Shobha Chakraborty

Pruritus vulvae is a symptom which is experienced by not less than 10% of women attending gynecological clinics. It presents a clinical problem of unusual difficulty because it has many possible causes and, unless the cause is found, the treatment is usually unsatisfactory.[1]

Pruritus means a sensation of itching and it is important to restrict the term to this. When a woman complains of "irritation", she often means that the vulva is painful, burning or tender—symptoms which differ from pruritus, not only in their nature but also in their underlying causes.

Irrespective of its etiology, pruritus vulvae is more troublesome at night when the women are in bed.

NATURAL DEFENCE MECHANISMS

The vaginal acidic pH allows only Doderlein's bacilli to survive. These organisms produce lactic acid, which makes the vagina self-sterilizing. When the pH rises and becomes alkaline, nonresident pathogens are able to grow. Apart from the acidic medium, the vagina has a tough stratified epithelium that presents as a barrier against pathogens, and there are no crypts unlike the endocervix where organisms can multiply.

WHAT IS VULVAL ITCH?

Itching of the vulva can result from irritation, allergy, inflammation, infection or cancer.

CAUSES OF VULVAL ITCH

Infections

- Bacterial vaginosis
- HSV type I or II
- Scabies
- Tinea cruris

- Trichomoniasis
- Yeast infection.

Noninfectious

- Allergic reactions
- Atopic dermatitis or eczema
- Atrophic vaginitis
- Chemical irritants
- Lichen simplex chronicus
- Precancerous lesions of the vulva
- Psoriasis
- Vulval cancer.

Infection is the commonest cause of pruritus. Sexually transmitted infections, such as herpes or Trichomoniasis can cause vulval itch, as can other infections, such as fungal infections and bacterial vaginosis. Fungal infection is caused by gram-positive fungus Candida albicans that flourishes in the acidic vagina. Candidiasis occurs when there is a change in the normal environment. This can occur after administration of broad-spectrum antibiotics, oral contraceptives, steroids, and in immunocompromised patients with HIV infection and diabetes. It causes intense vulval and vaginal pruritus with profuse curdy discharge. There is inflammation of the vulva, especially the labia minora and introitus, with excoriation. Vulval Candidiasis may produce erythema and edema as well as satellite lesions.[2] Trichomoniasis is the common infection in women. This is caused by a flagellate protozoan, Trichomonas vaginalis. Patients characteristically present with malodorous vaginal discharge and pruritus. Pruritus and inflammation of the vulva are present. Bacterial vaginosis produces a disturbance of the normal flora. The causative organism is *Gardnerella*. It is commonly stated that any type of vaginal discharge can cause pruritus vulva; this is not true. Purulent and mucopurulent discharges cause pain and tenderness. The only discharges associated with pruritus are those caused by vaginal infection with either Trichomonas vaginalis or Candida albicans; these account for at least 80% of all cases of pruritus vulva.[3]

"Crabs" (pubic lice) is a sexually transmitted disease that typically causes itching. Scabies, which can be spread sexually or through skin-to-skin contact, is a contagious skin disease that causes itching. Tinea cruris, a fungal infection, sometimes referred to as "jock itch" or "ringworm of the groin", can also cause infection of the vulva and the skin around it.

The only urinary condition associated with pruritus vulvae is glycosuria, and this is either a manifestation of diabetes or of a lowered renal threshold.

Irritation and allergy can occur as a result of exposure to soaps, feminine hygiene products, perfumes, lubricants, douches, creams or latex. Contact dermatitis from all sorts of cosmetics is a possibility. Sometimes antiseptic preparations used in the treatment of vaginitis are the cause of pruritus. Preparations containing benzocaine or other local anesthetics are especially liable to produce skin reactions and should never be applied to the vulva or vagina. A relationship between pruritus and coitus can often be traced to an idiosyncrasy to chemical or rubber constituents of contraceptives. In this case, avoiding exposure to the irritant or allergen may be all that is needed for the itching to resolve.

Some noninfectious skin conditions, such as psoriasis, eczema and lichen simplex chronicus can involve the vulva. Other noninfectious causes of vulval itch include changes associated with decreased hormonal levels following menopause, as well as precancerous changes and cancer. The treatment of vulval itch is highly variable depending on the cause of itching.

The most intense and persistent pruritus is associated with benign epithelial disorders of the vulva. Conditions like senile atrophy, lichen sclerosus, vulval intraepithelial neoplasia and Paget's disease are all responsible for pruritus. Vulval cancers initially cause intractable pruritus.

Psychological factors—Many mental disturbances have a sexual basis. So it is not surprising that the skin of the vulva can become the site for manifestations of psychoneuroses. Pruritus is often limited to one area of the labium, the skin of which becomes thickened and hard as a result of scratching, to give rise to the lesions called neurodermatitis.

Vulval itch is unlikely to require emergent treatment; however, some causes can be easily treated and others that can ultimately lead to serious complications. If you have a persistent itch, not responding to any measures, seek prompt medical care.

SYMPTOMS

Symptoms of vulval itch may vary depending on the underlying disease, disorder or condition.

Symptoms that may occur along with vulval itch (affecting the genitals or skin) are as follows:
 1. Bleeding after coitus
 2. Increased sensitivity to irritants
 3. Increased susceptibility to genital infections
 4. Itching in other areas of the skin
 5. Pain during contact
 6. Pain or burning of the vulva
 7. Pain or burning with urination
 8. Raised, thickened red or white patches
 9. Redness or swelling of the vulva
10. Sores, blisters or scabs in the affected area
11. Vaginal discharge
12. Visible eggs or crabs in the pubic hair.

Symptoms that might indicate a serious condition are as follows:
 1. Abnormal discharge or bleeding
 2. Changes in appearance, color, thickness, or the texture of vulva

3. Itchy skin in other areas of the body
4. Pain during sexual contact
5. Pain or burning with micturition
6. Pain or burning of the genitals
7. Pelvic pain
8. Redness or swelling of the genital sores, blisters or scabs.

POTENTIAL COMPLICATIONS OF VULVAL ITCHING

Failure to seek treatment can result in serious complications and permanent damage. Once the underlying cause is diagnosed, it is mandatory to follow the treatment plan to reduce the risk of potential complications, including:

➲ Secondary skin infection
➲ Spread of infectious diseases to close contacts or the partner
➲ Spread of cancer.

INVESTIGATION

The more careful the investigation, the more likely is the cause of pruritus to be found and the treatment to be successful. Chronic epithelial changes necessitate skin biopsy to exclude precancerous conditions or vulval cancer.

TREATMENT

When a specific and clear cause is found and the treatment is directed to it, the pruritus is invariably cured or controlled. Parasitic or fungal infections can be eliminated, glycosuria can be controlled and deficiency states corrected. When an underlying cause is not discovered or is doubtful, as happens in at least 50% of the cases, the treatment has to be tentative or empirical and the results are less than satisfactory.

General measures include advice on proper hygiene, on wearing loosefitting cotton underclothes, and on keeping the vulva well aerated. It is important to refrain from scratching. Treatment is directed primarily to eliminate any etiological factor discovered. Anemia is corrected, folic acid or vitamin B_{12} administered if a deficiency is present, glycosuria controlled, Candidiasis eradicated and proven antigens avoided. Antihistaminic should be given orally to reduce itching. Even in cases of extragenital fungal infection, application of fungicidal ointments to the vulva gives good results. Clotrimazole 500 mg, given vaginally, gives relief from the symptoms. Combination of antifungicide and corticosteroids in ointment form is particularly helpful. Clobetasol propionate 0.05% ointment is the definitive treatment for lichen sclerosus.

Treat trichomoniasis with oral metronidazole 500 mg orally twice daily for 7 days.

The difficult and intractable case of pruritus vulvae leaves such an impression that it is easy to become pessimistic and overlook the cures.

When a proper investigation to find etiological factors is carried out, a cure or considerable relief can be achieved in nearly 90% of all the cases.

REFERENCES

1. Biggs WS, Williams RM. Common gynecological infections. Prim care. 2009 March;36(1):33-51.
2. Superficial fungal infections. In: Habif T.P., ed. Clinical dermatology. 5th ed. St. Louis, Mo: Mosby Elsevier; 2009:chap 13.
3. Eckerl LO, Lentz GM. Infections of lower genital tract: vulva, vagina, cervix, toxic shock syndrome, HIV infections. In: Katz VL, Lentz GM, Lobo RA, Gershenson DM, eds. Comprehensive gynecology. 5th edition. Philadelphia, Pa: Mosby Elsevier; 2007: chap 22.

Adnexal Masses

Roza Olyai, Prachi Renjhen

The term adnexa (Latin word) means "appendage". The adnexal mass usually refers to mass arising from the ovaries, fallopian tubes, and structures of the broad ligament as these organs form the adnexa of the uterus. Adnexal masses may also have a nongynecological source. They can be benign or malignant. Common adnexal masses seen in premenopausal females are ovarian in origin—polycystic ovaries, follicular and corpus luteal cyst, tubal pregnancies, benign and malignant tumors, endometriomas and tubo-ovarian masses.

In postmenopausal women, common adnexal masses are cancer, fibroids, fibromas and diverticular abscess.

The initial detection and evaluation of an adnexal mass requires a high index of suspicion, a thorough history and physical examination, and careful attention to subtle historical clues. Timely, appropriate laboratory and radiographic studies are required for making the diagnosis.[1] It is important to evaluate the other anatomical structures as sources of masses within the pelvis and also during surgical procedures to prevent damage to nearby organs and structures.[2]

Adnexal masses that need attention are those with complex internal structure, with solid components, which are associated with pain, or are present in prepubescent or postmenopausal women, or are large >10 cm in diameter.

INCIDENCE

The exact incidence of occurrence of adnexal masses can't be determined as most adnexal masses are asymptomatic and resolve without clinical detection. When present, the clinical significance and incidence are different in accordance with the age group. Adnexal masses in prepubertal and postmenopausal age groups tend to have a malignant potential compared to those in the reproductive age group.

DIFFERENTIAL DIAGNOSIS

Gynecological Causes

- Benign ovarian tumors
- Corpus luteum cyst
- Follicular cyst
- Luteoma of pregnancy
- Mature teratoma
- Ovarian torsion
- Polycystic ovaries
- Serous and mucinous cystadenoma
- Theca-lutein cyst
- Ectopic pregnancy
- Endometrioma
- Hydrosalpinx
- Leiomyoma
- Malignant ovarian tumors
- Borderline tumors
- Epithelial carcinoma
- Ovarian germ cell tumor
- Ovarian sarcoma
- Sex-cord or stromal tumor
- Tubo-ovarian abscess
- Malignant nonovarian
- Endometrial carcinoma
- Fallopian tube carcinoma.

Nongynecological Causes

- Benign
- Appendicular abscess/mucocele
- Bladder diverticulum
- Diverticular abscess
- Nerve sheath tumor
- Pelvic kidney
- Peritoneal cyst
- Urethral diverticulum
- Malignant
- Gastrointestinal carcinoma
- Krukenberg tumor
- Retroperitoneal sarcomas.

DIAGNOSIS

The clinical presentation of adnexal masses is variable. However, most patients with adnexal mass are asymptomatic and are detected at the time of either a surgical procedure or during ultrasonography for evaluation of another complaint or routine pelvic examination.

Common presentation in symptomatic patients include:

- **Acute pain in abdomen:** This usually indicates hemorrhage or torsion. Associated symptoms like nausea, vomiting, referred pain from peritoneal irritation, fainting episodes and bleeding per vagina may indicate ectopic pregnancy.
- **Pelvic pain** due to infected tubo-ovarian mass may also be associated with symptoms like fever and abnormal vaginal discharge.
- **Dysmenorrhea and deep dysparunia** are the presenting features in patients with endometriosis or pelvic inflammatory disease.
- **Progressive abdominal distension** due to ascites or enlarging mass associated with loss of weight, loss of appetite, altered bowel and bladder habits and malaise indicate adnexal malignancy.

A good history should include information about tubal ligation or other tubal surgery, PID, or use of an intrauterine device as these are risk factors for ectopic pregnancy.

Details of family history of ovarian, endometrial, breast, or colon cancer must be taken. History of breast and ovarian cancer, multiple cases of breast cancer in the family, and a male family member with breast cancer predisposes the patient to increased risk of ovarian malignancy.

Physical Examination

Based on the nature of adnexal masses, a physical examination may not be useful. However, women exhibiting pelvic or lower abdominal symptoms should undergo a targeted examination based on their presenting condition. Women with nonspecific abdominal or pelvic symptoms, particularly those that do not respond to conservative therapy and that persist for more than a few weeks, should be thoroughly evaluated.

The examination should include the following:

- **General examination** to assess the vital signs and a general assessment, which is important in patients with acute presentation, such as torsion, hemorrhage, ectopic pregnancy or tubo-ovarian abscess.

  Patients with advanced malignancy may present with pallor, jaundice, edema of lower limbs and enlarged cervical supraclavicular, axillary, and inguinal lymph nodes.

- **Chest auscultation** should be done to evaluate for pleural effusion.

- **Abdominal examination** should be performed to assess for ascites, characteristic of the mass (size, shape contour, consistency, and site), tenderness, hepatosplenomegaly, or increased girth.

- **Pelvic examination**, including speculum examination, should be done. A bimanual examination to assess the size, tenderness, location, consistency, and mobility of the uterus and both adnexa. A rectovaginal examination may be done to assess tenderness or nodularity of the uterosacral ligaments.

Laboratory Evaluation

- **A urine pregnancy test** should be performed in any woman of reproductive age who presents with an adnexal mass. If the pregnancy test is positive, a quantitative beta subunit of human chorionic gonadotropin (β-hCG) level and transvaginal ultrasonography should be obtained. If the quantitative β-hCG level is greater than 2,000 mIU per mL (2,000 IU per L) and no intrauterine pregnancy is visible on transvaginal ultrasonography, an ectopic pregnancy should be suspected.

- **A complete blood count** with differential count is useful if PID or tubo-ovarian abscess is suspected. Patients with these conditions usually have an elevated white blood cell count with a predominance of neutrophils. A low hematocrit in a premenopausal woman could indicate an ectopic pregnancy, abnormal uterine bleeding (e.g. menorrhagia, metrorrhagia), or a blood dyscrasia. In a postmenopausal woman, a low hematocrit may be caused by colon cancer or anemia of chronic disease.

Tumor Markers

CA 125 Serum Marker Screening

CA 125 antigen is the most common serum marker used for distinguishing benign from malignant pelvic masses. It has a sensitivity of 61 to 90 percent, a specificity of 71 to 93 percent, a positive predictive value (PPV) of 35 to 91 percent, and a negative predictive value (NPV) of 67 to 90 percent for distinguishing between benign and malignant masses. Specificity and positive predictive value are consistently higher in postmenopausal women; CA 125 antigen elevations in these women should be considered highly suspicious for malignancy.

Its level should be estimated in postmenopausal patients with an adnexal mass to guide treatment options. A value greater than 35 U per mL should prompt further evaluation. If ovarian cancer is diagnosed, CA 125 level should be used to monitor the patient's response postoperatively.

The CA 125 antigen level is elevated in 80 percent of patients with epithelial ovarian cancer; however, it is elevated in only 50 percent of patients with stage I disease. For this reason, CA 125 level should not be used as a screening tool or when a mass is not identified, and should not be routinely used during the diagnostic workup of an adnexal mass in a premenopausal patient.

Inhibin A and B levels are done if a granulosa cell tumor is suspected, and are followed postoperatively.

Serum α-fetoprotein and quantitative β-hCG levels are done if germ cell tumors are suspected.

Hereditary ovarian cancer accounts for only a small percentage of overall cancer cases. Patients should have genetic counseling before undergoing *BRCA* mutation testing.

Imaging

Transvaginal ultrasonography remains the standard for the evaluation of adnexal masses. Advantages of transvaginal ultrasonography include ease of availability, cost-effectiveness, and patient tolerability. Also no other imaging technique has been found to be superior to ultrasonography for overall accuracy. Due to lack of specificity and low positive predictive value for cancer, transvaginal ultrasonography may be used in conjunction with abdominal ultrasonography to provide more accurate images of pelvic and abdominal masses.

Ultrasonography helps in assessing the size, mass characteristics (cystic, solid, or both), complexity (internal septae, excrescences and papillae), and the presence or absence of abdominal or pelvic fluid (ascites or blood).

Color Doppler ultrasonography allows measurement of blood flow in and around the mass. Its aim is to increase the specificity of ultrasonography. Though combination of ultrasonography and Doppler flow studies is superior to either alone, its use is controversial because the values of these indices overlap considerably between benign and malignant masses.[3]

Computed tomography (CT), magnetic resonance imaging (MRI), and positron emission tomography (PET) are not recommended for initial evaluation of adnexal masses, and their use after transvaginal ultrasonography is of limited value. These modalities should be used only in special circumstances.

Other Investigations

Mammography, gastrointestinal endoscopy and breast and digital rectal examinations should be done in all postmenopausal women with pelvic masses to rule out metastases from breast, colorectal, and gastric cancers. **Gastrointestinal endoscopy** is indicated in all patients who are anemic or older than 50 years, or who have a positive fecal occult blood test.

The US Preventive Services Task Force recommends against routine screening for ovarian cancer, including use of transvaginal ultrasonography, cancer antigen (CA) 125 levels, and screening pelvic examination.

TREATMENT

Most adnexal masses resolve spontaneously over time. It is good practice to avoid surgery for small, asymptomatic masses as it creates more pathology than the cure. Any surgery performed on adnexal structures can result in impaired fertility. However, asymptomatic masses can be early ovarian cancers that require immediate attention. The use of radiologic testing (transvaginal ultrasonography) helps to triage these cases and plan clinical management.

If a nongynecologic diagnosis is made, the patient should be treated appropriately.

For many gynecologic causes, specific medical or surgical treatment should be offered. Nonsteroidal anti-inflammatory drugs can be used for pain relief. Oral contraceptives are not effective in reducing the size of cyst.

Clinical, laboratory, or radiographic findings that suggest malignancy are:

- Family history of first-degree relative with ovarian or breast cancer
- CA 125 level greater than 35 U per mL in postmenopausal women and 200 U per mL in premenopausal age group
- Evidence of abdominal or distant metastasis
- Nodular or fixed pelvic mass (postmenopausal)
- Ultrasonography findings-including a solid component, thick septations (greater than 2 to 3 mm) including bilateral involvement
- Doppler flow to the solid component of the mass, and presence of ascites.

Cases with these feature should be referred to Gyne-oncologist for management:

- **All prepubescent girls** with an adnexal mass should be referred to a specialist with experience in pediatric gynecology
- Management of adnexal masses **in women of reproductive age** depends on pregnancy status and the size and complexity of the mass.

- If the pregnancy test is positive, ectopic pregnancy must be ruled out
- Adnexal masses detected during pregnancy are most often benign and have a low risk of becoming symptomatic during pregnancy, therefore, they may be observed until the postpartum period. In case additional imaging is needed, MRI is the modality of choice because it does not expose the fetus to radiation
- CA 125 antigen levels are elevated during preganancy and so low elevation in its level is not used as indicator of malignancy
- About 51 to 70 percent of masses spontaneously resolve during pregnancy and complications occur in less than 2 percent of pregnant patients with adnexal masses, therefore, expectant management is advised
- **Nonpregnant, premenopausal** women with an adnexal mass most likely have a follicular cyst. Simple cysts 10 cm or smaller can be managed conservatively with serial ultrasonography. These cysts have a very low incidence of malignancy. The optimal interval for repeat ultrasonography is controversial, and varies from 4 to 12 weeks.
- **Complex masses in premenopausal women** can also be followed conservatively if they are 10 cm or smaller or if they persist for less than 12 weeks. However, it is good to have opinion of Gyne-oncologist.

Postmenopausal women with a complex adnexal mass of any size or a simple cyst larger than 10 cm should be referred to a Gyne-oncologist

Postmenopausal women with a simple cyst 10 cm or smaller should have a CA 125 level drawn. If the level is greater than 35 U per mL, they should be referred. If it is less than 35 U per mL, the patient can be monitored with close follow-up and serial ultrasonography every 4 to 6 weeks.

Aspiration of non-unilocular cyst fluid for diagnosis and treatment of adnexal masses is typically contraindicated in postmenopausal women, especially in patients with potentially malignant masses. Aspiration is not always therapeutic and can induce spillage or seeding of cancer cells into the peritoneal cavity, changing the stage and prognosis. However, in patients who are unfit to undergo surgery and who have clinical and radiographic evidence of advanced ovarian cancer, aspiration can be performed to confirm the cancer diagnosis.

SURGICAL MANAGEMENT

The extent of surgery usually depends on the diagnosis, patient's age, and the patient's desire for ovarian function or fertility.

- **Laparotomy** is indicated in patients with high suspicion for malignancy, with large cysts, morbid obesity, history of or risk factors for abdominopelvic adhesions, hypovolemia, hemodynamically unstable patient, or those with significant cardiopulmonary disease
- **Hysterectomy with bilateral salpingo-oophorectomy and staging procedures** are standard management of gynecological cancer
- **Cystectomy** is the operation of choice in premenopausal women.

- **Hysterectomy or bilateral salpingo-oophorectomy** are appropriate after completion of childbearing, and may reduce the risk of future pelvic surgery. It is unknown if the benefits for preserving the ovaries outweigh the risk of leaving them in situ.
- In those cases where ovarian tissue cannot be preserved unilateral oophorectomy or salpingo-oophorectomy is done. Peri-menopausal and postmenopausal women can also undergo cystectomy or unilateral salpingo-oophorectomy
- The patient should be informed of the risk of bilaterality, which is approximately 2 to 3 percent for benign mucinous tumors, 15 percent for benign teratomas, and up to 25 percent for benign serous tumors.
- Laparoscopy is typically considered to be contraindicated in patients with masses suspicious for cancer based on transvaginal ultrasound findings, CA 125 antigen levels, and clinical assessment.[3]

REFERENCES

1. Adnexal Masses. Vanessa Givens, Gregg Mitchell, Carolyn Harraway-Smith, Avinash Reddy, David L. Maness, American Family Physician www.aafp.org/afp Volume 80, Number 8. October 15, 2009.
2. http://emedicine.medscape.com/article/258044.
3. Lisa Graham. ACOG Releases Guidelines on Management of Adnexal Masses Am Fam Physician. 2008;77(9):1320-3.

Missing IUD Threads

Sushma Pandey, Seema Pandey Choudhary, Rita Kumari Jha

INTRODUCTION

IUD is a convenient, highly effective, relatively safe, rapidly reversible and most cost effective contraceptive device. Worldwide, it is second in popularity as a contraceptive method only to the pill and its continuation rate is higher to that of the pills. About 85 million women are using it all over the world.

A correctly positioned IUD should be located at the fundus of the uterus with the arms fully expanded and extending towards the uterine cornua. The vertical portion of the 'CuT' should extend straight down in the uterine corpus (Fig. 1).

As with any medication or medical advice, there are a few side-effects and risks associated with IUD also and migration of it from its normal position with missing threads is one of them.[1] Besides, with frequent use of pelvic USG to evaluate gynecological complaints, the discovery of malpositioning of the device has become an increasingly common occurrence. About 10% of the IUDs are malpositioned.

ETIOPATHOGENESIS

Malpositioning of IUDS with missing threads may be due to:

i. Threads coiled inside either in endocervical canal or uterine cavity.
ii. Threads torn through.
iii. Device rotated with retraction of strings.
iv. Device embedded in the myometrium (one or both arms): It refers to IUD penetration into the endometrium or myometrium without an extension into the serosa. It may occur in about 18% of women with an IUD. It is more common in females with smaller fundal endometrial diameter.
v. Device expelled outside: In the first year of use, expulsion occurs in about 3 to 10% of women with CuT 380 A and 6% of women with LNG IUS. Risk factors for expulsion include[2] nulliparity, anatomical distortion of uterus, prior expulsion, insertion immediately after a second trimester abortion, postpartum, or early in menstrual cycle.
vi. Device protruding through the uterine serosa or completely outside the uterus and within the abdominal cavity:[3] Perforation usually occurs

during insertion and complicates about 1 in 1000 insertion procedures. Risk factors include clinical inexperience in IUD placement, an immobile and retroverted uterus, lactating women within six months of childbirth and presence of a myometrial defect. IUD perforation is variable in extent and symptomatology ranges from incomplete to complete.[4] Incomplete perforation may not be recognized immediately. Mild abdominal pain and uterine bleeding may pass unnoticed. In incomplete perforation, the most common complication is omental adhesion formation. Complete perforation is a more serious one perforating through all three layers of the uterus and may be associated with injury either to the bowel, bladder or blood vessels, presenting with severe abdominal pain and vaginal bleeding. Perforation is thought to be related to low estrogen levels.

vii. Device pulled up by the growing uterus in pregnancy:[5] It does occur in approximately two of every 100 females per year of IUD insertion. The risk of pregnancy is highest in the first year after insertion. Malpositioned device is a risk factor. None of the available studies is able to clarify whether it is the malposition that leads to increased risk of pregnancy or pregnancy itself causes malpositioning of the device.[6] Type of IUD also makes a difference. LNG IUS does not possess the same risk of pregnancy as CuT IUDs. These patients have a greater risk of adverse pregnancy outcome.[7] Risk includes miscarriage, preterm labor, chorioamnionitis and septic abortion.[8] Miscarriage rate is 40 to 50%, which is twice the rate in general female population. These risks are reduced with the removal of IUD early in pregnancy.

COMMON PRESENTATION OF MISSED IUCD

Patients having missing threads may have no symptoms and diagnosis may be at a routine follow-up examination. It occurs in about 40% of the cases. She may present with the following symptoms:

i. Abdominal cramping—being the leading symptom. It occurs in about 30% of the cases. Pain may occur either due to intrauterine displacement and stretching of uterine wall, infection or associated complication of pregnancy.

ii. Intermenstrual or postcoital bleeding or spotting—in about 9% of the cases.

iii. Associated pregnancy with bleeding—in about 2% of the cases.

iv. Recurrent urinary symptoms—in about 2% of the cases.

v. Others are—vaginal discharge and dyspareunia.

The triad of abdominal pain, intermittent diarrhea and fever associated with missing strings is indicative of complete perforation with bowel injury.

DIAGNOSIS

i. Diagnosis of missing thread is usually made by speculum examination.

ii. Various imaging modalities[9] are used in the evaluation of IUDs and USG is appropriate for initial evaluation. It is widely available and does not

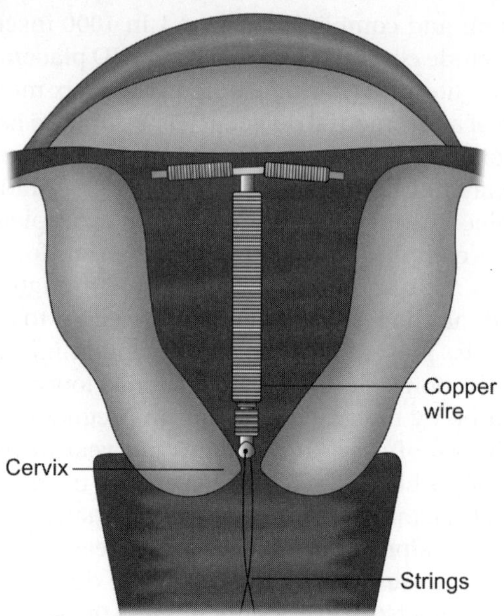

Fig. 1: Normal positioning of IUD

involve radiation. It easily helps to determine whether IUD is correctly positioned and can often help identifying IUD related complications.

iii. IUD displacement and myometrial perforation can be fully evaluated by performing US alone. Three-dimensional (3D) US is often helpful for further characterizing these findings and its use is becoming a standard practice in the routine evaluation of IUDs. Copper IUDs are visualized as an ecogenic stem and both the arms are seen entirely on saggital and transverse views. LNG IUS appears as an acoustic shadow between its proximal and distal ends, so the precise location is hindered. Both types of IUDs appear more conspicuous at 3D ultrasound than at 2D.

iv. Abdominal radiography, more specifically AP, and lateral views can be helpful in demonstrating an extrauterine IUD (Figs 2A to C) and is required for the diagnosis of IUD expulsion. A definite diagnosis of complete perforation is made if IUD is located above the pelvic brim. Conventional radiography exposes the patient to only minimal radiation and the radio-opaque IUD is easily identified if it has not been expelled.

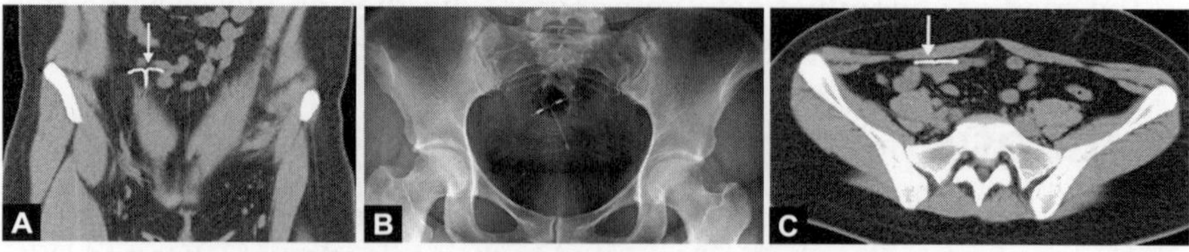

Figs 2A to C: Malpositioning of IUD with the missing threads

v. Occasionally, computed tomography (CT) scanning is used for the assessment of IUDs. It is the best modality for the evaluation of complications associated with intra-abdominal IUDs, such as visceral perforation. However, it exposes the patient to more radiation.

vi. MRI is not commonly used, but modern IUDs are safely imaged with both 1.5 T and 3.0 T magnets and appear as signal voids, if required.

MANAGEMENT

Different sites of IUD translocation vary in terms of their clinical significance and subsequent management.[10,11]

1. To start with, if the IUD strings are not visible on speculum examination, pregnancy should be excluded first.

2. If the woman is not pregnant, proper investigation should be done to locate the IUD.

3. If IUD is in situ and strings are retracted, initial exploration of endocervical canal with a cytobrush or uterine sound is done and the string is teased into the correct position.

4. If strings are in the uterine cavity and the IUD in the proper position, women may continue to use the device followed by routine periodic ultrasound checkup if they are asymptomatic. In symptomatic women, uterine cavity is explored and IUD is taken out either with a curette or IUD hook under sedation or paracervical block. Blind manipulation with artery forceps may be potentially dangerous, producing cervical and uterine injuries.

5. When IUD is embedded either in endometrium or myometrium, hysteroscopy is the ideal method of locating and removing it.[12] Recently, retrieval of IUDs under direct fluoroscopic control has been advocated.

6. It is important to teach all the IUD users to check strings periodically. Any woman with the symptoms suggestive of expulsion should be evaluated promptly. In incomplete expulsion, IUD is visible either in endocervical canal or vagina. It should be removed. Complete expulsion requires X-ray documentation and supportive USG. A new IUD can be inserted, if desired. The risk of re-expulsion appears to be higher than the risk of expulsion after initial insertion.

7. Management of uterine perforation by an IUD is controversial.[13] Some data suggest that surgical treatment should be reserved for the symptomatic patients. However, surgical removal of an intra-abdominal IUD is recommended by the World Health Organization (WHO) and is generally accepted as an appropriate treatment due to the potential for adhesion formation.[14] Laparoscopic surgery is preferred, but laparotomy is indicated when bowel perforation or severe sepsis is present.[15] Laparoscopy may be converted to laparotomy in the presence of adhesions that preclude safe laparoscopic removal. In symptomatic patients or patients with related complications, urgent surgical intervention may be appropriate. Antibiotics must be started once perforation is suspected or

diagnosed. IUD perforation is not a contraindication to future labor and vaginal delivery, as the uterine defect is small.

8. Management in pregnant patients with IUDs: We first determine whether the pregnancy is intrauterine or extrauterine. Ectopic or extrauterine pregnancy is managed accordingly. Management in a patient with an intrauterine pregnancy depends on gestational age and IUD location.

During the first trimester pregnancy: Removal of the IUD under US guidance using an IUD hook or alligator forceps is recommended.[16] However, if the location makes the removal difficult or will disrupt the pregnancy in future, the risks of IUD removal outweigh the benefits. Antibiotic prophylaxis is given when instruments' removal is performed during pregnancy. If a woman desires pregnancy termination, IUD removal is performed at the time of termination.

During the second trimester pregnancy: We counsel these women about the risk of preterm delivery, second trimester fetal loss and infection. No proven risk of birth defects has been reported. Given this information, for pregnancy after 12 weeks, removal of IUD by pulling on the strings can be done under ultrasound guidance. If the strings are not visible by USG and they appear located behind the placenta or protruding into the gestational sac, IUD should be left in situ. In the case of late second trimester, IUD should be left in place, and the patient should be counseled accordingly.[17]

RECOMMENDATIONS

i. Proper case selection, care with fitting, and access to experts in case of complications are required to maintain the acceptability and usefulness of this method.

ii. While insertion, the distance of IUD from uterine fundus should be 3 mm or less. A distance greater than 4 mm is often associated with high risk of expulsion/displacement. Besides enough length of the string, i.e. 3 cm should be left in the vagina and avoidance of tight pulling of the string during cutting will prevent its retraction inside the uterus.

iii. USG-guided insertion should be considered in the previous difficult insertion, obesity, adenomyosis and suspected abnormal or distorted uterine cavity.

iv. Awareness about its proper insertion through the trained experts is still needed at mass level; otherwise few complicated cases can limit the usefulness of the contraceptive method.

REFERENCES

1. Vasquez P, Schreiber CA. The missing IUD. Contraception. 2010;82:126.
2. Zhang J, Feldblum PJ, Chi IC, Farr MG. Risk factors for copper T IUD expulsion: an epidemiologic analysis. Contraception. 1992;46:427.
3. Kaislasuo J, Suhonen S, Gissler M, et al. Uterine perforation caused by intrauterine devices: clinical course and treatment. Hum Reprod. 2013;28:1546.

4. Heinberg EM, McCoy TW, Pasic R. The perforated intrauterine device: diagnosis and therapy. Contraception. 2004;69:289.

5. Braaten KP, Benson CB, Maurer R, Goldberg AB. Malpositioned intrauterine contraceptive devices: risk factors, outcomes, and future pregnancies. Obstet Gynecol. 2011;118:1014.

6. Moschos E, Twickler DM. Intrauterine devices in early pregnancy: findings on ultrasound and clinical outcomes. Am J Obstet Gynecol. 2011;204:427.

7. Ganer H, Levy A, Ohel I, Sheiner E. Pregnancy outcome in women with an intrauterine contraceptive device. Am J Obstet Gynecol. 2009;201:381.

8. Brahmi D, Steenland MW, Renner RM, et al. Pregnancy outcomes with an IUD in situ: a systematic review. Contraception. 2012;85:131.

9. Peri N, Graham D, Levine D. Imaging of intrauterine contraceptive devices. J Ultrasound Med. 2007;26:1389.

10. Ber A, Seidman DS. Management of the malpositioned levonorgestrel-releasing intrauterine system. Contraception. 2012;85:369.

11. Marchi NM, Castro S, Hidalgo MM, et al. Management of missing strings in users of intrauterine contraceptives. Contraception. 2012;86:354.

12. Zakin D, Sterm WZ, Rosenblatt R. Complete and partial uterine perforation and embedding following insertion of intrauterine devices. Diagnostic methods, prevention, and management. Obstet Gynecol Surv. 1981;36:401.

13. Adoni A, Ben Chetrit A. The management of intrauterine devices following uterine perforation. Contraception. 1991;43:77.

14. Markovitch O, Klein Z, Gidoni Y, et al. Extrauterine mislocated IUD: is surgical removal mandatory? Contraception. 2002;66:105.

15. Ozgun MT, Batukan C, Serin IS, et al. Surgical management of intra-abdominal mislocated intrauterine devices. Contraception. 2007;75:96.

16. Assaf A, Gohar M, Saad S, et al. Removal of intrauterine devices with missing tails during early pregnancy. Contraception. 1992;45:541.

17. Koetsawang S, Rachawat D, Piya-Anant M. Outcome of pregnancy in the presence of intrauterine device. Acta Obstet Gynecol Scand. 1977;56:479.

Chapter 46

Approach to an Infertile Couple

Pragya Mishra Choudhary

Infertility is defined as the inability of a reproductive age woman to conceive after 1 year of unprotected vaginal intercourse.[1] Based on this definition, the worldwide prevalence of infertility is about 16 %,[1] being slightly higher in the developing countries. It is estimated that one in seven to one in six couples have difficulty in conceiving at some point in their reproductive life.[1] The prevalence of fertility problems is on the rise which may reflect an increasing willingness of couples to seek advice and treatment which may be the result of increasing publicity of available treatments.

The approach to an infertile or a subfertile (being gentler terminology) couple should be patient-centered with treatment and care taking into account individual needs and preferences with couples having the opportunity to make informed decisions about their care and treatment. After 1–2 years of infertility, a couple should be offered further clinical assessment and investigations, earlier where the age of the woman is greater than 36 years or there is a known cause for infertility or a predisposing factor such as a history of ectopic pregnancy, PID or endometriosis.[1] It is ideal to refer people with fertility problems to a specialist as it improves the effectiveness and efficiency of the treatment and also increases patient's satisfaction.[1]

The approximate prevalence of the main causes of infertility are:[2]

- Unexplained—25%
- Male factors—30%
- Ovulatory disorders—25%
- Tubal damage—30%
- Uterine or peritoneal disorders—10%
- Combination of both male and female factors—40%.

PRINCIPLES OF MANAGEMENT

- The infertile couple should be dealt together
- No one is 'at fault' or 'to blame'; it is a shared problem.[3]
- Investigations and treatment should be carried out consistently in proper sequence.

- Counseling should be offered before, during and after investigation and treatment as fertility problems themselves and the investigation and treatment of fertility problems can cause psychological stress.[1]

Prior to embarking upon investigations some initial advice is central to the management of infertility problems. The couple should be seen together at the initial consultation and the following points are advised.[1]

- Majority (80%) of couples in the general population tend to conceive in the first year if the age of the woman is under 40 years and they are using regular unprotected intercourse. Fifty percent of those who fail to conceive in the first year will conceive in the second year.
- A couple's relationship can be affected by stress in the male or female partner and is likely to reduce libido and frequency of intercourse which can contribute to fertility problems.
- Couples should be advised that timed intercourse causes additional stress and hence, regular intercourse every two to three days optimizes the chance of pregnancy.
- So far it was known that fertility problems increase with increasing age of the female partner but recently it has been shown that male age also has an impact on fertility and offspring health.[4] The impact of male age is more noticeable after the age of 50 years with studies showing a concomitant increase in adverse outcome in the offspring.
- Women who smoke should be advised that smoking can reduce the chance of conceiving and passive smoking can also reduce fertility. Men who smoke should be informed that smoking has an association with poor semen quality.
- Men who indulge in excessive drinking should be informed that it is detrimental to semen quality.
- Obesity has an impact on infertility and women with BMI greater than 30 should be advised to lose weight. Losing at least 10% of the original body weight can remarkably increase the chances of ovulation and thereby conception.
- Some occupations can affect both male and female fertility as a result of exposure to hazardous chemicals and hence, change in occupation should be advised in such circumstances.
- Recreational drugs can also have an impact on both male and female infertility.
- Folic acid should be recommended in a dose of 0.4 mg per day in women trying to conceive and continued up to 12 weeks of pregnancy in order to prevent neural tube defects. A higher dose of 5 mg per day is recommended in women who have previously had a baby with neural tube defect (NTD) or women on antiepileptic medication or known to have diabetes.[1]
- Women who are nonimmune to Rubella should be advised about vaccination and avoidance of pregnancy for 1 month after the rubella vaccine.
- Screening for *Chlamydia trachomatis* should be carried out prior to any uterine instrumentation and appropriate treatment given.

➲ Screening for cervical cancer: Specific inquiry about the timing and the result of the most recent cervical smear should be made if the woman is above 25 years.

INVESTIGATIONS

The best approach for investigations is to carry out the ones felt most relevant for the couple at the initial consultation and to start with the least invasive first.

Semen Analysis

There is evidence of declining trend in sperm count and motility in the last one and a half decades and this has been linked to the theory of testicular dysgenesis syndrome (TDS), which comprises a developmental disorder with increased rates of testicular cancer, undescended testis and congenital malformations.[5] This may be due to environmental factors. Semen for analysis should be collected after 72 hours of abstinence and not longer as sperm motility tends to fall with prolonged periods of abstinence.

The results of semen analysis should be compared with the following World Health Organization reference values (5th edition):[6]

➲ Semen volume: 1.5 mL or more
➲ pH: 7.2 or more
➲ Sperm concentration: 15 million spermatozoa or more
➲ Total sperm number: 39 million spermatozoa per ejaculate or more
➲ Total motility (% of progressive motility and nonprogressive motility): 40% or more motile or 32% or more with progressive motility
➲ Vitality: 58% or more live spermatozoa
➲ Sperm morphology (% of normal forms): 4% or more.

In case of any abnormal result, a repeat confirmatory test should ideally be carried out after 3 months as the entire spermatogenic process including transit in the ductal testicular system takes 3 months. In cases where gross spermatozoa deficiency (azoospermia or severe oligospermia) has been detected the repeat test should be carried out as soon as possible.[5] Screening for antisperm antibodies should not be offered because there is no evidence to improve fertility.

Additional investigations on the male partner are indicated if any abnormality is detected while taking history, physical examination or initial semen analysis. These may include:[5]

➲ **Endocrine tests:** FSH, LH, testosterone, prolactin should be measured in men with sperm counts of < 5 million/mL. Other indications for serum endocrinology testing include evidence of impaired sexual function (e.g. impotence, reduced libido) and clinical symptoms of endocrine disease (e.g. hypothyroidism, diabetes).
➲ **Genetic evaluation:** Karyotyping to rule out abnormalities in the structure or number of sex chromosomes and autosomes such as Klinefelter's syndrome or microdeletions of Y chromosomes.

- **Imaging**: Scrotal ultrasound if an abnormality such as a testicular tumor is detected on physical examination.
  Colour-flow Doppler: For diagnosis of varicocele.
- **Testicular biopsy** can aid the diagnosis of severe oligospermia and azoospermia and facilitate sperm recovery for intracytoplasmic sperm injection (ICSI)
- A number of tests have been developed to assess the functional ability of sperm such as the postcoital test, sperm penetration assay (SPA) and the hemizona assay (HZA) but the general consensus is that they are of limited value from a practical point of view.
- **Sperm DNA fragmentation** has been shown to be a robust predictor of assisted reproductive outcomes.

Tests for Assessing Ovulation[7]

- **Basal body temperature chart**: Based on the fact that rise in progesterone after ovulation increases the body temperature slightly (approx. 0.5°C). However, it does not reliably predict ovulation and is not recommended.
- **Serial vaginal ultrasound scan** in a spontaneous or an ovulation induction cycle helps tracking the follicular growth and the time of ovulation.
- **LH surge detection** using urinary LH test kits.
- **Serum progesterone in the mid-luteal phase** (day 21 of a 28-days cycle or day 28 of a 35-days cycle): Value > 4 ng/mL indicates ovulation and > 10 ng/mL indicates adequate luteal phase.

Tests for Ovarian Reserve[7]

These tests predict the likely ovarian response to gonadotropin stimulation in IVF and the potential for successful IVF.

- **Baseline day 2/3 serum FSH and LH**: A day 2/3 FSH >10 mIU/mL indicates poor ovarian reserve. A high LH or LH/FSH ratio > 2 indicates PCOS. Low LH, FSH, estradiol indicates hypogonadotropic hypogonadism.
- **Antral follicle count day 2/3**: It is one of the best predictors of response to ovarian stimulation with count < or equal to 4 for a poor response and > 16 for a high response.
- **Serum anti-Müllerian hormone (AMH)**: Serum AMH is a useful marker for predicting ovarian aging and the potential for successful IVF. Reduced serum AMH indicates diminished ovarian reserve and associated with poor response to IVF. Normal values range from 0.7 to 3.5 ng/mL.
- **Ovarian volume and stromal blood flow**: Decreased ovarian volume is indicative of ovarian ageing and can sometimes be seen before rise in FSH.
- **Serum inhibin B**: Levels less than 45 pg/mL indicates poor ovarian reserve. Decrease in inhibin B may precede rise in FSH.
- **Baseline day 3 estradiol** less than 80 pg/mL indicates good ovarian reserve. However tests such as ovarian volume, ovarian blood flow, inhibin B, estradiol (E2) should not be used individually to predict outcome of infertility treatment.[1]

Other Hormonal Tests

- **Serum prolactin**: Done in women with ovulatory disorders, galactorrhea or a pituitary tumor. Derangement in prolactin can lead to anovulatory cycles.
- **Thyroid function tests**: Approximately 5% of women attending infertility clinic are diagnosed to have thyroid dysfunction. Derangement can lead to anovulatory cycle.
- Fasting serum insulin, fasting and postprandial blood sugars, DHEAS, androstenedione, testosterone in case of patients with PCOS diagnosed by USG or symptomatology or having features of androgenization.

Pelvic Ultrasound

It is an important tool for evaluating the uterus, uterine cavity, adnexae, presence or absence of PCO pattern, ovarian volume and antral follicle count.

Tests for Tubal Patency[7]

- **Hysterosalpingogram (HSG)**: It is one of the most reliable, inexpensive and less invasive tests for tubal patency. It helps to assess the uterine cavity at the same time. It can detect uterine malformations, adhesions (Asherman's), submucosal fibroids. Women not known to have comorbidities such as PID, previous ectopic pregnancy or endometriosis should be offered HSG.
- **Hysterosalpingo-contrast-sonography (HyCoSy)**: It is an inexpensive and well-tolerated method of detecting tubal patency with the additional advantage of giving information about the uterine cavity, pelvic adhesions and fimbrial movement.
- **Laparoscopy and dye test**: Women who are thought to have comorbidities should be offered this test as a pelvic assessment can be carried out along with tubal patency.
- **Hysteroscopy**: Women should only be offered hysteroscopy if clinically indicated and not as part of the initial investigation because the effectiveness of surgical treatment of uterine abnormalities on improving pregnancy rates has not been established.[1]
- **Endometrial biopsy**: It should not be used to evaluate the luteal phase. Its main role is in ruling out endometrial tuberculosis through DNA/RNA polymerase chain reaction test in the developing countries.

TREATMENT

Depending on the diagnosis, treatment can fall into one or more categories in order to restore fertility:

- Medical
- Surgical
- Assisted reproductive technologies (ART)

Medical

Induction of Ovulation[8]

Hypogonadotropic hypogonadism (WHO 1)

Ovulation is induced using pulsatile GnRH agonist if the pituitary gland is functional. If the pituitary gland is functionally absent or in case of treatment failure with pulsatile GnRH, direct stimulation of the ovaries with exogenous gonadotropins (FSH and LH) results in follicle growth and ovulation. In cases where anovulation is caused due to extreme weight loss restoration of normal weight can lead to regular ovulatory cycle.

Normogonadotropic anovulation (WHO 2)

- **Lifestyle interventions such as weight reduction, stopping of smoking, diet restriction and exercise are paramount in induction of ovulation in normogonadotropic anovulation.**
- Clomiphene citrate (CC) is one of the oldest drugs used for ovulation induction. It is an antiestrogen, a nonselective E_2 receptor antagonist and interferes with negative endogenous estrogen feedback at the hypothalamic-pituitary level resulting in gonadotropin release by the pituitary and ovulation induction. CC is given in a dose of 50 mg/day and can be increased in two steps to 150 mg/day. It is generally started on day 3. Restoration of ovulation occurs in 80% of patients with a cumulative live birth rate between 40 to 60%. Uncommon side effects are hot flushes, nausea and visual disturbances. Multiple pregnancy rate is between 2% and 16%. However, severe ovarian hyperstimulation is rare with CC. The use of CC is not recommended for a period longer than 12 months as there is a theoretical risk of ovarian cancer.
- Aromatase inhibitors such as letrozole were previously used for ovulation induction but have now been withdrawn from the Indian market after reporting of fetal toxicity resulting in official warning by the producer not to use letrozole for ovulation induction.
- **Gonadotropins (FSH and LH)** were initially derived from post menopausal urine. Later highly purified urinary preparations were made by removing non active proteins and a step further was the production of human FSH in Chinese hamster ovary cell lines using recombinant DNA technology. Gonadotropins act by direct stimulation of follicle growth in the ovary. The main treatment regimens are the step up protocol and the step down protocol. In the step up protocol, the starting dose of FSH is 37.5–50 IU/day which is increased by 37.5–50 IU/day till the FSH threshold is surpassed and ongoing follicle growth and ovulation occurs. In the step down protocol, the starting dose of FSH equals the response dose and from that point, the dose is lowered every 3 days by 37.5–50 IU resulting in the development of a single dominant follicle. Urinary or recombinant hCG is used to trigger ovulation when at least one follicle reaches the size of 18 mm. When more than 3 follicles >12 mm are present, stimulation should ideally be cancelled.

- **Insulin sensitizers**, the most commonly used one is metformin (biguanide) and pioglitazone/rosiglitazone (thiazolidinediones).

Metformin works by reducing hepatic gluconeogenesis and insulin concentration. Thiazolidinediones act by increasing glucose uptake in adipose and muscle tissue and decreasing hepatic glucose output. Lowering insulin resistance and hyperandrogenism normalizes FSH responsiveness and restoration of ovulation. Metformin is given in a dose of 500–1500 mg/day in daily divided doses. Ideally, metformin should be started in a dose of 500–850 gm/day and increased weekly to a maximum of 2000 mg/day in order to reduce gastrointestinal side-effects. Sustained release preparations help to reduce side-effects. Metformin is not considered superior to CC as first-line treatment of anovulation and neither is a combination of metformin and CC. Metformin should rather be added to CC as second-line treatment in clomiphene-resistant cases. It gives 50% ovulation rate in obese PCOS patients.

Newer insulin sensitizers are myo-inositol, D-chiro-inositol, n-acetylcysteine and melatonin. Study of 50 overweight women with PCOS has shown very good results after six months of combined administration of myo-inositol and D-chiro-inositol in a physiological plasma ratio of 40:1 in lowering the risk of metabolic syndrome.[9]

Surgical[1]

Prior to embarking upon ART, surgery to enhance fertility should be tried which is considered to be a more judicious use of resources. Surgery could involve the tubes, ovaries or the uterus.

Tubes: Where expertise is available, tubal microsurgery and laparoscopic tubal surgery should be tried for mild tubal disease such as peritubal adhesions. In cases with cornual block, selective salpingography plus tubal catheterization or hysteroscopic tubal cannulation are treatment options to improve fertility. Clipping of Fallopian tubes or salpingectomy for hydrosalpinges prior to IVF through laparoscopy have been shown to improve chances of a live birth.

Uterus: Women with intrauterine adhesions (Asherman's syndrome) benefit from hysteroscopic adhesiolysis which is likely to restore menstruation and also improve the chance of conception. Transcervical resection of submucous myoma, septum resection in case of septate/subseptate uterus, removal of endometrial polyp has all shown to improve fertility rate.

Ovaries: Laparoscopic ovarian drilling is a modern reintroduction of wedge resection of the ovaries. Small holes are drilled in the ovarian cortex using electrocautery or laser treatment. The whole idea is to reduce circulating serum androgens and restore ovulation. The main advantage is reduction in multiple pregnancy rates and no risk of ovarian hyperstimulation syndrome. The drawbacks besides the usual risks of laparoscopic surgery and anesthesia are intra-abdominal adhesion formation and potential accelerated decline of ovarian reserve.[8] Laparoscopic cystectomy for endometriotic cyst has also been shown to improve pregnancy rate.

Pelvis: Surgery on the pelvis to improve pregnancy outcome involves laparoscopic surgical ablation or resection of endometriotic implants for minimal to mild endometriosis and laparoscopic adhesiolysis.

Assisted Reproduction Techniques

Any treatment that deals with means of conception other than vaginal intercourse falls under this category.[1]

Intrauterine insemination (IUI) using washed fresh or cryopreserved semen of husband or partner is one of the simplest assisted reproductive techniques. The success rates for IUI range from 6% in natural cycle to 18–19% with ovulation induction using clomiphene citrate (CC) and or gonadotropins. The indications for IUI are innumerable.[7]

- **Mild male factor infertility:** Semen parameters are only mildly subnormal. Patients with severe male factor infertility should go directly for intracytoplasmic sperm injection (ICSI).
- **Ejaculatory failure** due to anatomical, neurological, psychological or drug-induced conditions
- **Ovulatory dysfunction**
- **Endometriosis (mild to moderate)**
- **Vaginismus**
- **Cervical factor**
- **HIV, Hepatitis B, C positive husband**
- **Allergy to seminal plasma**
- **Unexplained infertility**

However, NICE guidelines 2013 recommend IVF for people with unexplained infertility, mild endometriosis or mild male factor infertility if they are having regular unprotected intercourse for 2 years.[1]

The indications for using husband's cryopreserved sample are:
- Absentee husband
- Post antineoplastic treatment
- Vasectomy
- Poor semen parameters
- Drug therapy

Indications for AID (artificial insemination by donor) are:
- Severe abnormal semen parameters
- Azoospermia
- Hereditary disease in male
- Repeated failures at IVF/ICSI

In vitro fertilization: IVF was initially developed to overcome infertility from irreparable tubal damage. However, the indications have increased from the time of its first success in 1978 and can be broadly divided into tubal factor, unexplained infertility, ovulatory dysfunction, endometriosis, ovarian failure or diminished ovarian reserve and moderate oligoasthe-noteratozoospermia.[10] It is now estimated that up to 35% of subfertile couples could benefit from IVF.[3]

Intracytoplasmic sperm injection (ICSI):[10] Initially, ICSI was devised for severe male factor infertility and as an adjunct to sperm retrieval procedures such as PESA (percutaneous epididymal sperm aspiration) and TESE (testicular sperm extraction) but the indications for its use today are previous failed IVF, oocyte factors, age of the woman greater than 35 years and unexplained infertility. The success rate of ICSI is higher than IVF.

ART is a rapidly growing field with newer and costlier advances and better success rates–IVM (in vitro maturation), IMSI (intracytoplasmic morphologically selected sperm injection), embryo vitrification, laser assisted hatching and embryoscope to name a few.

TREATMENT OPTIONS FOR MALE INFERTILITY[5]

Medical

Men with known endocrine disorders such as hyperprolactinemia, hypothyroidism and congenital adrenal hyperplasia can benefit from specific hormonal treatments. Men with pretesticular cause (hypogonadotropic hypogonadism) for oligozoospermia and azoospermia can be successfully treated with GnRH or gonadotropins. Recent evidence suggests that antioxidant supplementation in subfertile males, including carnitines, vitamin C, vitamin E, selenium, zinc and coenzyme Q10, improves semen quality and live birth rates in couples undergoing fertility treatment.

The basis for above is that sperm DNA damage secondary to oxidative stress may be the cause of between 30% and 80% of male subfertility cases.

Urological Surgery

Reversal of vasectomy: The success rate of this procedure depends on the skill of the operating surgeon, surgical technique and the time from initial surgery and declines with increasing time.

Surgical sperm retrieval: Sperm can be retrieved from the testis or the epididymis for use in IVF/ICSI. Success rates of almost 100% have been reported for surgical sperm retrieval in obstructive cases and 50% in non-obstructive cases.

Surgery for varicocele: NICE recommends that men should not be offered surgery for varicocele as it does not improve pregnancy rates.

ART: It is mainly used for causes at the testicular level which are largely irreversible. Surgical sperm retrieval with assisted reproduction or donor sperm may be considered.

CONCLUSION

Management of a subfertile couple can be made relatively less complicated with a methodical approach, starting with the most appropriate and the least invasive investigations for the couple being treated or one can say a 'tailor-made' approach may be most ideal. Counseling at every step is essential and can alleviate anxiety of the already stressed subfertile couple. Prior to embarking upon any ART technique ethical issues should always be considered and discussed with the couple concerned.

REFERENCES

1. NICE clinical guideline 156. Fertility: Assessment and treatment for people with fertility problems. (guidance.nice.org.uk/cg156).
2. Human fertilisation and embryology authority. Fertility treatment in 2010-trends and figures. London:HFEA; 2010.
3. Stirrat GM, Mills MS, Draycott TJ. Notes on Obstetrics and Gynaecology. 5th Edition. Chapter 18 Fertility and Subfertility.
4. Royal College of Obstetricians and Gynaecologists. Reproductive Ageing. SAC Opinion Paper 24. London: RCOG; 2011.
5. Assessment of the infertile male. The Obstetrician and Gynaecologist. 2013;15:1-9.
6. WHO manual of examination and processing of human semen. 5th Edition.
7. Palshetkar N (Ed). Advanced infertility management. FOGSI FOCUS November 2011.
8. Aboulghar M, Rizk B. Ovarian Stimulation. Ovulation induction for anovulatory patients. Cambridge University Press.
9. European Review for medical and pharmacological sciences. 2012;16: 575-81.
10. Fritz MA, Speroff L. Clinical gynaecologic endocrinology and infertility, 8th Edition. Assisted Reproductive Technologies. Lipincott Williams and Wilkins.

Intrauterine Insemination

Neelam

INTRODUCTION

Intrauterine insemination (IUI) is one of the commonest procedures done in assisted reproductive technology. This is because it is simple, safe, painless and extremely cost-effective. It entails deposition of morphologically normal, washed, motile sperms in the uterus near fundus.

A pair of normally functioning ovaries, hormonally responsive endometrium, and at least one patent tube in the female partner and a minimum of 10 million/mL sperm in the male partner are mandatory pre-requisites for this procedure.

IUI has received a boost recently with the advent of controlled ovarian hyperstimulation (COH) and newer, modern methods for sperm preparation becoming easily available due to an increase in in vitro fertilization and embryo transfer (IVF-ET) procedures. Seminal plasma contains prostaglandin, debris, leukocytes and nonmotile cells. Insemination with unwashed semen results in severe uterine cramps due to the presence of prostaglandin while also increasing the risk for contacting infections.

INDICATIONS

The main indications for doing the procedure can be divided into the following groups:
 A. Unexplained infertility
 B. Male factor as a cause of infertility
   1. Ejaculatory failure (hypospadias, impotency, retrograde ejaculation)
   2. Sperm factor (oligozoospermia, asthenozoospermia, oligoasthenozoospermia, teratozoospermia, oligoasthenoteratozoospermia)
   3. Excessively viscous semen
 C. Female factors as a cause of infertility
   1. Ovarian causes (endometriosis, polycystic ovarian syndrome or PCOS)
   2. Cervical causes (cervical stenosis due to previous surgery, cervical mucus hostility)
   3. Vaginismus
 D. Immunological infertility

ABSOLUTE CONTRAINDICATIONS

The absolute contraindications for the procedure are:
A. Bilateral tubal block
B. Severe oligoasthenoteratozoospermia
C. Unexplained bleeding per vagina
D. Severe PID
E. Pregnancy is contraindicated

BASIC SETUP FOR IUI

It consists of:
1. Semen collection room: The male partner is under a considerable amount of duress while attempting to produce the semen sample on demand. Provision of a quiet and comfortable room with privacy can help to alleviate some of the stress. Here, both the partners could benefit from the privacy. Erotic magazines, literature and videos should be made available for their use in the semen collection room.
2. Ultrasound machine: A modern, dedicated ultrasound machine with or without color Doppler is an indispensable part of the infertility clinic.
3. Makler's chamber: It is used for determining the count and motility of semen samples and thus helps in semen analysis.
4. IUI room: This can be a separate chamber or the operating room may also work as the insemination room.
5. Laboratory: The laboratory for intrauterine insemination should be a dedicated laboratory with standard precautions for maintenance of a sterile environment. Under no circumstances, should it be an extension to or share premises with the histopathological or other laboratory within the hospital. This is the place where sperm preparation could be carried out, it could house a cryopreservation unit, which is utilized for keeping cryopreserved donor semen samples.
6. Counselor and record maintenance room.

Besides the above, a laminar flow and an incubator are important tools for keeping the environment sterile and maintaining the media and prepared sperm at 37 degree Celsius.

STEPS IN INTRAUTERINE INSEMINATION

Intrauterine insemination consists of five steps:
- Patient selection
- Controlled ovarian hyperstimulation
- Follicular monitoring
- Sperm preparation
- Insemination.

Patient Selection

Patient selection is extremely important for optimizing results in IUI. Any couple who is being considered for IUI should have been thoroughly evaluated by means of history, clinical examination, and basic laboratory investigations comprising of hemoglobin estimation, ABO grouping and Rhesus typing, and screening for common sexually transmitted illnesses (STIs) like syphilis with a venereal disease research laboratory (VDRL) test, Hepatitis B, C, and HIV status. Apart from these, fasting and postprandial blood sugar estimation ought to be done to rule out hyperglycemia. For the male partner, same serological tests, blood sugar estimation, ABO grouping and Rh typing and seminal fluid analysis should be done.

Apart from these, to confirm ovulation, quantitative estimation of serum progesterone on day 20 (or 7 days before next menses in case of irregular cycles) should be done. A hysterosalpingography (HSG) is an effective test to rule out tubal blockage. If HSG is abnormal, a laparoscopy and dye procedure is done under general anesthesia as the next step to confirm tubal patency and to investigate peritoneal factors, if any. HSG should be performed between day 6 to day 11 under standard perioperative antibiotic cover. Another tool which is utilized to assess pelvic anatomy for structural abnormalities of the uterus, Fallopian tubes and the ovaries is the trans vaginal sonography (TVS) which shows them in detail and may also show corpus luteum or developing follicles according to proliferative or secretory phase of menstrual cycle.

The single most important factor which determines the success of IUI and IVF is the age of the female partner,, as there is a well-documented decline in pregnancy rate (PR) after 35 years of age.[1]

Controlled Ovarian Hyperstimulation

Intrauterine insemination can be carried out in natural as well as in stimulated cycles but the pregnancy rate has been found to increase when controlled ovarian hyperstimulation (COH) is used which, however, increases the risks of multiple pregnancy and ovarian hyperstimulation syndrome as well as the cost of treatment.[2]

Controlled ovarian hyperstimulation can be done with:
A. Clomiphene citrate: 50–150mg/day for 5 days (day 2 to day 6).
B. Clomiphene citrate and gonadotropins (follicle stimulating hormone/ human menopausal gonadotropin 75–150 IU)
C. Gonadotropins only
D. Gonadotropin releasing hormone analog (GnRHa) with gonadotropins (urinary or recombinant).

Other pharmacological adjuvants such as metformin, corticosteroids and bromocryptins may be added when required. It has been seen that 4–6 cycles of IUI gives the best cumulative pregnancy rates as PR becomes drastically reduced after 6 cycles. So it should be taken into account and stimulation protocols should be tailor-made for individual patients. Considerations should also be given if the patient has undergone IUI previously at another center and the stimulation protocol used.

The Royal College of Obstetricians and Gynecologists guidelines have recommended that not more than 12 cycles of clomiphene citrate should be offered to a woman as PR plateau.[3] Clomiphene citrate has been found to adversely affect endometrial thickness as well as cervical mucus production/quality. Optimal response has been found with a combination of CC together with gonadotropin administration and this regimen is also cost-effective. Thus when using CC alone in doses 50–150 mg, gonadotropin HMG or FSH (75/150 IU) is added on day 7, 8 or 9 and an ultrasound scan is done on day 10 to ascertain the size and number of dominant follicles and endometrial thickness. To achieve the optimum goal of getting one or two follicles of 18–20 mm and an endometrial thickness of $\geq$ 7 mm more gonadotropins can be added on a daily or an alternate day basis as needed.

GnRH antagonists have also proved useful in IUI procedures as when used in fixed (day 6 onwards) or flexible (when follicle size is >14 mm) protocol; it reduces the incidence of premature LH surge and luteinization (from 20–2%) and results in oocyte of better quality and hence better pregnancy rate (53.8 vs 30.8%).[4] Since GnRH antagonist suppresses LH level instantaneously by blocking its receptors in the pituitary, it also gives time to delay hCG administration for triggering ovulation. It has been seen that if GnRH antagonist is added in patients with elevated serum luteinizing hormone (LH) pregnancy rate increases (23.1%).[5] Stimulation with gonadotropins gives better PR (cumulative PR 30–60% in patients <40 years),[6] but it has to be balanced against the high cost of treatment, frequent monitoring with USG, the risk of multiple pregnancy and OHSS.

Follicular Monitoring

Ultrasound is an integral part of infertility workup and treatment. For IUI, first ultrasound is done on day 2–3 to rule out any overt abnormality of the ovary and uterus, antral follicles (AF, follicles between 6–8 mm of size) are counted and endometrial thickness is measured. There should be normally 4–6 AF in each ovary and the presence of more than 8 follicles in each ovary creates suspicion of polycystic ovaries.

If gonadotropins are not being used in COH, the next ultrasound is done on day 10, when one or more follicle of >12 mm can be seen and the endometrial thickness should be 7 mm or more. It should be followed by repeating the scan 1–2 days later to get matured follicles of 18–20 mm or more. Endometrial thickness when measured from outer to outer wall in the widest part should be between 8–10 mm and of triple line pattern, clear central line and echogenicity of outer lines is less than half of echogenicity of myometrium. When only gonadotropins are used (either in step up or step down protocol) for stimulation, the second scan is done on day 6 of stimulation, to check for the presence of lead follicles, and the doses are adjusted accordingly. Endometrial thickness is also noted. Then, according to the response of stimulation, third and fourth scan is done 2–3 days apart so that 2 dominant follicles of 16–18 mm or larger and a triple line pattern endometrium is reached by day 12–14, when HCG 5000–10000 IU is administered for ovulation. On day 12, the endometrial thickness of ≥9 mm showing triple line gives the best pregnancy rate.

Sperm Preparation

Ideally a sperm washing technique should be quick, easy and cost-effective as well as should not damage the sperm and should also remove toxic/bioactive substance and reactive oxygen species from semen.[7]

Segregating and collecting the morphologically normal, motile sperm and capacitating for IUI (or fertilization) is very important. So there are following steps in sperm preparation:

A. Semen collection
B. Pre-wash checking of number and motility
C. Semen wash
D. Post-wash check

Semen Collection

After having abstained for 2–3 days, the male partner is asked to produce a semen sample by masturbation and collect in a sterile wide-mouth pot after washing the penis and hands with soap and water and drying them. After liquefaction at 37°C, a drop of semen is taken in Makler's chamber and pre-wash examination is done to confirm count and motility.

Semen Wash

There are two commonly used methods:

A. Swim-up
B. Discontinuous density gradient

Swim up technique (Fig. 1): This method is used for preparation of normal semen samples or of mild asthenozoospermia (40–50% motility) or with mild teratozoospermia (8–14% normal morphology). The male partner should be asked to collect semen in the collection pot labeled with the patient's name in the standard way. The collected specimen is put in the incubator at 37°C

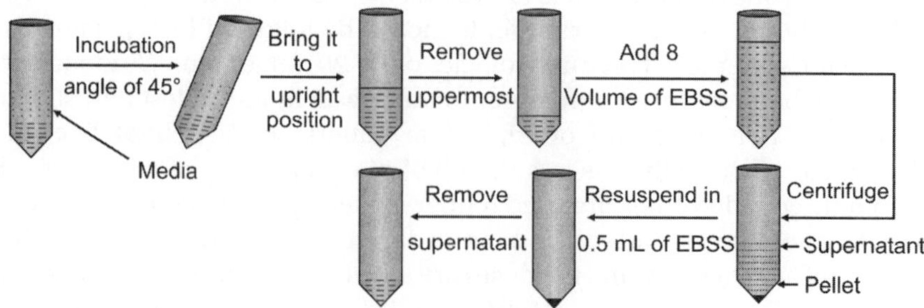

Fig. 1: Swim up technique

for liquefaction. After 20–30 minutes sample is checked for liquefaction and a pre-wash analysis of count and motility is done. The semen sample should never be mixed with a pipette or vigorously syringed with 17G needle even if its viscous, as this may severely damage the spermatozoa.[8]

1.2 mL of sperm wash media is gently layered over liquefied semen (1 mL) in a labeled sterile conical test tube. Tube is inclined (45 degree) and incubated for 1 hour at 37 degree Celsius. It is then gently returned to upright position and uppermost 1 mL is removed. 8 mL of sperm wash media is added to it in another test tube and centrifuged at 1500 rpm for 5 minutes. The pellet is resuspended in 5 mL of media and post-wash sperm concentration and motility is assessed before insemination (WHO, 1999).

Advantages and disadvantages of swim up method: This method is easy to perform, cost effective and gives high motile fractions but it gives low yield and can only be used in semen with high sperm counts.

Discontiuous density gradient: It selects sperm on the basis of their density as motile sperms are denser than either non-motile or dead sperm and debris. As previously, all the material should be labeled meticulously with the patient's name.

3 mL of 80% pure sperm or alternate media is pipetted into 10 mL labeled sterile conical bottom test tube. 3 mL of 40% pure sperm (alternate media) is gently overlaid on 80% layer so that interface between the two remains intact. Now gently 1–2 mL of liquefied semen is overlaid on the gradient and it is centrifuged at 1500 rpm for 20 minutes. Supernatent is discarded and the pellet is resuspended in another conical bottom test tube in 5–10 mL sperm wash media and centrifuged at 1500 rpm for 5 minutes. Pellet is resuspended in 0.5 mL of sperm wash media and concentration and motility is assessed before insemination (WHO).[9]

Advantages and disadvantages of density gradient: With this a clean and highly motile fraction of sperm, is recovered, leukocytes are eliminated, reactive oxygen species are reduced. The main disadvantage is its being expensive and there is a risk of endotoxins.[7]

IUI TECHNIQUE

The technique of IUI is equally important as the sperm preparation (Fig. 2).

The patient is asked to empty her bladder and lie in the lithotomy position. The vulva and vagina are cleaned with normal saline and sterile draping applied in the usual fashion. A sterile cusco's speculum is inserted in the vagina to provide adequate exposure of the cervix and to fix it. Mucus is cleaned with gauze and plenty of saline, then preloaded 0.3–0.5 mL of prepared semen in IUI catheter is gently introduced through external and internal os till it reaches just below the fundus. The prepared sperm is injected inside the cavity very slowly. This process may be done under ultrasound guidance too. The IUI catheter is kept inside the cavity in the same position for a few minutes before withdrawing, to avoid negative suction effect and immediate reflux. IUI should be done very gently to avoid release of prostaglandins which could

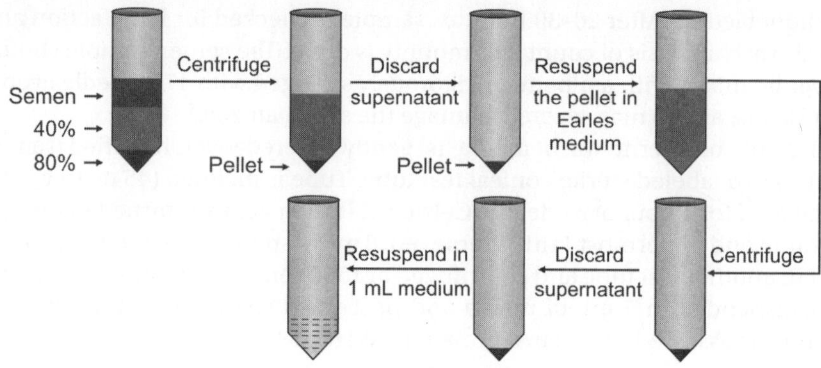

Fig. 2: IUI technique

initiate uterine contractions causing cramps in abdomen and reflux. Patient is kept in the supine position for 15–20 minutes before discharge. Luteal support with natural micronized progesterone 200 mg twice daily for internal application for ten days may be given before discharge.

LIMITATIONS OF IUI

Though IUI is a simple procedure and is used widely, it has its limitations which the couple should be counseled about while taking consent. The maximum success rate is observed in the first 4–6 cycles. After that, the couple should be encouraged to try an in vitro fertilization (IVF) cycle rather than continuing with IUI cycles, which will then have very poor yield. A major limitation of IUI is that the quality of oocyte or embryo or whether fertilization occurred, or whether an embryo formed—all these cannot be seen under direct vision.

COMPLICATIONS OF IUI

The major complications of this simple procedure are:
A. Infection
B. Bleeding
C. Pain
D. Trauma
E. Ovarian hyperstimulation syndrome
F. Multiple pregnancy

Patients should always be counseled about all possible complications. OHSS if untreated, may become life-threatening and the patient may even need ICU care. Care should also be taken regarding maintaining absolute sterility and careful handling at all times. If 3 or more mature follicles are present, then the cycle may be converted to an IVF cycle or extra follicles can be aspirated or cancelled.

RESULTS IN IUI

Results in IUI depend upon the age of female partner, cause and duration of infertility, ovarian stimulation protocols, endometrial thickness, number of IUI cycle and previous failures at IUI cycles. Before taking the patient for IUI, they should be counseled about the expected success rate of IUI. This helps the patients to overcome failures later and also does not set the bar unreasonably high. Expected clinical pregnancy rate per treatment cycle with ovulation induction is 15–20%. However, this declines with the age of the woman and other factors which have been mentioned above. In highly selective cases, utilizing clomiphene citrate for induction, about 40% of the patients become pregnant and PR per induced cycle is about 20–25%.[10] Results of donor insemination is high, around 40–45% when done with COH.[11] Many RCT conducted in the UK, USA, and Netherlands have found that super-ovulation plus IUI significantly increases the pregnancy rate compared to IUI alone (OR 1.7, 95% CI 1.2 to 2.6).[12] However, ovarian stimulation increases multiple conceptions too.[12]

REFERENCES

1. Dorey S, Sneelinger RM, Penzias AS. Study on Clomiphene citrate and intrauterine insemination: Analysis of more than 4100 cycles. Department of Gynecology, Boston, Massachusetts, USA. 2008;90(6):2281-6.
2. Leven MI, Wild J, Steer P. Higher multiple births and the modern management of infertility in Britain. The British Association of Perinatal Medicine. Br J Obstet Gynaecol. 1992;99:607-13.
3. RCOG guideline for infertility. Fertility assessment and treatment in people with fertility problems, Clinical Guideline. RCOG press. February 2004;57-8.
4. Allegra A, et al. Hum Reprod. Epub 2006 Oct10. GnRH antagonist induced inhibition of the premature LH surge increases pregnancy rates in IUI stimulated cycles. A prospective randomized trial. 2007;22(1);101-18.
5. Martinez-Salazar J, Cerrillo M, Quea G, Pacheco A, Garcia-Velarco JA. GnRH antagonist ganirelix prevents premature luteinization in IUI cycles: Rationale for its use. Reprod Biomed Online. 2009;19(2):156-61.
6. Nuojua-Huttunem S, et al. Intrauterine insemination treatment in subfertility; an analysis of factors affecting outcome. Human Reproduction. 1999;14(3):698-703.
7. Henkel R, Kierspel E, Hajimohammad M, Staff T, Hoogendijk C, Mehvert C, et al. DNA fragmentation of spermatozoa and assisted reproduction technology. RBM online, Comp. 2003;1:44-51.
8. Knuth UA, Neuwinger J, Nieschlag E. Bias to routine semen analysis by uncontrolled changes in laboratory environment – detection by long term sampling of monthly means for quality control. Int J Androl. 1989;12;375-83.
9. WHO laboratory manual for the examination and processing of human semen; Fifth ed. 2010:164-5.
10. Dickey RP, Manual of Intrauterine Insemination and Ovulation Induction. Dickey RP, Brinsden PR, Pyrzak R (Eds). Cambridge Univ Press. 2010;7:78.
11. Kanthi Bansal, A hand book of intrauterine insemination and in vitro fertilization, Jaypee Brothers. 2003;5:18.
12. Gunick DS, Casson SA, Contifaris C,Overstreet JW, Factor Litvac P, Steikampt MP, et al. Efficacy of superovulation and intrauterine insemination in the treatment of infertility. National Cooperative Reproductive Medicine Network. N Engl J Med. 1999;340:177-83.

Chapter
48

Carcinoma Vulva

Sunesh Kumar, Sandeep Mathur, DN Sharma

Cancer of vulva ranks fourth among female genital tract cancers. It comprises approximately 2–4% of all genital tract cancers.[1] Most busy hospitals and departments of obstetrics and gynecology come across one or two new cases per year. Majority of women suffering from vulval cancer tend to be elderly more than 70 years of age. Recently increasing trend is seen in occurrence of disease among younger women[2] related to human papillomavirus (HPV) infection. In the past treatment comprised of radical surgical excision in the form of radical vulvectomy and bilateral inguino-femoral lymphadenectomy. However, while managing disease in younger women a less radical treatment in the form of local wide excision or hemi-vulvectomy with ipsilateral lymphadenectomy is a preferred approach. A great majority of vulvar cancer tend to be squamous cell carcinoma.

INCIDENCE

Exact incidence of carcinoma vulva in India remains unknown. However, data from Delhi Cancer Registry shows an incidence of 0.5% in year 2004. In United States of America an estimated 4,340 new cases are seen with 940 deaths annually.[1,36]

ETIOLOGY AND PREDISPOSING CONDITIONS

Exact etiology remains unknown, however, chronic vulval irritation, chronic vulval skin condition such as lichen sclerosus and immune suppression are thought to be some of the predisposing factors.

Lately HPV infection with serotype 16 and 33 has been implicated with occurrence of disease in younger women.[38]

Lichen Sclerosus

A long associated vulval non-neoplastic condition associated with chronic itch and scratch is found in a large number of squamous cell carcinoma of vulva. Exact mechanism of development of carcinoma vulva in long-standing lichen sclerosus remains unknown. Onset of cracks or fissure or discharge may indicate development of carcinoma in long-standing lichen sclerosus.

Vulval Intraepithelial Neoplasia (VIN)

Similar to intraepithelial neoplasia seen in cancer cervix, a preinvasive state called as vulval intraepithelial neoplasia (VIN) has been described with approximately 9% risk of progression to invasive lesion if left untreated. VIN usually tends to be present as hyperemic lesion, raised above surface and present for a significant time. Only a biopsy from suspicious area confirms the diagnosis.

Other Known Predisposing Conditions

- Recurrent sexually transmitted disease of vulva.
- Immunosuppression either due to drugs or infection.
- Smoking.
- Paget's disease of Vulva: Similar to Paget's disease of breast, Paget's disease of vulva has a risk of adenocarcinoma of vulva in the underlying tissue. Local wide dissection with inclusion of underlying dermal tissue is needed to rule out coexisting malignancy.

  Repeated evaluation is needed as recurrences are common with Paget's disease.

PATHOLOGY OF VULVAR CARCINOMA

Vulvar Intraepithelial Neoplasm (VIN)

It is a range of morphological alterations from mild to severe dysplasia or carcinoma in situ. Like cervical intraepithelial neoplasia, it is also divided from VIN I to VIN III.[3]

Morphology

- VIN I: Atypical or dysplastic cells at all levels of epithelial majority restricted to basal layers
- VIN II: Majority of dysplastic cells confined to the lower 2/3rd of epithelium
- VIN III or squamous cell carcinoma in situ: All layers of epithelium showing dysplastic keratinocytes and lack of maturation of epithelium towards the surface. The earlier term bowenoid papulosis is referred by most pathologists now as VIN III.

  The three tier grading may lack reproducibility especially for VIN I and II lesions. There is greater agreement for the VIN III/Ca in situ lesions.[4] However, it is in concordance with the concept of multistep progression of carcinoma. There is a rising incidence of these lesions due to increased infection with human papillomavirus (HPV).[5]

INVASIVE CARCINOMA

Microinvasive Squamous Cell Carcinoma

It is now defined as a carcinoma in which the invasive component measures less than 1 mm in depth. It is most commonly associated with a VIN III lesion. Grossly, it is identical to appearance of VIN III lesion.

Morphology

It can be differentiated from VIN III by the irregular out pouch of tumor cells from the basal layer infiltrating to the underlying stroma. There may be a desmoplastic stromal response around the invasive zone. The edges of a VIN III lesion on the other hand are smooth and rounded unlike that of microinvasive carcinoma. Desmoplastic stromal response is lacking.

Invasive Squamous Cell Carcinoma (SCC)

It is a malignant neoplasm that arises from vulvar keratinocytes and has potential for metastasis. This is the most common of all vulvar malignancies. SCC can arise in association with a pre-existing VIN or in the setting of inflammatory vulvar dermatosis.[6,7] The SCC arising in association with VIN occurs in women less than 60 years, are associated with HPV infection and may be associated with preneoplastic or invasive carcinoma of the cervix.[8] The inflammatory dermatoses associated with SCC are lichen sclerosis or chronic lichen planus.[9]

Morphology

Both basaloid and warty types of SCC can be seen. The basaloid variant has more regular, rounded compact cells with minimal pleomorphism and may be associated with a basaloid VIN III lesion. The warty pattern of SCC has more pleomorphic tumor cells with obvious keratinized squamous differentiation. It is more often exophytic in growth pattern and has many koilocyte like cells. HPV association can be found in both variants and hence p16, which is a surrogate marker of high-risk HPV infection is found in all layers of the tumor and can be detected by immunohistochemistry in histologic sections[10] (Figs 1 and 2).

The SCCs associated with vulval dermatoses tend to be well differentiated and lack p16 expression. Larger tumor size, local invasion and lymph node involvement are poor prognostic signs.[11,12]

Verrucous Carcinoma[13]

It is an extremely well-differentiated, exophytic of SCC associated with excellent prognosis. It presents as a slow growing but exophytic, disfiguring mass, which may obscure the normal vulva completely.

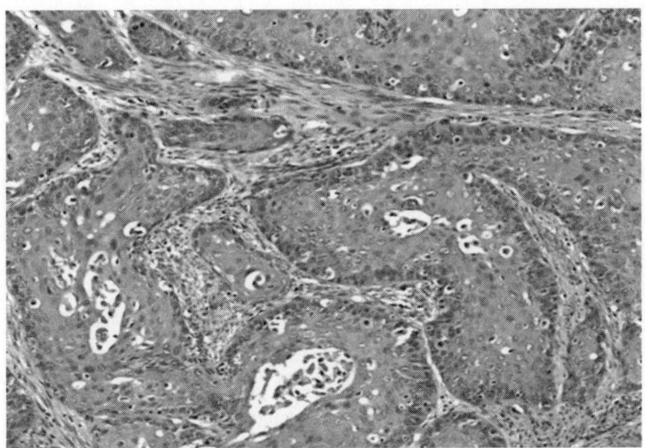

Fig. 1: Keratinizing squamous cell carcinoma
(For color version, see Plate 5)

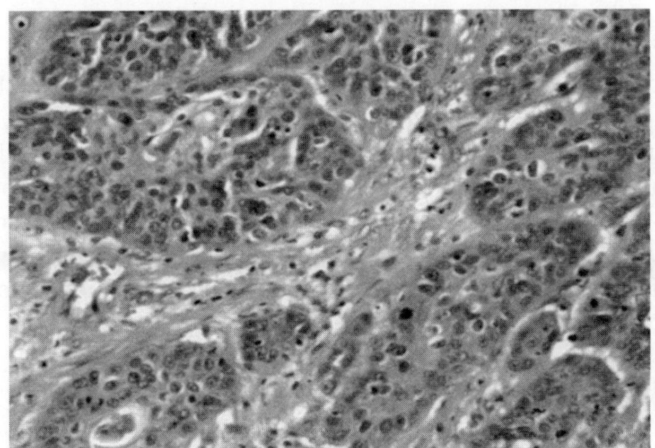

Fig. 2: Basaloid squamous cell carcinoma composed of islands of smaller basaloid cells
(For color version, see Plate 5)

Morphology

The tumor displays verruciform architecture. There is marked hyperkeratosis and acanthosis with elongation of rete ridges. The rete ridges have a typical bulbous contour. They have pushing margins and a destructive stromal invasion is lacking. As a rule there should be absence of frank nuclear atypia or brisk mitotic activity. A superficial biopsy is not appropriate for diagnosis of this entity as the diagnostic features are in the lower layers of the epithelium (Fig. 3).

Extramammary Paget's Disease[14]

It is an intraepidermal/in situ adenocarcinoma occupying the squamous epithelium. After breast vulva is the commonest site of Paget's disease.

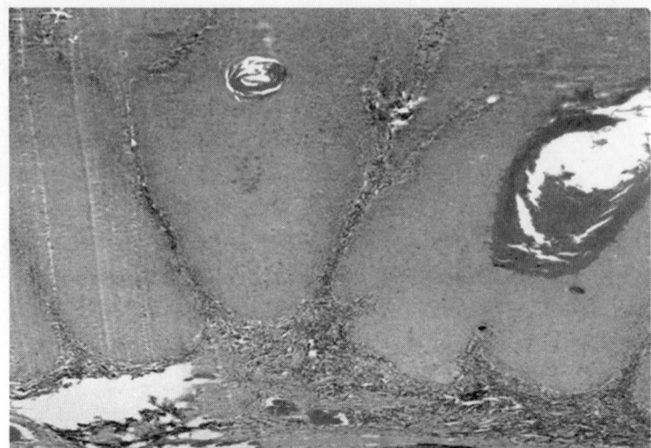

Fig. 3: Verrucous carcinoma displaying broad based rete ridges
(For color version, see Plate 6)

Morphology

It is characterized by presence of cells with clear cytoplasm having fine granules in cytoplasm. These clear cells are seen in the basal layers in early lesions but may occupy any position within squamous mucosa in later stages. Unlike breast, there is usually an absence of an underlying adenocarcinoma. These cells express CK7, Carcinoembryonic antigen (CEA) and MUC5AC by immunohistochemistry.[15] The exact origin of Paget's disease of vulva is unknown. However, it is postulated to arise from cutaneous sweat ducts or pluripotential stem cells of vulvar epidermis.[16]

Basal Cell Carcinoma[17,18]

It is an indolent, slow growing neoplasm presents as superficial, well-defined skin colored papules. It has tendency for local invasion, which may be destructive. However, distant metastases are not seen (Fig. 4).

Morphology

The tumor comprises of islands of basaloid cells having a peripheral palisaded arrangement. The islands of tumor are retracted from the surrounded stroma as defined by a clear space. Mitosis and apoptotic bodies are usually easily found. Melanotic pigment and desmoplastic stroma may be seen.

Malignant Melanoma[19-21]

It is an aggressive tumor of the vulva exhibiting melanocytic differentiation. It commonly occurs in labia majora and minora in older women. Uerthral and vaginal involvement in melanomas of the labia minora are associated with a very poor prognosis.

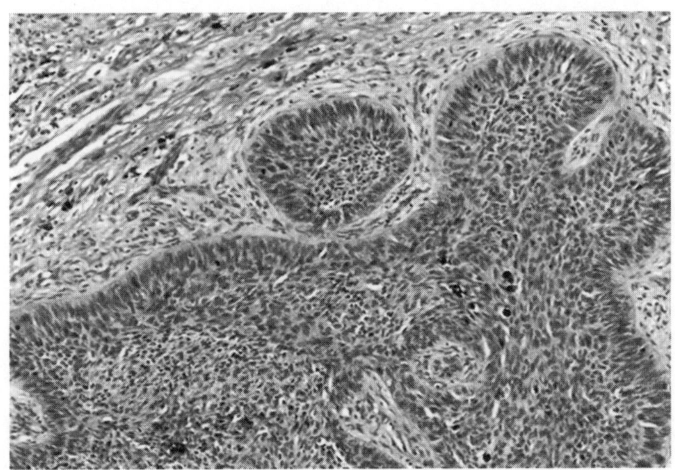

Fig. 4: Basal cell carcinoma composed of islands of basaloid cells with peripheral palisading of nuclei and scant pigment
(For color version, see Plate 6)

Morphology

Histologically, it is divided into subtypes like superficial spreading, nodular, acral-lentiginous, mucosal-lentiginous, verrucous and lentigo-maligna. They pertain to the patterns of the in-situ component of the melanoma. From pathological view point, the most important information that needs to be incorporated in the report is the Breslow thickness as it determines the treatment and outcome. It measures the distance from the top of the granular layer of the epidermis to the deepest melanoma cells in the dermis or subcutis. The Clark levels are not easily applicable for mucosal melanomas and vulval melanomas. Higher Breslow thickness, vertical growth phase, ulceration, intralymphatic spread and satellite lesions are histologic features associated with worse prognosis (Fig. 5).

Merkel Cell Carcinoma[22]

It is primary malignant and highly aggressive tumor of the vulva displaying neuroendocrine differentiation. It is postulated to arise from epidermal Merkel cell. It is located in dermis and comprises of small round cells with hyperchromatic nuclei and high nucleus to cytoplasmic ratio. It may show pseudorosette formation and displays abundant mitotic activity. The tumor cells display dot positivity for CK 20 by immunohistochemistry. Vascular and lymphatic invasion is commonly seen.

Bartholin Gland Tumors[23,24]

Glandular hyperplasia, adenomas, adenocarcinomas and squamous cell carcinomas are rarely seen to originate from Bartholin glands. The adenocarcinomas can be papillary, mucinous or colloid subtypes. Adenoid

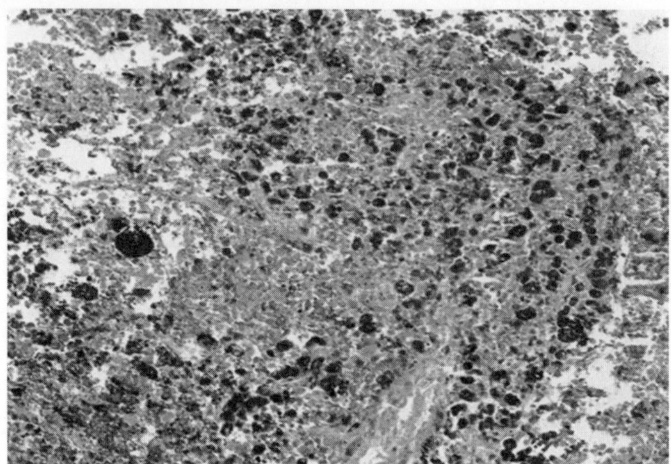

Fig. 5: Malignant melanoma composed of islands of densely pigmented tumor cells
(For color version, see Plate 6)

cystic carcinomas similar to salivary counterparts also arise in Bartholin glands.

Urethral Carcinoma[25]

Majority are SCCs arising from squamous epithelium in anterior 1/3rd of urethra. Pure transitional cell carcinomas are extremely uncommon.

CLINICAL PRESENTATION

Symptoms

Pruritus vulvae is the most common presenting symptoms present in more than 50% cases. Duration of pruritus may be several months to years.

Ulcer on Vulva

Presence of a nonhealing ulcer or a growth on vulva may be noted in 30–40% cases. Discharging ulcer or a lesion on vulva may be other presenting symptom.

At the time of presentation most patients have symptoms for 3–6 months or even longer. Old age and fear of seclusion often delays in bringing symptoms to the notice of care-taker in the family.

Signs

Lesion may be present in the form of a growth or ulcer present most often in labia majora. However, disease can present involving clitoris or perineum. Simultaneous presence of enlarged inguinal lymph nodes may be noted in advance cases. As disease spreads, it tend to involve lower 1/3rd of vagina or

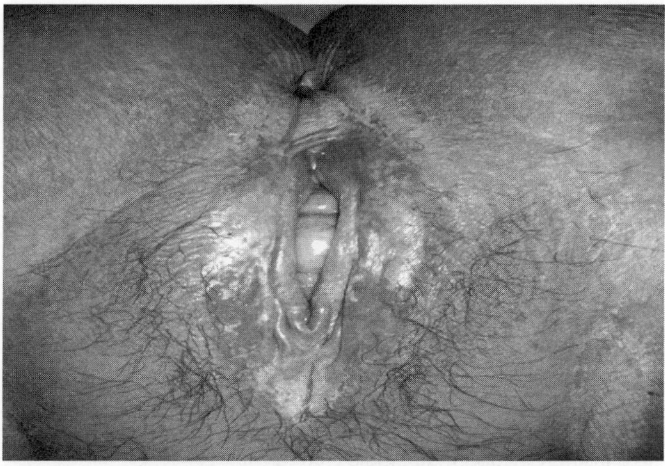

Fig. 6: Vulval intraepithelial neoplasia
(For color version, see Plate 7)

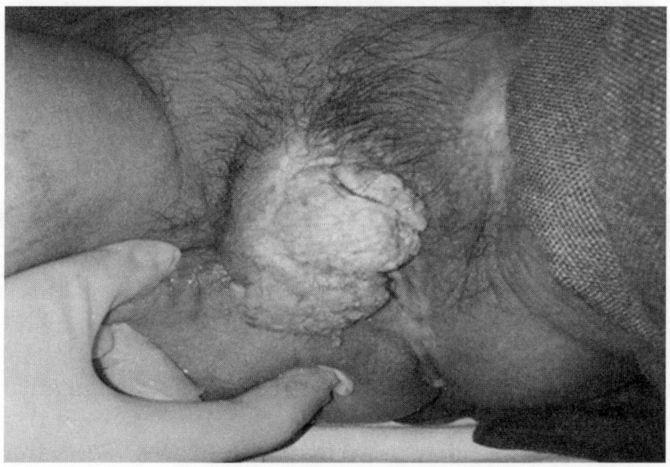

Fig. 7: Carcinoma vulva
(For color version, see Plate 7)

urethra and rarely anal canal. It is not uncommon to have multiple lesions involving bilateral labia (Figs 6 and 7).

DIAGNOSIS

Diagnosis can be established by obtaining a biopsy with the help of Keyes' biopsy forceps or with the help of a knife. Most biopsy can be obtained under local anesthesia in outpatient setting.

STAGING OF CARCINOMA VULVA[26]

Latest revized staging of Carcinoma Vulva by FIGO in 2009 is given in Table 1.

Table 1: FIGO staging criteria for carcinoma of the vulva (2009)	
Stage I:	Tumor confined to the vulva
IA	Lesions < 2 cm in size, confined to the vulva or perineum and with stromal invasion < 1 mm, no nodal metastasis
IB	Lesions > 2 cm in size or with stromal invasion > 1.0 mm, confined to the vulva or perineum, with negative nodes
Stage II:	Tumor of any size with extension to adjacent perineal structures (1/3 lower urethra, 1/3 lower vagina, anus) with negative nodes
Stage III:	Tumor of any size with or without extension to adjacent perineal structures (1/3 lower urethra, 1/3 lower vagina, anus) with positive inguinofemoral lymph nodes
IIIA	i. With 1lymph node metastasis (> 5 mm), or ii. 1–2 lymph node metastasis (> 5 mm)
IIIB	i. With 2 or more lymph node metastasis (> 5 mm), or ii. 3 or more lymph metastasis (< 5 mm)
IIIC	With positive nodes with extracapsular spread
Stage IV:	Tumor invades other regional (2/3 upper urethra, 2/3 upper vagina), or distant structures
IVA	Tumor invades any of the following: i. Upper urethra and/or vaginal mucosa, bladder mucosa, rectal mucosa, or fixed to pelvic bone, or ii. Fixed to ulcerated inguinofemoral lymph nodes
IVB	Any distant metastasis including pelvic lymph nodes.

TNM Staging[1,34]

Tumor Extent (T)

- T is: The cancer is not growing into the underlying tissues. This stage, also known as carcinoma in situ, is not included in the FIGO system.
- T1: The cancer is growing only in the vulva or perineum.
  - T1a: The cancer has grown no more than 1 mm into underlying tissues (stroma) and is 2 cm or smaller in size.
  - T1b: The cancer is either more than 2 cm or it has grown more than 1 mm into underlying tissue (stroma).
- T2: The tumor can be any size. The cancer is growing into the anus or the lower third of the vagina or urethra (This is called stage 2/3 in the FIGO system).
- T3: The tumor can be any size. The cancer is growing into the upper urethra, bladder or rectum or into the pubic bone (This is called stage 4 in the FIGO system).

Lymph Node Spread of Cancer (N)

- N0: No lymph node spread
- N1: The cancer has spread to 1 or 2 lymph nodes in the groin with the following features:
  - N1a: The cancer has spread to 1 or 2 lymph nodes and the area of cancer spread are both less than 5 mm in size

- N1b: The cancer has spread to one lymph node and the area of cancer spread is 5 mm or greater.
- N2: The cancer has spread to groin lymph nodes with the following features:
  - N2a: The cancer has spread to 3 or more lymph nodes, but each area of spread is less than 5 mm
  - N2b: The cancer has spread to 2 or more lymph nodes with each area of spread 5 mm or greater
  - N2c: The cancer has spread to lymph nodes and has started growing through the outer covering of at least one of the lymph nodes (extra-capsular spread)
  - N3: The cancer has spread to the lymph nodes causing open sores (ulceration) or causing the lymph node to be stuck (fixed) to the tissue below it.

Distant Spread of Cancer (M)

- M0: No distant spread
- M1: The cancer spread to distant sites (includes spread to pelvic lymph nodes).

Stage Grouping

The grouping of T, N and M determines the stage:
Stage 0 (T, N0, M0)
Stage I (T1, N0, M0)
Stage IA (T1a, N0, M0)
Stage IB (T1b, N0, M0)
Stage II (T2, N0, M0)
Stage IIIA (T1 or T2, N1a or N1b, M0)
Stage IIIB (T1 or T2, N2a or N2b, M0)
Stage IIIC (T1 or T2, N2c, M0)
Stage IVA (T1 or T2, N3, M0) or T3, any N, M0)
Stage IVB (any T, any N, M1).

TREATMENT

Surgery remains the most common mode of treatment. Most cases in spite of advanced age, co-morbidities such as diabetes mellitus, hypertension or coronary artery disease can be managed by surgery. Only advanced stages such as stage III or stage IV need the alternative line of treatment in the form of chemoradiation followed by limited surgical excision.

In the past, most commonly used surgical procedure has been en-block excision of skin with deeper tissue over mons and vulva (Radical Vulvectomy) combined with inguinofemoral lymph node dissection. Such an extensive dissection is associated with high rates of wound breakdown, local infection, lymphedema of legs and other postoperative complications. Recently, there have been changing trends in surgical treatment with less extensive dissection and early ambulation of patient. While managing disease in younger patients local wide surgical excision with 1–2 cm tumor free margin is indicated to preserve coital and sensory sexual function.

Following section describes stage wise surgical management of carcinoma vulva.

Stage IA (Tumor less than 2 cm in Diameter, Depth of Invasion less than 1 mm)

This stage is associated with a very risk of lymph node metastasis. Local wide excision with 1–2 cm tumor free margin or hemivulvectomy is considered adequate surgery. Since, chances of lymph node involvement are low, it is omitted in surgical management. In this case, final histology reveals greater than 1 mm invasion of dermis, a thorough inguinofemoral node dissection is needed.

Stage IB (Tumor more than 2 cm in Diameter and Depth of Dermal Invasion more than 1 mm)

With depth of dermal invasion more than 1 mm, there is a significant chance of lymph node metastasis. Therefore, surgery comprises of inguinofemoral lymph node dissection along with radical vulvectomy. For lesions situated more than 2 cm away from midline contralateral lymphadenectomy can be avoided. However, there is a frequent crossing over of lymphatics to opposite site clitoral area and perineum.

Surgical Procedures[27-29,37] for Radical Vulvectomy with Inguinal Femoral Lymphadenectomy

1. Butterfly incision (Ways and Taussing)
2. Longhorn incision
3. Triple incision
4. Hemivulvectomy.

Butterfly Incision (Fig. 8)

It was originally described by Ways from UK in 1951 and Taussing from USA. This technique became very popular and remained in use for next 30 years. It consisted of en bloc resection of wide area of skin with deeper tissue over symphysis pubis, lower abdomen and median aspect of thigh. Although, ensuring wide tumor free margins, the technique was associated with wound gaps, frequent breakdown of suture line, exudation of serum from raw area, prolong healing time and long hospital stay.

Slowly people realized the futility of such a large incision and modifications were suggested.

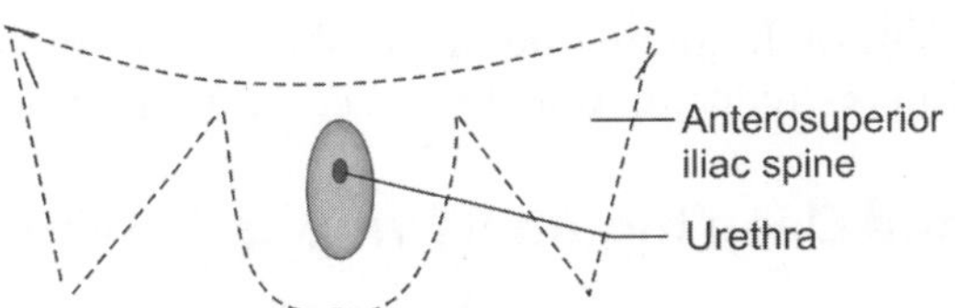

Fig. 8: Butterfly incision

Longhorn Incision

This incision limits the portion of skin removed over groin area. Superiorly incision extends over mons pubis and laterally up to labiocrural folds and posteriorly over perineum depending upon locations of lesion (Fig. 9).

Triple Incision Technique

Two separate incisions are made parallel to inguinal ligament giving access to superficial inguinal lymph nodes on either side. Third incision is made over vulva in a circular fashion to remove growth with a 1–2 cm tumor free margin (Fig. 10).

Wound break down rate is considerably less with triple technique. Currently, this is more commonly used for radical vulvectomy.

Hemivulvectomy/Local Wide Excision

In young patients with invasive disease a less radical procedure in the form of hemivulvectomy or local wide excision with at least 1–2 cm tumor margin can be employed. This limits amount of vulval skin removed and also limits

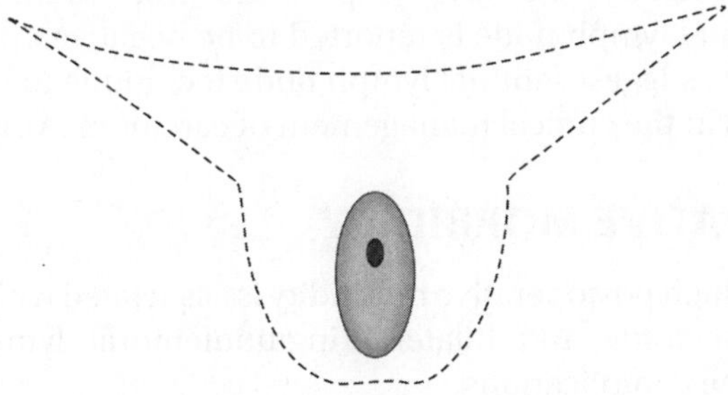

Fig. 9: Longhorn incision

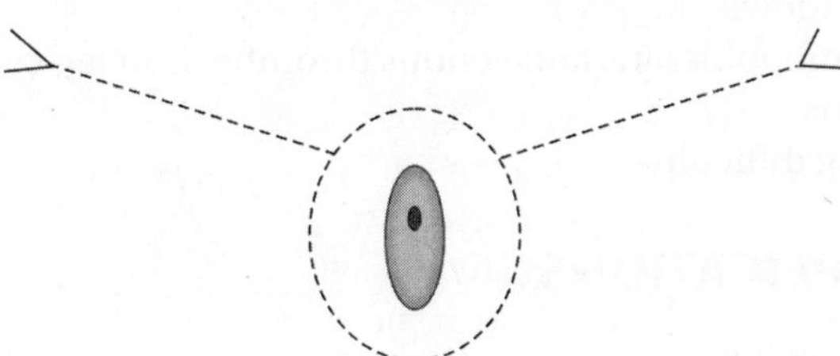

Fig. 10: Triple incision techniques

disfigurement of vulva. Inguinofemoral lymphadenectomy can be limited to same side if lesion is small and more than 2 cm from midline.

Superficial and Deep Inguinal Lymphadenectomy

Essential part of surgery for carcinoma vulva is adequate removal of superficial and deep inguinal lymph nodes. Prognosis depends a great deal on involvement of lymph nodes. Superficial inguinal lymph nodes are present in the form of a chain, running parallel to inguinal ligament. Deep inguinal lymph node (gland of Clouquet) is present in the femoral canal medial to femoral vessel.

Most surgeons do not remove pelvic lymph nodes. In case deep inguinal LN turns out to be positive, patient is treated with irradiation to pelvic lymph node. However, if deep inguinal lymph node is not involved then chances of pelvic lymph node being involved are very low.

Sentinel Lymph Node Sampling for Carcinoma Vulva

Since, major morbidity in a surgical procedure for carcinoma vulva is associated with extensive dissection to remove lymph nodes, a new approach has been adopted to limit dissection. In this technique, either a blue colored dye is injected around vulval lesion before start of procedure or a radioisotope (Technetium 99) is injected around the lesion 30 minutes to 2 hours before the procedure and search is made for first lymph node from the draining area which shows presence of blue colored dye or presence of radioactivity in case of use of T99 isotope.[30-32]

Sentinel LN is immediately subjected to frozen section. Extensive lymph node dissection removing all the lymph nodes from draining area can be avoided if sentinel lymph node is reported to be negative on frozen section. Available reports suggest sentinel lymph node technique to be sensitive and is being utilized in the clinical management of carcinoma vulva cases.[33,35]

POSTOPERATIVE MORBIDITY

A considerably high postoperative morbidity is associated with the procedure of radical vulvectomy and bilateral inguinofemoral lymphadenectomy. Following are the complications:

- Serous exudation from wound site
- Wound breakdown
- Venous thrombophlebitis and venous thrombosis in leg veins
- Local cellulitis
- Urine voiding difficulties

LATE COMPLICATIONS

- Introital narrowing
- Lymphedema legs

➲ Coital difficulties
➲ Recurrence of disease

RECURRENCE

Risk of recurrence in a case of carcinoma vulva correlates best with lymph node involvement. Both local recurrences and distant recurrences in lymph nodes can occur in a case of carcinoma vulva. Prognosis becomes guarded following recurrence. Recurrences are usually treated with radiation therapy and chemotherapy (Cisplatin and 5-FU).

Stage-wise treatment of carcinoma vulva is summarized in Table 2.

RADIATION THERAPY IN CARCINOMA VULVA

The landscape of radiation treatment in carcinoma vulva has evolved much over the past decade. With the evolution of multimodality treatment, radiation has now an increasingly important role to play in the "organ and function preserving" management of carcinoma vulva which at many times require radical surgery. Though earlier not thought to be radiosensitive disease, radiation therapy has now shown excellent results particularly in combination with concurrent chemotherapy.

Radiation therapy can be employed as definitive therapy in selected patients, as adjuvant treatment after radical or conservative surgery, as preoperative therapy, and for palliation of locally advanced disease.

Radical vulvectomy with bilateral inguinofemoral lymph node dissection has been the standard of care for most vulvar cancers in the past. The morbidities of the surgery have been reduced with the use of "Triple incision" and the advancement in postoperative management of these patients. Nevertheless, the late term squeal and psychosexual effects of the surgery have urged the clinicians to explore treatment options in these patients. Definitive radiation therapy remains an option in patients with advanced stage disease not amenable for surgery due to medical comorbidities or local extent of disease requiring extensive surgery, those with recurrent disease after surgery and early stage disease involving midline structures. This has been employed in the form of either external beam radiotherapy or brachytherapy (Fig. 11) or a combination of both. Typically, the radiation treatment volumes include the primary vulvar site in early lesions and also

Table 2: Stage-wise treatment of carcinoma vulva	
Stage Ia	Local wide excision
Stage Ib	Local wide excision + inguinal lymphadenectomy/radical vulvectomy with complete inguinofemoral lymphadenectomy
Stage II	Radical vulvectomy with bilateral inguinofemoral lymphadenectomy
Stage III	Surgery or chemoradiation followed by surgery
Stage IV	Chemotherapy, chemoradiation

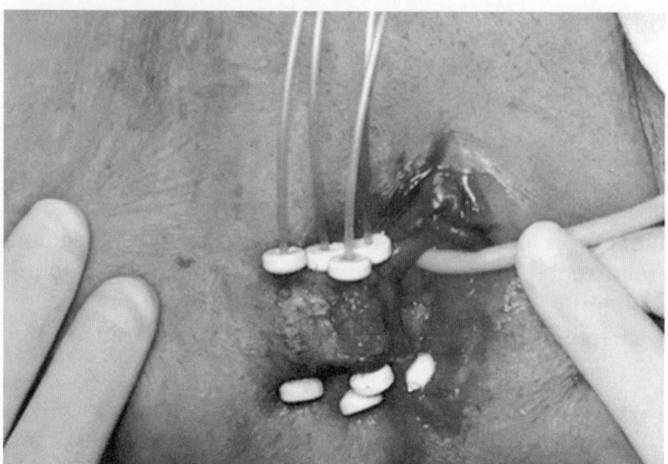

Fig. 11: Clinical image showing the brachytherapy implant for vulvar carcinoma
(For color version, see Plate 7)

includes bilateral inguinal with or without pelvic nodes for advanced lesions. A radiation dose in the range of 60–70 Gray for the gross disease and 45–50 Gray for the microscopic disease is employed.

Concurrent chemoradiation has now emerged as another option in both preoperative and definitive management of vulvar cancers. In a prospective multi-institutional study (GOG 99), Moore et al[39] reported results of 73 unresectable patients of squamous cell carcinoma of vulva (FIGO stage III and IV) treated with a split course concurrent chemoradiation followed by surgical excision of residual tumor and bilateral inguinofemoral lymph node dissection. Radiation therapy consisted of 47.6 Gray in two courses of 23.8 Gray each separated by a gap of 1.5–2.5 weeks along with concurrent cisplatin and 5-Flurouracil. Seventy one patients completed their treatment and 48% of patients had complete clinical response and 70% of these patients had complete pathological response. However, Grade 3–4 skin toxicity was found in 53% of patients. Encouraging results from this and other trials[40] stimulated interest in further study on this treatment approach. In a prospective multi-institutional study (GOG-205) by Moore et al[41] 58 patients of unresectable squamous cell carcinoma of vulva were treated with concurrent chemoradiotherapy followed by surgical biopsy or excision and bilateral inguinofemoral lymph node dissection. Radiation was delivered to a dose of 57.6 Gray to the primary tumor and gross disease and 45 Gray to nodes and pelvis. Concurrent chemotherapy with cisplatin and with or without amifostine was employed. No split was used during the treatment. Forty patients completed treatment and 64% overall had complete clinical response and 27.5% of patients had Grade 3 or more radiation dermatitis and a significant proportion of patients (> 60%) developed Grade 3 or more hematological toxicity. The results of the study demonstrated the higher response of chemoradiotherapy with escalated dose schedule but at a price of higher toxicity. The advancements in the radiation therapy techniques in the recent times might help us in optimizing the treatment outcomes in this regard. With modern RT facilities like IMRT, one can expect better tolerance to chemoradiotherapy regimes. Beriwal et al[42] reported their experience of 18 patients with locally advanced vulvar cancers treated with concurrent chemoradiotherapy with intensity modulated radiotherapy (IMRT). About 70% of the patients achieved pathological complete response rate and no patient developed acute or late grade 3 radiation toxicity. The results of the study indicate the use of concurrent chemoradiation in patients with unresectable primary or nodal disease and also in patients with disease encroaching midline structures, where the surgical morbidity could be profound and debilitating.

Adjuvant radiotherapy is indicated in patients with adverse pathological factors like close surgical margins (<8 mm),[43] depth of invasion more than 5 mm and lymphovascular space invasion.[2] In a study by Faul et al[43] postoperative radiation therapy reduced local recurrence from 58 to 16% in patients with close surgical margins (<8 mm) or with positive margins and improved survival in patients with positive margins. Patients with margins less than 5 mm or positive margins should be assessed for re-surgical excision if possible or else should be offered adjuvant postoperative radiotherapy. After dissection of the lymph nodes, adjuvant radiation is recommended in patients with more than one involved nodes, extracapsular extension or gross residual nodal disease.[44] Adjuvant radiotherapy is not warranted in patients with only one node positive without extracapsular extension.[45] Based on the results of GROINSS-V[46] (Groningen International Study on Sentinel nodes in Vulvar cancer), patients with unifocal tumors < 4 cm, not encroaching on midline structures (away at least by 1.5–2 cm) and negative on sentinel lymph node biopsy might be spared of inguinal lymph node dissection and can be addressed with radiotherapy alone. The use of radiation therapy to address nodes in cases of clinically node negative and positive only on sentinel lymph node biopsy is still investigational.[47] Despite the results from recent studies, however, inguinofemoral lymph node dissection still remains the standard of care for most of the patients.

Palliative radiotherapy is indicated in patients with advanced incurable disease, in patients with distant metastasis and to palliative symptoms like bleeding, fungation, ulceration, etc. A dose of 20 Gray in 5 fractions is usually recommended for this.[48]

Overall, radiation therapy has now a central role to play in the management of carcinoma vulva. A multidisciplinary approach and individualized treatment plan gives the best functional and survival outcome.

LEARNING POINTS

- Vulval carcinoma is an uncommon gynaecological malignancy mostly seen in elderly women.
- Recently occurrence of disease is being noted in younger women related to HPV Infection (HPV 16, 18)
- A number of predisposing factors have been noted such as Lichen Sclerosus, Chronic Vulval Irritation, VIN, HIV infection
- Diagnosis is made by vulval biopsy in symptomatic patients.
- Squamous cell carcinoma is the most common histology, other being basal cell carcinoma, malignant melanoma, adenocarcinoma and Paget's disease of vulva.
- FIGO staging (2009) and TNM classification are used for staging.
- Surgery is the first line treatment for most cases of carcinoma vulva.
- Advanced stages, elderly patient unfit for anaesthesia and recurrent tumors are managed by radiation alone or chemoradiation.
- Radical vulvectomy with bilateral inguinofemoral lymphadenectomy is the most commonly used procedure by triple incision technique.
- In younger patients a less radical approach such as hemivulvectomy with ipsilateral lymphadenectomy can be used.
- Lymph node metastasis is the most important prognostic marker.

REFERENCES

1. American Cancer Society. Vulvar Cancer. Available at : http://www.cancer.org/acs/groups/cid/documents/webcontent/003147-pdf.pdf. Accessed August 10, 2011.
2. Lanneau GS, Argenta PA, Lanneau MS, et al. Vulvar cancer in young women: demographic features and outcome evaluation. Am J Obstet Gynecol. 2009;200:645e1-5.
3. Kaufman RH. Intraepithelial neoplasia of the vulva. Gynecol Oncol. 1995;56:8-21.
4. Preti M, et al. Inter-observer variation in histopathological diagnosis and grading of vulvar intraepithelial neoplasia: results of a European collaborative study. BJOG. 2000;107:594-9.
5. Iversen T, Tretli S. Intraepithelial and invasive squamous cell neoplasia of the vulva; Trends in incidence, recurrence and survival rate in Norway. Obstet Gynecol. 1998; 91: 969-72.
6. Toki T, et al. Probable nonpapilloma virus etiology of squamous cell carcinoma of the vulva in older women: a clinicopathological study using in situ hybridization and polymerase chain reaction. Int J Gynecol Pathol. 1991;10:107-25.
7. Trimble CL, et al. Heterogenous etiology of squamous carcinoma of the vulva. Obstet Gynecol. 1996;87:59-64.
8. Hording U, et al. Human papilloma viruses and multifocal genital neoplasia. Int J Gynecol Pathol. 1996;15:230-4.
9. Franck JM, Young AW. Squamous cell carcinoma in situ arising within lichen planus of the vulva. Dermatol Surg. 1995;21:890-4.
10. Santos M, et al. p16 overexpression identifies HPV- positive vulvar squamous cell carcinomas. Am J Surg Pathol. 2006;30:1347-56.

11. Ndubisi B, et al. Staging and recurrence of disease in squamous cell carcinoma of the vulva. Gynecol Oncol. 1995;59:34-7.

12. Piurab, et al. Squamous cell carcinoma of the vulva in the south of Israel: a study of fifty cases. J Surg Oncol. 1998;67:174-81.

13. Gualco M, et al. Morphologic and biologic studies on ten cases of verrucous carcinoma of the vulva supporting the theory of a discrete clinic-pathologic entity. Int J Gynecol Cancer. 2003;13:317-24.

14. Molini V, et al. Paget disease of the vulva. Thirty six cases. Ann Dermatol Venereol. 1993;120:522-7.

15. Lundquist K, Kohler S, Rouse RV. Intraepidermal cyto keratin 7 expression is not restricted to Paget cells but is also seen in Toker cells and Merkel cells. Am J Surg Pathol. 1999;23:212-9.

16. Teixeira MR, et al. Karyotypic findings in tumors of the vulva and vagina. Cancer Genet Cytogenet. 1999;111:87-91.

17. Benedet JL, et al. Basal cell carcinoma of the vulva: clinical features and treatment results twenty eight patients. Obstet Gynecol. 1997;90:765-8.

18. Mulayim N, et al. Vulvar basal cell carcinoma: Two unusual presentations and review of the literature. Gynecol Oncol. 2002;85:532-7.

19. Dunton CJ, Berd D. Vulvar melanoma, biologically different from other cutaneous melanomas. Lancet. 1999;354:2013-4.

20. Panizzon RG. Vulvar melanoma. Semin Dermatol. 1996;15:67-70.

21. Sugiyama VE, et al. Large series of 359 vulvar melanoma patients-a multivariate analysis. Obstet Gynecol. 2007;109(4Suppl):121S.

22. Hierro I, et al. Merkel cell (neuroendocrine) carcinoma of the vulva. A case report with immunohistochemical and ultrastructural findings and review of the literature. Pathol Res Pract. 2000;196:503-9.

23. Obermair A, et al. Primary Bartholin's gland carcinoma: a report of seven cases. Aust NZ J Obstet Gynecol. 2001;41:78-81.

24. Yang SYV, et al. Adenoid cystic carcinoma of the Bartholin's gland: report of two cases and review of the literature. Gynecol Oncol. 2006;100:422-5.

25. Dalbagni G, et al. Female urethral carcinoma: an analysis of treatment outcome and a plea for a standardized management strategy. Br J Urol. 1998;82:835-41.

26. Pecorelli S. Revised FIGO staging for carcinoma of the vulva, cervix, and endometrium. Int J Gynecol Obstet. 2009;105:103-4.

27. Moore DH, Koh WJ, McGuire WP, et al. Vulva. In: Barakat RP, Markman M, Randall ME (eds). Principles and practice of gynecologic oncology. 5th edition. Baltimore (MD) : Lippincott Williams and Williams. 2009;p. 555-90.

28. Hacker NF, Leuchter RS, Berek JS, et al. Radical vulvectomy and bilateral inguinal lymphadenectomy through separate groin incisions. Obstet Gynecol. 1981;58:574-9.

29. Siller BS, Alvarez RD, Conner WD, et al. T2/3 vulva cancer : a case-control study of triple incision versus en bloc radical vulvectomy and inguinal lymphadenectomy. Gynecol Oncol. 1995;57:335-9.

30. Levenback C, Burke TW, Gershenson DM, et al. Intraoperative lymphatic mapping for vulvar cancer. Obstet Gynecol. 1994;84:163-7.

31. Oonk MH, van de Nieuwenh of HP, de Hullu JA, et al. The role of sentinel node biopsy in gynaecological cancer: a review. Curr Opin Oncol. 2009;21:425-32.

32. van der Zee AG, Oonk MH, de Hullu JA, et al. Sentinel node dissection is safe in the treatment or early-stage vulvar cancer. J Clin Oncol. 2008;28:884-9.

33. Levenback CF, van der Zee AG, Rob L, et al. Sentinel lymph node biopsy in patients with gynaecologic cancers: expert panel statement from the International Sentinel Node Society Meeting. Gynecol Oncol. 2009;114:151-6.

34. American Joint Committee on Cancer. Vulvar Cancer. AJCC Cancer Staging Manual 7th ed. New York, NY: Springer. 2010:379-86.

35. Levenback CF, van der Zee AG, Rob L, et al. Sentinel lymph node biopsy in patients with gynaecologic cancers. Expert panel statement from the international sentinel node society meeting, February 21, 2008. Gynecol Oncol. 2009 Aug;114(2):151-6.

36. PDQ database. Vulvar Cancer. Bethesda, Md : National Cancer Institute; 9/7/2012. Accessed at http://www/cancer.gov/cancertopics/pdq/treatment/vulvar/Health Professional on September 12, 2012.

37. Rouzier R, Haddad B, Atallah D, et al. Surgery for vulvar cancer. Clin Obst Gyn. 2005;48:869-78.

38. van der Avoort IAM, Shirango H, Hovenaars BM, et al. Vulvar squamous cell carcinoma is a mutlifactorial disease following two separate and independent pathways. Int J Gyn path. 2005;25:22-9.

39. Moore DH, Thomas GM, Montana GS, et al. Preoperative chemoradiation for advanced vulvar cancer: a phase II study of the gynecologic oncology group. Int J Radiat Oncol Biol Phys. 1998;42:79-85.

40. Montana GS, Kang SK. Carcinoma of the vulva. In: Halperin EC, Parez CA, Brady LW (eds). Perez and Brady's principles and practice of radiationoncology. 5th Edition. Philadelphia: Lippincott Williams and Wilkins. 2008;p. 1692-707.

41. Moore DH, Ali S, Barnes M, et al. A phase II trial of radiation therapy and weekly cisplatin chemotherapy for the treatment of locally advanced squamous cell carcinoma of the vulva: A gynecologic oncology group study. Gynecologic Oncology. 2012;124:529-33.

42. Beriwal S, Coon D, Heron DE, et al. Preoperative intensity-modulated radiotherapyand chemotherapy for locally advanced vulvar carcinoma. Gynecol Oncol. 2008;109:291-5.

43. Faul cm, Mirmow D, Huang Q, et al. Adjuvant radiation for vulvar carcinoma: Improved local control. Int J Radiat Oncol Biol Phys. 1997;38:381-9.

44. Homesley HD, Bundy BN, Sedlis A, et al. Radiation therapy versus pelvic noderesection for carcinoma of the vulva with positive groin nodes. Obstet Gynecol. 1986;68:733-40.

45. Fons G, Groenen SM, Oonk MH, et al. Adjuvant radiotherapy in patients with vulvar cancer and one intracapsular lymph node metastasis is not beneficial. Gynecol Oncol. 2009;114:343-5.

46. Van der Zee AG, Oonk MH, De Hullu JA, et al. Sentinel node dissection is safe in the treatment of early-stage vulvar cancer, J Clin Oncol. 2008;26:884-9.

47. Groningen International Study on Sentinel nodes in Vulvar cancer II (GROINSS-V-II) 2009. http://www.esgo.org/Research/Documents/groins.pdf.

48. Sharma DN, Rath GK, Kumar S. Treatment outcome of patients with carcinoma of vulva: experience from a tertiary cancer center of India. J Cancer Res Ther. 2010;6:503-7.

Chapter 49

Management of Abnormal Pap Smear

Usha Didwania

Cervical cancer is the second most common cancer in women worldwide and most common cause of death in the developing world. Cervical cancer mortality is about 40% higher in younger than 65 years and 150% higher in older than 65 years of age in black women than for white women.

According to the World Health Organization (WHO), by 2025 the number of new cancer cases in India will be approximately 2,26,084.

The incidence of precancerous lesions of cervix is 100 times higher than frank cancer of cervix. Thus, the screening for precancerous cervical lesions as well as early cervical cancer, when it can be treated, is essential.

Since the introduction of cervical cytology by Dr Papanicolaou in 1940 for the screening of cervical cancer, its incidence has drastically come down. This test is called 'Pap smear test'. It tests the exfoliated cells of the cervix.

The causal relationship of human papillomavirus (HPV) with cancer cervix was established by Zur Hausen in 1984. There are more than 100 types of HPV viruses, out of which mainly 16, 18, 31, 33, 35, 39, 45, 51 are high-risk HPV and have been linked to the carcinoma cervix. Although the incidence of infection is high, most infections resolve but those who remain persistently infected, develop precursor lesions. It was also established that there is a long time gap between HPV infection and acquisition of cervical cancer.

There are risk factors for the development of cervical cancer, i.e. immunosuppression, smoking, vitamin deficiency, Chlamydial infection, long use of OCP, teenage pregnancy, DES exposure in utero, etc.

If detected at the preinvasive stage, cervical cancer can be prevented. On this basis, the benefits of screening are proved and Pap smear is being used as a primary screening test around the world.

For this purpose, **New Cervical Cancer Screening Guidelines** were announced in March 2012 by United States Preventive Services Task Force (USPSTF) and American Cancer Society (ACS), American Society for Colposcopy and Cervical Pathology, and American Society for Clinical Pathology. These recommendations apply to women who have cervix and regardless of her sexual history but these recommendations do not apply to women who had high-grade precancerous and cancer cervix lesions, women within utero exposure to diethylstilbestrol or immunocompromised women.

USPSTF recommendations are as follows:

- Women of any age should not be screened annually by any screening method.
- Screening of women of 21–65 years of age with cytology, every 3 years.
- Screening of women of 30–65 years of age with cytology, every 3 years. Women who want to lengthen the screening interval, co-testing of cytology and HPV is done every 5 years.
- Recommendation is against the screening of women under 21 years of age.
- Recommendation is against the women aged above 65 years of age, who had adequate prior screening and they are not of high-risk category for cervical cancer.
- Recommendation against screening of women who have had a hysterectomy with the removal of cervix and with no history of CIN 1/CIN 2/CIN 3.

  Women, who have had subtotal hysterectomy, should continue screening according to the guidelines.
- Recommends against screening for cancer cervix using HPV testing alone or in combination with cytology in women under 30 years of age.
- Women with a history of HPV vaccination should be screened according to the age-specific recommendation for the general population (The possibility of reduced need for screening in vaccinated women is not yet established.)

  National Cancer Institute, Bethesda developed the Bethesda system for **reporting the results of cervical cytology** as a uniform system of terminology that would provide clear guidance for clinical management. The "Squamous Intraepithelial Lesion" term is used by the Bethesda system for abnormal growth on cervix referring squamous cell type on the cervix. "Dysplasia" and "Cervical Intraepithelial Neoplasia" are the terms with the same meaning. This recommendation received widespread acceptance in the world after the workshop held in 1988 and in 1991. In the Bethesda workshop in 2001, participants supported the view that cervical cytology is primarily a screening test. However, a patient's final diagnosis and management must integrate the clinical and laboratory results. Thus, the term "Interpretation" is used for cervical cytology findings.

THE BETHESDA SYSTEM

Specimen Adequacy

- Satisfactory for evaluation
- Unsatisfactory for evaluation (specify the reason)
- Specimen rejected or not processed (specify the reason)
- Specimen processed, examined but unsatisfactory for the evaluation of epithelial abnormality.

General Catagorization

- Negative for Intraepithelial lesion or malignancy
- Epithelial cell abnormality.

Others

Interpretation/Result

- Negative for intraepithelial lesion or malignancy organisms:
  - Trichomonas vaginalis
  - Fungal organisms, e.g. Candida
  - Shift in flora suggesting bacterial vaginosis
  - Bacteria morphologically consistent with Actinomycosis
  - Cellular changes consistent with HSV
- Other non-neoplastic findings:
  - Reactive cellular changes associated with inflammation, radiation, intrauterine contraceptive device, glandular cell status
  - Posthysterectomy atrophy.

Epithelial Cell Abnormality

- Squamous cell:
  - Atypical squamous cell (ASC)
  - Atypical squamous cell of undetermined significance (ASC-US)
- ASC—Cannot exclude HSIL (ASC-H):
  - Low-grade squamous intraepithelial lesion (LSIL)—encompassing: HPV, mild dysplasia/CIN 1
  - High-grade squamous intraepithelial lesion (HSIL)—encompassing: moderate and severe dysplasia, carcinoma—in situ, CIN 2 and CIN 3
  - Squamous cell carcinoma
- Glandular cell
  - Atypical glandular cells (AGC) (specify endocervical, endometrial, or not otherwise specified (NOS)
  - Atypical glandular cells favor neoplastic (specified endocervical or NOS)
  - Endocervical adenocarcinoma—in situ
  - Adenocarcinoma

Others (list not comprehensive): Endometrial cells in women > 40 years of age.

Best time for smear collection is from tenth to twentieth days of the cycle. The woman should avoid sex, vaginal medication, pessary or douching for 2–3 days before the test.

Adequacy of the Sample

For a satisfactory evaluation of the specimen, presence of endocervical/ transformation zone component with adequate squamous cells should be there. Partially obscuring inflammatory or blood cells may be added to satisfactory group. If 50–75% of the epithelial cells cannot be visualized, it is considered partially obscured. If more than 75% of the epithelial cells are obscured, specimen is unsatisfactory. It may be because of poor fixation, paucity of cells, air-drying artifact, thick smear, and covering of blood, inflammatory exudates or other contaminants.

For a satisfactory specimen type, there should be an estimated 8000 to 12000 well-visualized squamous cells for conventional smears and 5000 squamous cells for liquid-based preparations. There should be at least 10 well preserved endocervical or metaplastic cells. LBC is 80% sensitive.

Management Protocol for negative malignant cell smear is shown in Flow chart 1.

Negative for malignant cells—It is the smear showing no cervical intraepithelial neoplasia, glandular dysplasia or malignancy. The category includes those where cells show reactive changes and also those where the micro-organisms are identified. Clinically suspicious looking cervix must be referred for colposcopy.

Management protocol for unsatisfactory smears is shown in Flow chart 2.

Management protocol for abnormal Pap smear as primary screening is shown in Flow chart 3.

Flow chart 1: Management protocol for "negative for malignant cells" smear

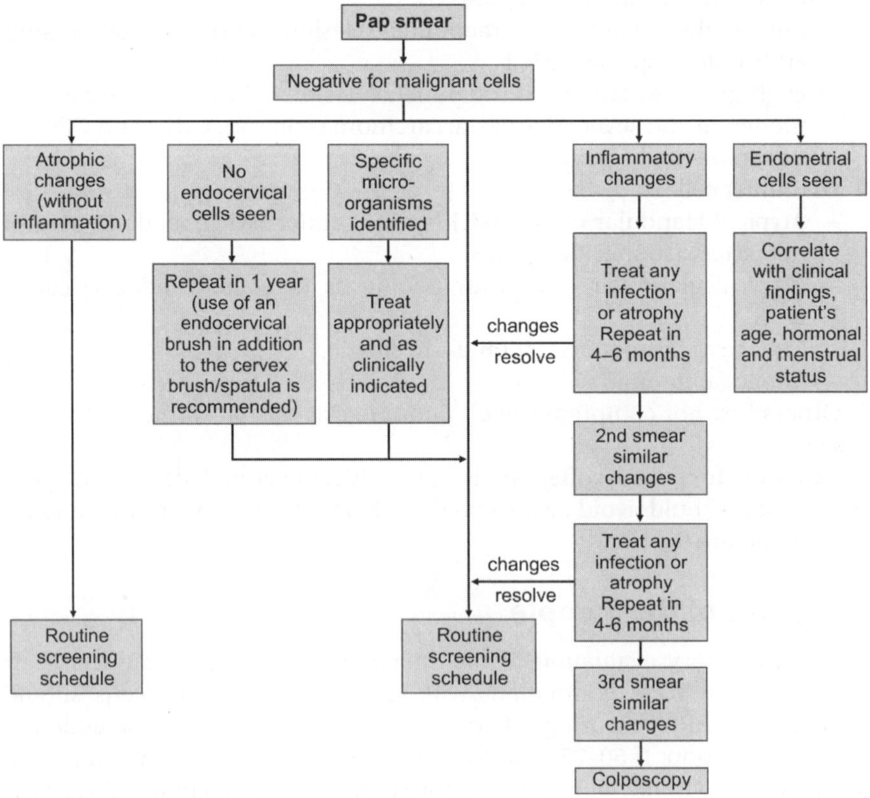

Flow chart 2: Management protocol for unsatisfactory smears (Smear is unreliable for detection of any abnormality)

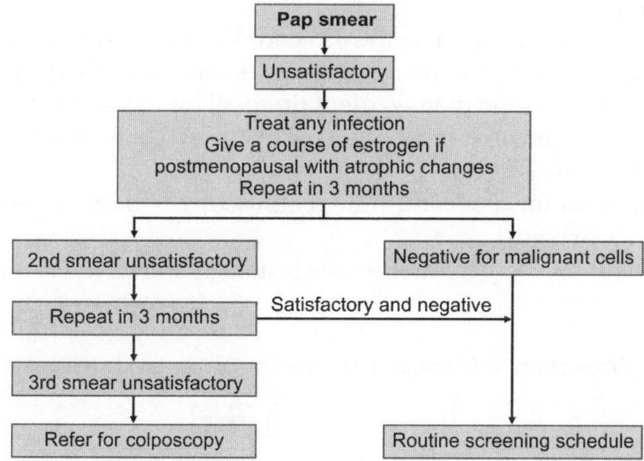

Atypical squamous cells of undetermined significance (ASC-US). This means that the smear shows cells which are not typical squamocolumnar cervical cells or endocervical glandular cells. This abnormality is not sufficient to constitute "dysplasia". The aim is to find out if the abnormality is "significant" by seeing what happens over time. If the lesion is due to dysplasia, it may clear up spontaneously due to the host's immune defence system or it may persist and show itself again as ASC-US, or it may progress to dysplasia. So, a Pap smear should be repeated after every 6 months.

Flow chart 3: Management protocol for abnormal Pap smear (primary screening)

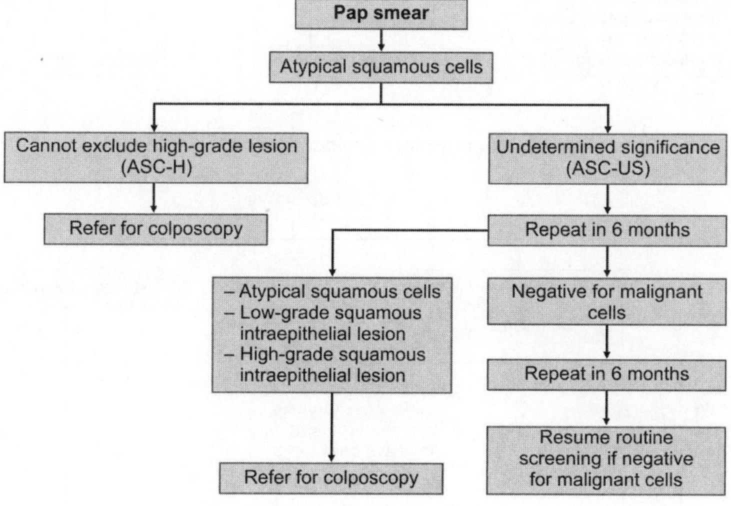

If a repeat smear again shows ASC-US, it may well represent a dysplastic lesion which is not clearly seen in specimen. This case should be evaluated by colposcopy.

In postmenopausal patients, ASC-US could be due to the lack of estrogen. Pap smear should be repeated after treatment with vaginal estrogen.

Flow chart 4 shows the management protocol for low-grade lesions.

LSIL lesion is a sign of dysplasia due to HPV infection. It usually disappears in about eight months.

If LSIL appears for a second time, colposcopy is done to see if a more severe lesion is present.

Management protocol for high-grade lesions is shown in Flow chart 5.

Flow chart 4: Management protocol for low-grade lesions

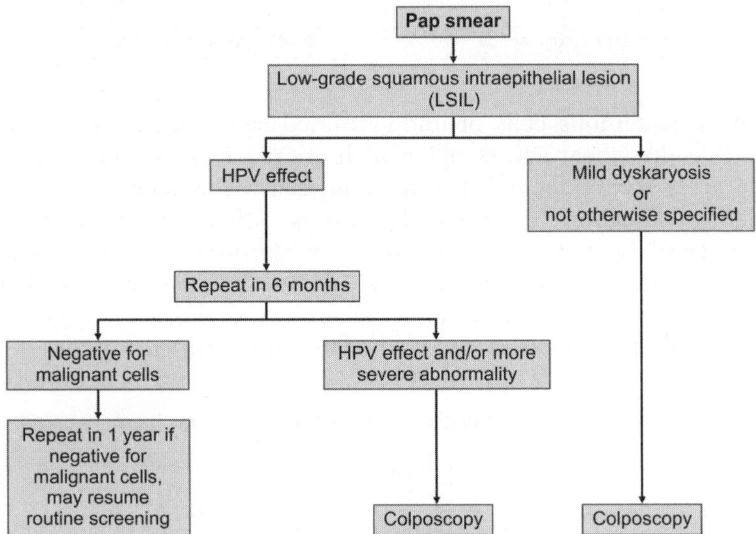

Flow chart 5: Management protocol for high-grade lesions

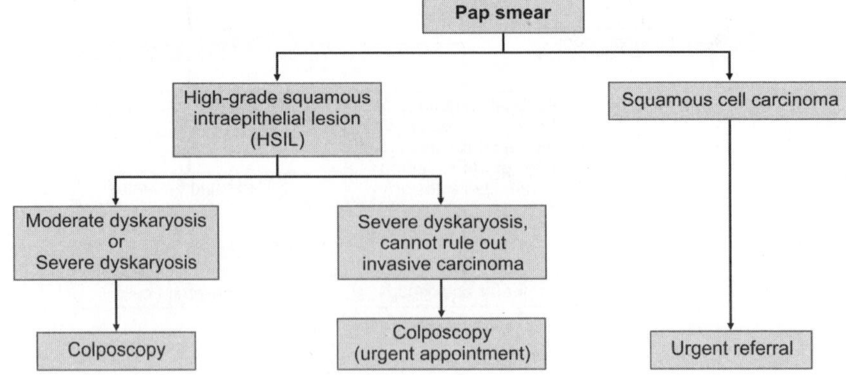

Moderate dyskaryosis—CIN 2.

Severe dyskaryosis—CIN 3. Invasive carcinoma is not ruled out.

When a lesion is seen on cervix clinically, it should be evaluated by colposcopy and directed biopsy regardless of the Pap smear result.

Management of abnormal glandular cells is shown in Flow chart 6.

Undetermined significance means that cell changes exceed the criteria for reactive process but lack the criteria for dysplasia.

Favor neoplastic means that cytological changes suggest dysplasia or adenocarcinoma-in-situ or adenocarcinoma but lack criteria for definite interpretation.

AGC-US may be a precursor of this or it may also be found in association with squamous cell dysplasia. Colposcopy is suggested in these situations (Flow chart 7).

Flow chart 6: Abnormal glandular cells lesions management

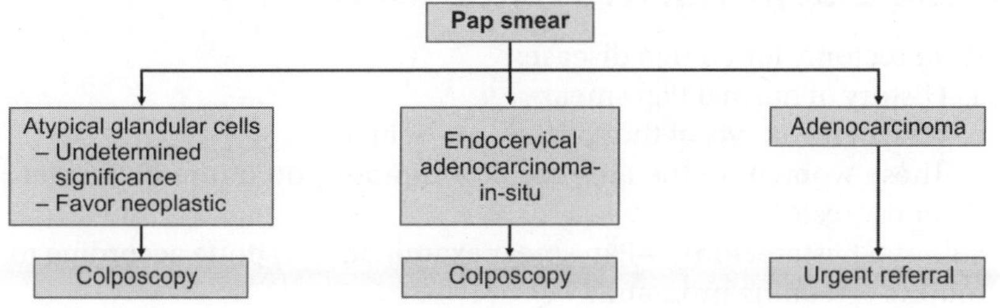

Flow chart 7: Management protocol for abnormal smears (following treatment for CIN or CGIN)

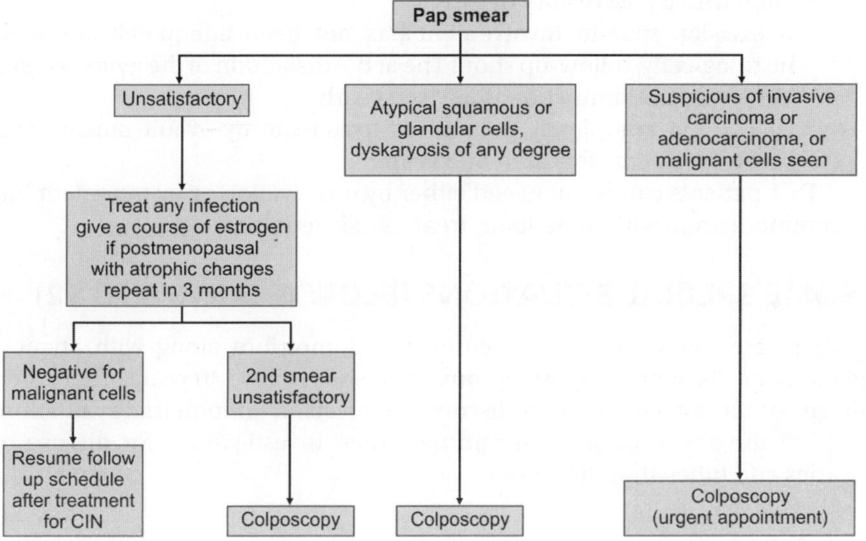

Clinically suspicious-looking cervix irrespective of pap smear result must be referred for colposcopy.

MANAGEMENT OF ABNORMAL SMEARS AND CIN IN PREGNANCY

1. Colposcopic evaluation done to exclude invasive disease.
2. If high-grade lesion is suspected on colposcopy, a biopsy is indicated to exclude the invasive disease. Cervical biopsy is safe in pregnancy.
3. In case of CIN 2/CIN 3, Colposcopic review should be done in 2nd/3rd trimester to exclude the progression of the disease.
4. Treatment of CIN should be deferred till 8 weeks postpartum. Then the lesion should be re-assessed. In breastfeeding mothers, local application of estrogen before colposcopy may help in accurate assessment.

Management of labor is not influenced by the presence of CIN of any severity.

PAP SMEAR AFTER HYSTERECTOMY

1. Hysterectomy for benign disease:
    a. History of normal Pap smear
    b. HPE of the cervix of the specimen is benign
       These women, in the absence of symptoms, do not need further Pap smear tests.
2. Subtotal hysterectomy—Pap smear examination is done according to the routine screening program.
3. Hysterectomy where HPE of the specimen is not known.
   One baseline Pap smear is taken from the vault. If this is normal, no further tests are required.
4. Immunosuppressed women—Pap smear test each year
5. Women with a past history of CIN:
    – If excision margin involvement has not been adequately assessed histologically, follow-up should be at the discretion of the gynecologist. Vault smear examination is advised yearly.
    – CIN 1/2/3 completely excised at hysterectomy—vault smear tests yearly for 5 years followed by 2 yearly.

CIN 1 patients can be managed either by observation or by treatment but in immunocompromised patients, treatment is required.

SOME SPECIAL SITUATIONS (FLOW CHARTS 8 TO 12)

If there are risk factors for Carcinoma endometrium along with atypical glandular cells or patient is symptomatic or she is above 40 years of age, then diagnostic curettage with hysteroscopy is advised for endometrial evaluation.

If all the above findings are normal, then investigations for disease in ovaries and tubes should be done.

Flow chart 8: Abnormal smears (ASCUS/LSIL) colposcopy—normal/unsatisfactory

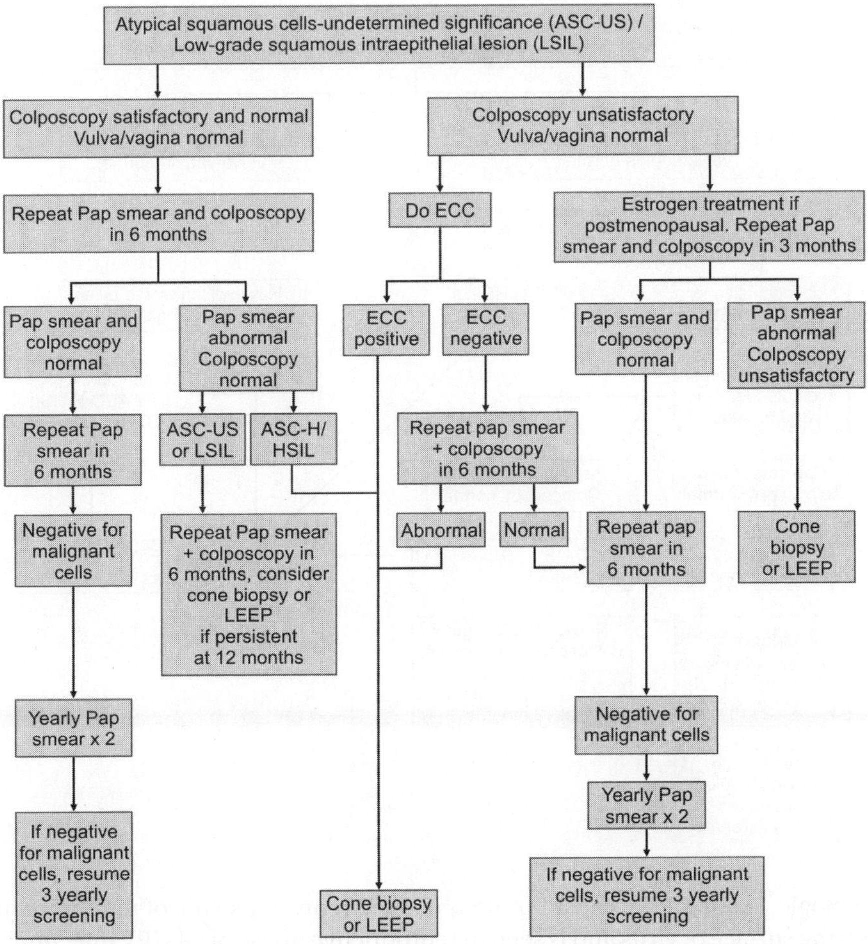

Atypical squamous cells-undetermined significance (ASC-US) / Low-grade squamous intraepithelial lesion (LSIL)

- Colposcopy satisfactory and normal Vulva/vagina normal
  - Repeat Pap smear and colposcopy in 6 months
    - Pap smear and colposcopy normal
      - Repeat Pap smear in 6 months
        - Negative for malignant cells
          - Yearly Pap smear x 2
            - If negative for malignant cells, resume 3 yearly screening
    - Pap smear abnormal Colposcopy normal
      - ASC-US or LSIL
      - ASC-H/HSIL
        - Repeat Pap smear + colposcopy in 6 months, consider cone biopsy or LEEP if persistent at 12 months

- Colposcopy unsatisfactory Vulva/vagina normal
  - Do ECC
    - ECC positive
      - Cone biopsy or LEEP
    - ECC negative
      - Repeat pap smear + colposcopy in 6 months
        - Abnormal
        - Normal
  - Estrogen treatment if postmenopausal. Repeat Pap smear and colposcopy in 3 months
    - Pap smear and colposcopy normal
      - Repeat pap smear in 6 months
        - Negative for malignant cells
          - Yearly Pap smear x 2
            - If negative for malignant cells, resume 3 yearly screening
    - Pap smear abnormal Colposcopy unsatisfactory
      - Cone biopsy or LEEP

FUTURE PROGRESS

The dilemma is that neither cytology, colposcopy nor HPV DNA testing indicates whether regression or progression of the precursor lesion will occur. It is well-known that HPV infection is present in more than 99% of cases. However, not all HPVs give rise to cervical dysplasia. Therefore, some more specific tests like prognostic markers would be of value in differentiating between patients who will progress to cancer from precursor lesion and those who will not. HPV-L1 capsid protein is one of the eight known HPV, specific proteins, a marker which could have prognostic information about the evolution of early dysplastic changes and could be useful in predicting their

Flow chart 9: Abnormal smears (ASC-H/HSIL) and unsatisfactory or normal colposcopy

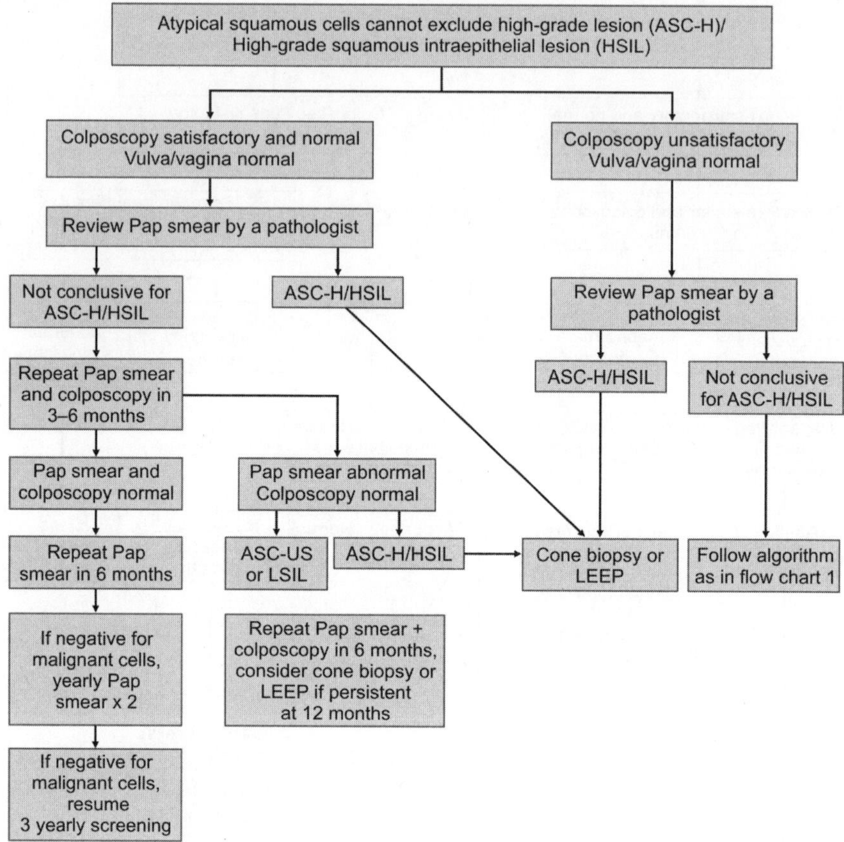

biologic potential. L1 capsid protein of HPV represents 90% of total protein on the surface of virus and is seen in reproductive phase of all HPV infections. L1 is usually negative in normal pap smears and positive in mild to moderate dysplasia, rarely positive in severe dysplasia and negative in carcinoma cervix. It was shown that high-risk HPV infection causing mild and moderate dysplasia without the detected HPV-L1 capsid protein is significantly more likely to progress (76%) than HPV-L1 positive cases (24%).

Studies are underway to investigate the possibilities of using routine HPV testing as a primary screening method with follow-up by Pap tests in HPV-positive women.

CONCLUSION

Any abnormal smear must be followed by careful clinical examination, colposcopy and biopsy. Although the whole procedure causes psychological

Flow chart 10: Atypical glandular cells

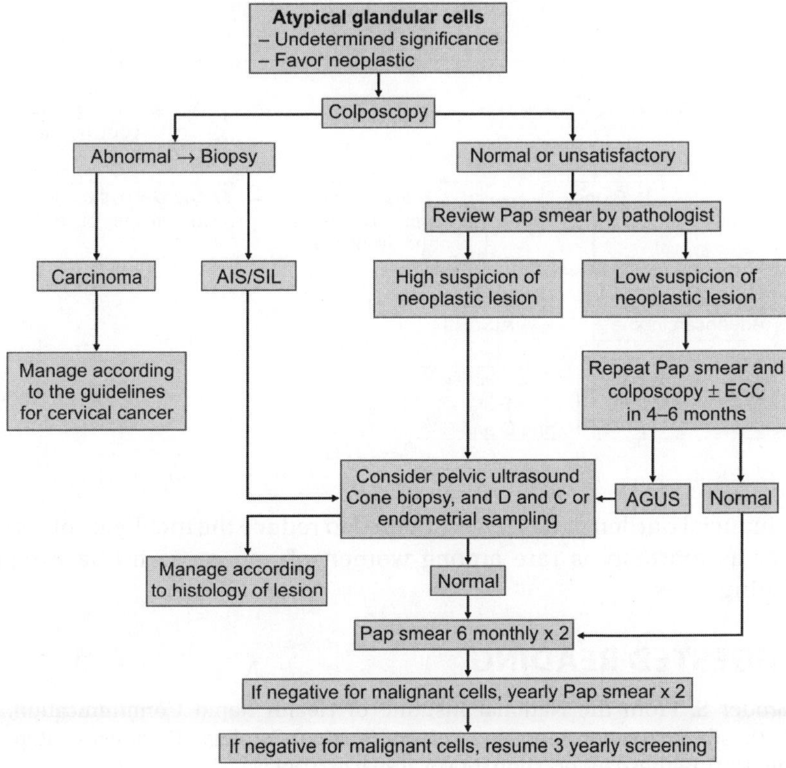

Flow chart 11: Management of endocervical adenocarcinoma on Pap smear

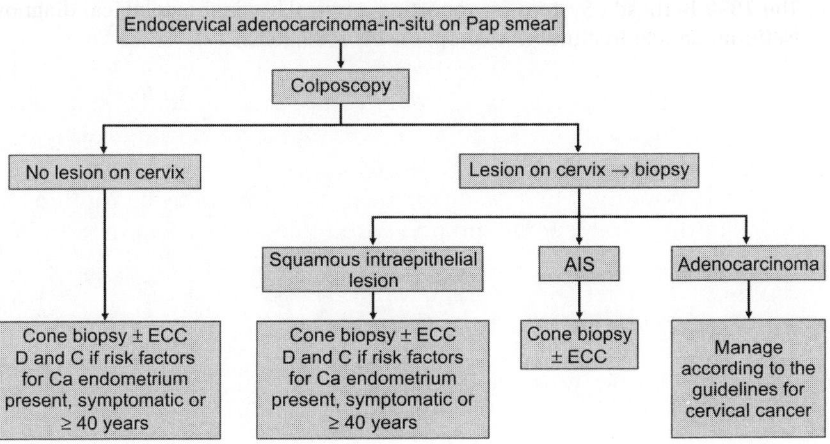

Flow chart 12: Management of adenocarcinoma on Pap smear

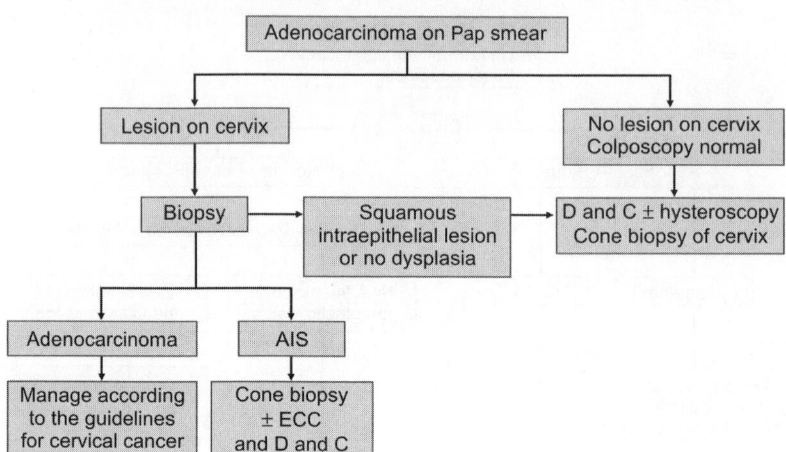

and financial burden, it has largely helped to reduce the incidence of cervical cancer as mortality is rare among women of any age, who have regular screening.

SUGGESTED READING

1. Broder S. From the National Institute of Health Rapid Communication. The Bethesda System for Reporting Cervical/Vaginal Cytologic Diagnoses—Report of the 1991 Bethesda Workshop. JAMA. 1992;267:1892.
2. Cervical cancer screening (PDQ), National Cancer Institute. Feb 26, 2013(37).
3. Management Guidelines for Abnormal Pap Smear (E)-Health-(PDF) The Cervical Screen, Singapore.
4. Pap and HPV Testing, National Cancer Institute.
5. Pap Smear—Medicine, Medscape. Nov 7, 2012.
6. The 1998 Bethesda System for reporting cervical/vaginal cytological diagnoses. National Cancer Institute workshop, JAMA. 1989;262:931-4.

Chapter 50

Benign Ovarian Tumors

Nisha Singh

Ovary is the gonadal organ for women. It produces all important sex hormones to sustain womanhood and germ cells to maintain continuity of human life. Thus, a healthy functioning ovary is essential for human life. The ovary is prone to develop various disorders ranging from streak ovaries to infections to endometriosis to benign and malignant tumors. Certainly, tumors of the ovary are the most dreaded disorders. The late diagnosis, poor prognosis and effect on fertility further add to the misery. We shall be dealing with benign ovarian tumors in this chapter.

ETIOPATHOGENESIS (TABLE 1)

The etiology of ovarian tumors is unknown. Several hypotheses have been proposed based on epidemiological, histological, immunohistochemical, genetic and experimental studies.

PATHOLOGY

Histologically, the ovary is divided into cortex and medulla and surrounded by a simple cuboidal surface epithelium. Ovarian tumors may arise from all three components. The WHO classification of ovarian tumors (Table 2) is based on their basic histological characters.

Table 1: Risk modifiers of ovarian tumors

Risk factors	Protective factors
❖ Nulliparity	❖ Oral contraceptive
❖ Infertility	❖ Pregnancy
❖ Early menarche	❖ Breastfeeding
❖ Late menopause	❖ Tubal ligation
❖ Endometriosis	❖ Hysterectomy
❖ Family history of cancers (ovary, breast, colon, endometrium)	❖ Salpingo-oophorectomy.
❖ Talc use	
❖ Prolonged use of ovulation inducing drugs	
❖ HRT (Human replacement therapy)	

Table 2: WHO histological classification of tumors of the ovary

SURFACE EPITHELIAL STROMAL TUMORS

	Malignant	Borderline	Benign
Serous tumors	Adenocarcinoma Surface papillary adenocarcinoma Adenocarcinofibroma	Papillary cystic tumor Surface papillary tumor Adenofibroma Cystadenofibroma	Cystadenoma Papillary cystadenoma Surface papilloma Adenofibroma Cystadenofibroma
Mucinous tumors	Adenocarcinoma Adenocarcinofibroma	Endocervical type Intestinal type	Cystadenoma Adenofibroma cystadenofibroma Mucinous cystic tumor with mural nodules and pseudomyxoma peritonei
Endometroid	Adenocarcinoma Adenocarcinofibroma Malignant mullerian mixed tumor Adenosarcoma Endometroid stromal sarcoma Undifferentiated ovarian sarcoma	Cystic tumor Adenofibroma Cystadenofibroma	Cystadenoma Adenofibroma and cystadenofibroma
Clear cell tumors	Adenocarcinoma Adenocarcinofibroma	Cystic tumor Adenofibroma and cystadenofibroma	Cystadenoma Adenofibroma and cystadenofibroma
Transitional cell tumors	Transitional cell carcinoma Malignant Brenner tumor	Borderline Brenner tumor	Benign Brenner tumor

Squamous cell tumors—Squamous cell carcinoma epidermoid cyst

Mixed Epithelial tumors—Malignant borderline benign

Undifferentiated and unclassified tumors—Undifferentiated carcinoma adenocarcinoma,

SEX CORD STROMAL TUMORS

Granulosa—stormal cell tumors

Granulosa cell tumor group	Thecoma-fibroma group
Adult granulosa cell tumor Juvenile granulosa cell tumor	Thecoma-typical, luteinized Fibroma cellular fibroma Fibrosarcoma Stromal tumor with minor sex cord elements Sclerozing stromal tumor Signet ring stromal tumor Unclassified (fibrothecoma)

Contd...

Contd...

Sertoli stromal cell tumors

Sertoli-Leydig cell tumor group (androblastomas)
❖ Well differentiated
❖ Of intermediate differentiation
❖ Variant with heterologous element (specify type)
❖ Poorly differentiated (Sarcomatoid)
❖ Variant with heterologous element (specify type)
❖ Retiform variant with heterologous element (specify type)
Sertoli cell tumor
Stromal leydig cell tumor

Sex cord—stromal tumors of mixed or unclassified cell types)
Sex cord tumor with annular tubules
Gynandroblastoma (specify components)
Sex cord—stromal tumor, unclassified

Steroid cell tumors
Stromal luteoma
Leydig cell tumor group—Hilus cell tumor, Leydig cell tumor (non hilar)
Steroid cell tumor, not otherwise specified-well differentiated, malignant

GERM CELL TUMORS

Primitive germ cell tumor	**Germ cell sex-cord stromal tumor**
Dysgerminoma Yolk sac tumor Embryonal carcinoma Polyembryoma Non-gestational choriocarcinoma Mixed germ cell tumor (specify components)	Gonadoblastoma Variant with malignant germ cell tumor Mixed germ cell-sex cord-stromal tumor Variant with malignant germ cell tumor
Biphasic and triphasic teratoma	**Monodermal teratoma and somatic-type tumors associated with dermoid cysts**
Immature teratoma Mature teratoma Solid Cystic Dermoid cyst Fetiform teratoma (homunculus)	Thyroid tumor group-struma ovarii Carcinoid group Neuroectodermal tumor group Carcinoma group Melanocytic group Pituitary-type tumor group

TUMORS OF THE RETE OVARII

Adenocarcinoma
Adenoma
Cystadenoma
Cystadenofibroma

MISCELLANEOUS TUMORS

Small cell carcinoma, hypercalcemic type
Small cell carcinoma, pulmonary type
Large cell neuroendocrine carcinoma
Hepatoid carcinoma
Primary ovarian mesothelioma
Wilms tumor

Contd...

Contd...

Gestational choriocarcinoma
Hydatidiform mole
Adenoid cystic carcinoma
Basal cell tumor
Ovarian wolffian tumor
Paraganglioma
Myxoma
Soft tissue tumors, not specific to the ovary
Others

Tumor like conditions
Lymphoid and hematopoitic tumors
Secondary tumors

Ovarian tumors may also be classified into benign, borderline and malignant variants depending upon their clinical behavior and ability to metastasize.

Benign epithelial tumors: 60% of all ovarian tumors are epithelial in origin. Almost all epithelial ovarian tumors have benign, borderline and malignant variants.

Serous cystadenoma: Constitute 30% of all ovarian tumors and are the most common benign epithelial tumors. They are uniloculated or multiloculated cysts lined with columnar or cuboidal epithelium and filled with serous fluid as shown in Figure 1. Occasionally, polypoidal excrescences can be seen on the inner cyst wall. Only 10% are bilateral. They are commonly seen in reproductive years.

Mucinous cystadenoma: They are the second most common benign epithelial tumors. They are multiloculated cysts filled with mucoid material (Fig. 2). They are the largest in size, may exceed 30 cm in diameter. The lining epithelium has columnar mucus secreting cells and papillary projections are rare. Only 5% are bilateral. They may be associated with a rare condition called pseudomyxoma peritonei, wherein mucoid fluid is present in the peritoneal cavity without rupture of the tumor.

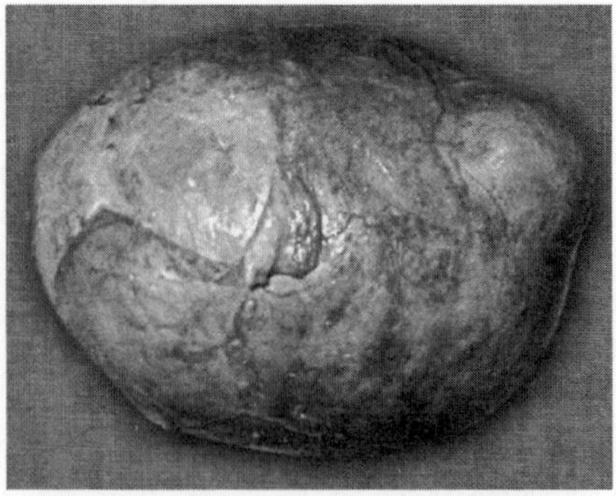

Fig. 1: Benign serous cystadenoma
(For color version, see Plate 8)

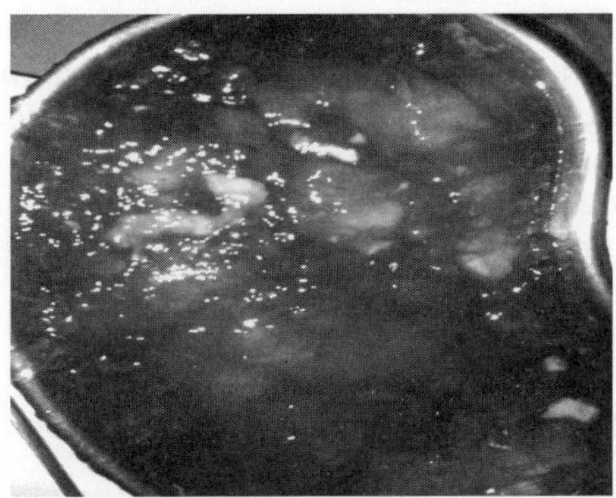

Fig. 2: Mucin from a benign mucinous cystadenoma
(For color version, see Plate 8)

Endometroid cystadenoma: May be associated with endometriosis or endometrial hyperplasia. The cyst is lined by well-differentiated cells of endometrial type. They are unilateral. Only 5% of epithelial tumors are endometroid.

Brenner (Transitional) tumors: These are mostly small, solid, unilateral and occur in 6th–7th decade of life. The epithelial element resembles uroepithelium.

Clear cell (Mesonephroid) tumors: They arise from serosal cells, are lined by clear cells (hobnail cells) and are rarely benign.

Sex cord stromal cell tumors: These are grey-brown, solid tumors that originate from ovarian matrix and produce sex hormones.

Thecoma, fibroma, sclerozing stromal tumor and sertoli cell tumors are mostly benign.

Thecomas produce estrogen and are common in young women.

Sertoli cell tumors may produce both estrogen and androgen.

Fibroma occurs more commonly in postmenopausal women. Its association with ascites and hydrothorax is known as Meig's syndrome, a benign condition mimicking ovarian carcinoma. They are hormonally inactive.

Sclerozing stromal tumors are hormonally inactive and less common.

Granulosa cells tumors—have indolent growth pattern and low malignant potential. They are more common in menopausal women and 70% produce estrogen.

Germ cell tumors: They arise from germinal elements of the ovary and constitute 3–7% of all ovarian tumors. The germ cell tumors present at a younger age, in 2nd or 3rd decade of life.

The mature teratoma is the most common (95%) germ cell tumor tund is clinically benign. It originates from a single germ cell and may contain any of the three germ layers, i.e. ectoderm, mesoderm or endoderm. Size may vary from 0.5 cm to 40 cm in diameter. The ectodermal components include skin, hair, teeth and sebaceous material, endodermal components include thyroid tissue and mesodermal components include bone or smooth muscles.

Mature teratoma is further classified as mature cystic teratoma (dermoid cyst), mature solid teratoma, fertiform teratoma and monodermal teratoma depending upon its consistency, shape and type of tissue. The monodermal teratoma is composed of solely or predominantly one type of specialized tissue, the most common being struma ovarii which is composed of thyroid tissue, 1–3% of mature teratomas may undergo malignant transformation in women above 40 years of age.

Ovarian leiomyoma are rare solid tumors of ovary.

CLINICAL FEATURES

Most benign ovarian tumors present with some common symptoms like pain, abdominal swelling, bloating or pressure effects. Some of them produce special symptoms, based on hormones they secrete.

Pain

Ovarian tumors usually present with mild pain of gradual onset that persists throughout the day. This is because of the increasing size and pressure effects. Until the tumor is confined to the pelvis, it presents with vague heaviness in the lower abdomen.

Acute pain is seen in cases of hemorrhage, rupture or torsion of the ovarian tumor. Torsion gives rise to acute onset of sharp constant pain due to ischemia of the cyst. Hemorrhage in the cyst leads to stretching of the capsule that causes acute pain. Rupture of the cyst leads to intraperitoneal bleeding mimicking ectopic pregnancy.

Abdominal Swelling

The ovarian tumor is noticed as an abdominal swelling only when it is large and grows out of the pelvis.

Pressure Effect

Gastrointestinal symptoms of bloating or heaviness and urinary symptoms like frequency of micturition are common. In extreme cases, edema of legs, varicose veins and hemorrhoids may result.

Hormonal Effects

Estrogen secreting tumors (granulosa cell tumors, atheroma and Sertoli cell tumors) present with menstrual disturbances. Rarely other features like precocious puberty, glandular hyperplasia, breast enlargement and postmenopausal bleeding may be seen.

Androgen producing tumors (Sertoli-Leydig tumors and gonadoblastoma) may cause hirsutism and acne initially followed by deepening of voice or clitoromegaly. Very rarely thyrotoxicosis may result from struma ovarii.

DIFFERENTIAL DIAGNOSIS

All benign or malignant tumors of the ovary mostly present as an adnexal mass in the early stages of the disease. Thus, it is important to understand all differential diagnosis of an adnexal mass and reach the correct diagnosis with all clinical skills and diagnostic aids.

The differential diagnoses of adnexal mass with pain include non-tumorous conditions like ectopic pregnancy, pelvic inflammatory disease, endometriosis, appendicitis, and diverticulitis.

Pregnancy, fibroid uterus, full bladder, distended bowel, physiological ovarian cysts (follicular and corpus luteal cysts) and parovarian cysts may also present as adnexal mass without pain.

Follicular cyst: A simple follicular cyst is the most common ovarian cyst often found incidentally in young women. A follicle more than 3 cm, is called a follicular cyst. It is lined by granulose cells and results from non-rupture of a dominant follicle or failure of atresia of a non dominant follicle. It usually resolves over 3–6 months. Sometimes, it may enlarge and rupture leading to acute abdominal pain.

Corpus luteum cyst: A persistent corpus luteum forms a cyst due to hemorrhage into its lumen. It may enlarge to size of more than 8 cm and later present as acute abdomen with hemoperitoneum. Surgical intervention may be required in such cases.

Massive Edema of ovary: This is not a physiological cyst but presents as a tumor in young women. Torsion of the involved ovary may produce acute abdominal pain. Size may vary from 5–35 cm in diameter.

How to Reach the Diagnosis of Benign Ovarian Tumor

Detailed menstrual history and gynecological examination help to exclude pregnancy related conditions. Presence of normal menstrual cycles and normal size uterus excludes uterine pathology. A benign ovarian tumor is clinically felt as a solid cystic mass in the fornix. It is not tender and moves easily from side to side.

Some investigations are yet mandatory to confirm the diagnosis and plan further management.

INVESTIGATIONS

Ultrasonography (USG)

This is the single most important investigation to confirm the diagnosis with 81% sensitivity and 75% specificity. Transvaginal ultrasound provides better resolution than abdominal one. Unilateral cystic ovarian mass without septations or solid areas is suggestive of benign epithelial tumor and unilateral solid tumor in young women is suggestive of germ cell or stromal tumor. In contrast, complex, large (>8–10 cm), bilateral mass with irregular borders, solid components and multiple thick septations (>2–3 mm) favors malignancy. Ascites, enlarged lymph nodes and peritoneal masses suggest advanced malignancy.

USG is a component of risk of malignancy index (RMI) used to differentiate benign from malignant tumors. USG characteristics for ultrasound scan (U) score are multilocular cyst, solid areas, metastases, ascites and bilateral lesions. Scoring includes U score of 0 if no cyst is present, 1 if only one characteristic is found and 3 if two or more characteristics are found.

Tumor Markers

Cancer antigen (CA)-125 is the most common well studied tumor marker for epithelial ovarian tumors. A level above 30 U/mL is abnormal. It may be raised in some nontumor conditions like endometriosis, tuberculosis or pelvic inflammatory disease. Level above 300 U/mL is usually associated with ovarian or peritoneal malignancy.

Germ cell tumors are associated with very specific tumor markers (Table 3). Granulosa cell tumor shows raised serum inhibin A levels.

Risk of Malignancy Index (RMI)

The Royal College of Obstetricians and Gynecologists (RCOG) recommends the use of RMI to plan management of ovarian cysts. RMI = CA 125 X U Score X menopausal status.

Serum CA 125 level is used as it is, U score is determined by USG findings and menopausal woman is given a score of 3 while premenopausal woman is given a score of 1.

RMI score of 250 or more is suggestive of a malignant ovarian cyst which should be managed by a gynecological oncologist. RMI has specificity of 90% and sensitivity of 70%.

Table 3: Tumor markers in germ cell tumors

Types of Germ cell tumors	Types of tumor markers			
	β HCG	AFP	LDH	PLAP
Dysgerminoma			+	+ –
Endodermal sinus tumor		+		
Embryonal carcinoma	+	+		
Choriocarcinoma	+			
Immature teratoma				
Polyembryoma	+	+ –		
Mixed germ cell tumor	+ –	+ –	+ –	+ –

Doppler Study

The malignant ovarian tumor has neovascularization which is picked up as low resistance, high velocity flow on Doppler study. This characteristic has been utilized in differentiating benign ovarian cysts from malignant ones through various scoring systems. Scoring system by Alcazar et al involves scoring for papillary projections, solid areas, central vascularity and Doppler velocimetry. A study in our department evaluated this scoring system for differentiating benign and malignant ovarian tumors, and found a sensitivity of 94.4% and specificity of 95%.

USG Guided Cyst Aspiration

This diagnostic test has been tried by some for differentiating benign and malignant ovarian cysts. The degree of risk of dissemination of malignant cells in the peritoneal cavity along the needle track is not well established. It has a false positive rate of 2% and false negative rate of 71%. Due to its poor prognostic value, it is not a recommended test.

MANAGEMENT OF BENIGN OVARIAN TUMORS

The ovarian tumor is diagnosed as benign preoperatively by clinical, sonological and biochemical features. Confirmatory diagnosis is made only after surgicopathological evaluation. Treatment is based on age of the patient and desire for further childbearing.

Incidental finding—Young girls and infertile women are diagnosed to have ovarian cyst on USG examination for other reasons. Most of these cysts are functional cysts. A follicular cyst measuring 3–8 cm; with no solid areas or septations and normal CA 125 level may be followed up to 3–6 months. Persistence or enlargement of cyst indicates removal.

Cysts more than 8 cm are likely to cause pain due to stretching of ovarian capsule or pressure effects. They are also at increased risk of rupture or torsion. For these reasons, any ovarian cyst of more than 8 cm diameter needs surgical management in all age groups.

All symptomatic cysts should also be removed surgically.

Women over 50 years of age are more likely to have malignant ovarian tumors. Thus, any ovarian cyst warrants complete evaluation in these women. Only simple, echo free, unilateral cysts without solid areas or papillary formations, size less than 8 cm and normal CA 125 may be managed conservatively with 3–6 monthly USG and CA 125 estimation. All other ovarian tumors should be removed surgically.

Surgical Removal of Benign Ovarian Tumors

With increased availability and advantages of laparoscopic equipment, laparoscopic removal of benign ovarian cysts is the best treatment option in young adolescents and reproductive age women.

In the perimenopausal and menopausal women, laparoscopic removal may be undertaken if the facility of frozen section is available. If the frozen section examination of the removed cyst shows malignancy, complete surgery may be undertaken at the same time.

If the facility is not available or there is doubt about benign or malignant nature of the tumor, it is advisable to perform total abdominal hysterectomy with bilateral salpingo-oophorectomy with peritoneal washings and biopsy.

All the removed tissues must undergo histopathological examination.

SUGGESTED READING

1. Alcazar JL, Merce LT, Laparte C, et al. A new scoring system to differentiate benign from malignant adnexal masses. Am J Obstet Gynecol. 2003;188:685-92.
2. Hoffman BL. Pelvic Mass in Williams Gynecology 1st edition. Mc Graw Hill publication. 2008;197-224.
3. Uma S, Neera K, Nisha, Ekta. Evaluation of new scoring system to differentiate between benign and malignant adnexal mass. J Obstet Gynecol India. 2006;56(2):162-5.
4. Zanetto U, Downey G. Benign tumors of the ovary in Gynecology by Robert W Shaw, 4th edition. Elsevier Publication. 2011;668-77.

Malignant Ovarian Tumors

Nisha Singh

INTRODUCTION

Ovarian cancer is the sixth most common cancer and seventh leading cause of cancer death among women worldwide. The age standardized incidence is 6.6/100,000 and the mortality rate is 4/100,000 worldwide. In India, it is the third leading cancer in women after cancer of cervix and breast. A woman's lifetime risk of ovarian cancer is 1.7%.

ETIOLOGY

The etiology of ovarian cancer is presumed to be a complex process involving interaction of surface epithelial cells with ovarian stromal cells. The various hypothesis include:

- Incessant ovulation—cyclical ovulation causes damage to the surface epithelium. This is repaired by post ovulation mitosis and proliferation which has great potential for the formation of aberrant DNA and inactivation of tumor suppresser genes. Ovulation also leads to the formation of ovarian inclusion cysts due to the entrapment of surface epithelium in the stromal tissue. This leads to p53 over expression
- Hyperstimulation of ovarian tissue by pituitary gonadotropins—excessive stimulation of ovary by pituitary hormones (FSH and LH) may play a role in causation of ovarian cancer. Excess of estrogen and deficiency of progesterone could play a role in development of endometroid and clear cell tumors
- Inflammation has been suggested to be a major factor leading to ovarian cancer. Association of environmental toxins (asbestos, talc, napkins, etc.) and pelvic inflammatory disease with ovarian cancer is explained with inflammation hypothesis
- Endometriosis is also associated with increased incidence of endometroid ovarian cancer
- Genetic polymorphism—plays a role in pathogenesis of familial ovarian cancer. The high risk (20–25%) in women with BRCA1 and BRCA2 gene mutation supports the same

- Role of angiogenesis is well known in development of any cancer. Current research is evaluating serum vascular endothelial growth factor (VEGF) as a promising diagnostic marker and anti-angiogenesis drugs for treatment of refractory cases.

HISTOPATHOLOGY

Epithelial Ovarian Tumors

They constitute 60% of all ovarian tumors and 90% of ovarian cancers. There is wide variation from benign to borderline to malignant tumors and different characteristics are based on the type of surface epithelium.

Borderline Epithelial Tumors

They are tumors of low malignant potential; 80% remain localized and have good prognosis. The stromal invasion varies between 3–10 mm. They account for 15% of epithelial tumors. They occur more frequently in premenopausal women. Only 20% may be metastatic with poor prognosis. Diagnosis can only be confirmed by following histological features:

- Epithelial hyperplasia with pseudostratification, tufting, cribriform and micropapillary architecture
- Mild nuclear atypia and mild increased mitotic activity
- Detached cell clusters
- Absence of destructive stromal invasion.

Epithelial ovarian cancer can also be divided into low grade and high grade cancer. The low grade cancer is usually serous or mucinous, unresponsive to chemotherapy, frequently arise from borderline precursors, contain B-Raf and K-Ras oncogenes but have a significantly longer progression free survival. The high grade cancer is rapidly growing, aggressive neoplasm with p53 mutation and no precursor lesions.

- Serous cystadenocarcinoma—constitute 80% of epithelial ovarian cancer. The cells resemble tubal secretary cells and cysts are filled with serous fluid (Figs 1A and B). Papillary excrescences and laminated calcified 'psammoma bodies are common. Papillary and glandular structures predominate in low grade cancer while solid sheets of cells with high mitotic activity predominate in high grade cancer.
- Endometroid ovarian cancer—is the second most common type seen in 10% cases of epithelial ovarian cancer. The prognosis is better than the serous and mucinous counterparts.
- Mucinous cystadenocarcinoma—can be endocervical or intestinal type. Papillary excrescences indicate malignancy. They constitute 10% of epithelial ovarian cancer.

The other epithelial ovarian cancers make up less than 1%.
- Clear cell carcinoma—is characterized by clear, peg-like hobnail arrangement of malignant cells. They are invariably malignant and have poorest prognosis.

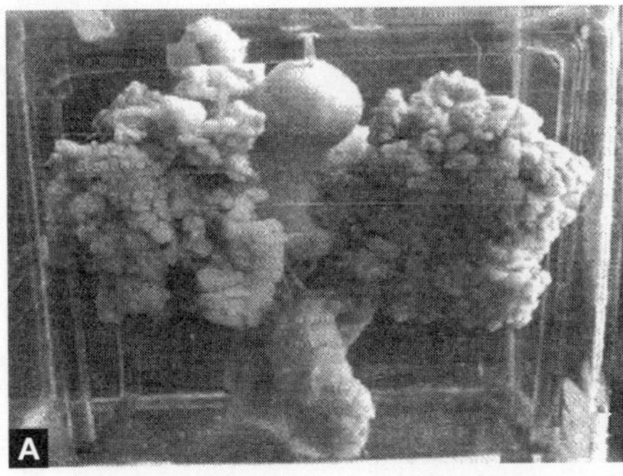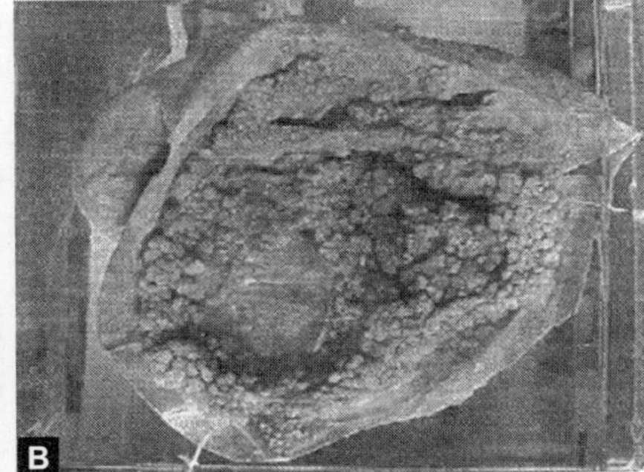

Figs 1A and B: (A) Specimen of uterus and ovaries covered with papillary excrescences. (B) Papillary projections within the cyst on cut section
(For color version, see Plate 8)

➲ Malignant brenner, transitional cell and undifferentiated carcinoma are the other rare subtypes.

Sex Cord Stromal Cell Tumors

They account for 7% of malignant ovarian tumors. The granulosa cell tumors are juvenile and adult type and both may be malignant. Fibrosarcoma and Sertoli-Leydig cell tumors are rarely malignant.

Germ Cell Tumors

Constitute 3–7% of all ovarian tumors and one-third of these can be malignant. Dysgerminoma (Fig. 2), yolk sac tumor, embryonal carcinoma and non gestational choriocarcinoma are the malignant tumors with specific tumor markers. Teratomas are germ cell tumors that can display an array of embryonic elements. Immature teratoma (Fig. 3) are malignant and are defined by the presence of neuroepithelium. Malignant change in a teratoma can produce a squamous carcinoma, sarcoma and other malignancies.

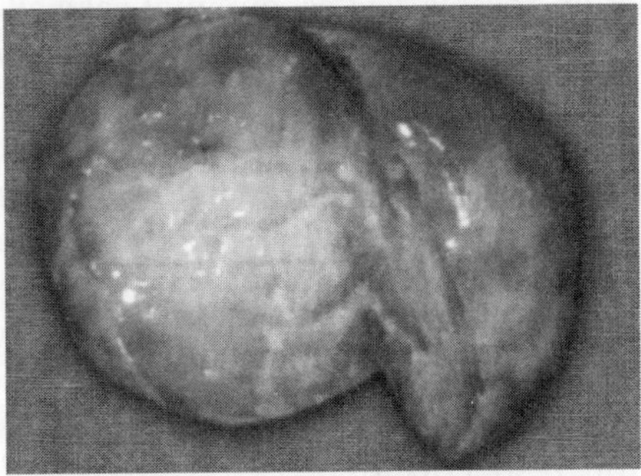

Fig. 2: Dysgerminoma
(For color version, see Plate 8)

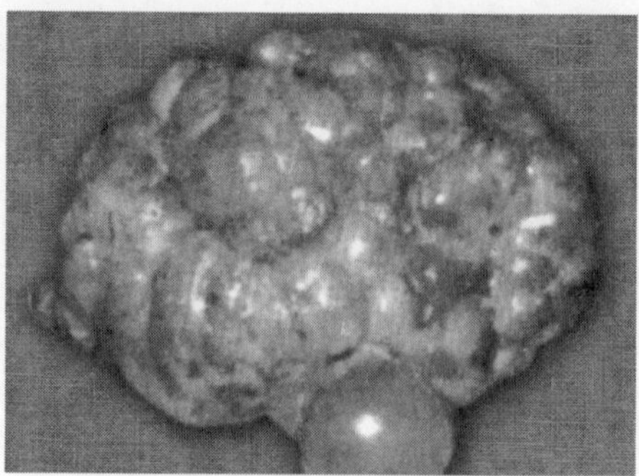

Fig. 3: Immature teratoma
(For color version, see Plate 8)

CLINICAL FEATURES

Ovarian cancer can occur at any age, the most common epithelial ovarian cancer is seen in women above 50 years of age, while germ cell tumors are common in women below 20 years. Signs and symptoms depend upon the stage of the disease which indirectly reflects the spread of disease.

In early stage of disease, most women are asymptomatic or may have vague problems like abdominal discomfort, bloating, early satiety and dyspepsia for which the women do not usually consult a gynecologist. This is the reason that 70% cases of ovarian cancer are diagnosed in advanced stage. Symptoms of abdominal distension, feeling of heaviness or lump in abdomen, arise when the tumor bulk increases and ascites sets in. In late stage of disease, symptoms correlate with site of metastasis or local infiltration. Symptoms of weight loss and appetite loss are also common.

Important Points in Clinical Examination

A detailed examination should start from general and systemic examination. A woman with ovarian cancer is generally cachexic, pale and emaciated. Cervical inguinal lymph nodes and breast should be palpated for metastasis. Abdominal examination reveals ascites, omental cake and abdomino pelvic mass. The mass is unilateral or bilateral, irregular, has variable consistency and restricted mobility.

On bimanual pelvic examination, uterus may or may not be palpated separate from the mass. Rectovaginal examination gives better idea of disease spread in the pouch of Douglas and adjacent bowel. Extension to the rectal wall may also be appreciated.

In advanced stages, the pressure of the mass on lymphatics may produce unilateral or bilateral pedal edema. Some sex cord stromal tumors may produce features of estrogen-androgen excess like irregular menstrual bleeding or virilization, respectively.

Modes and Pattern of Spread of Ovarian Cancer

Ovarian cancer may spread by various routes:

- Direct extension—tumor spreads from the ovary to adjacent organs by breaking the capsule. Fallopian tube, uterus, bladder, rectum and sigmoid colon are involved by direct extension.
- Peritoneal dissemination—this is the most common method of spread characterized by shedding and seeding of cancer cells on all peritoneal surfaces. Peritoneal dissemination leads to involvement of omentum, intestines, liver, stomach and diaphragm.
- Lymphatic spread—the common iliac and para aortic nodes are primarily involved. Later the retroperitoneal and obturator lymph nodes may also be involved.
- Blood borne metastasis—this leads to involvement of distant organs like liver and lungs.

Role of Tumor Markers in Ovarian Cancer

They are used for screening, diagnosis, prognosis, recurrence and response to therapy.

CA 125—this is the most commonly used tumor marker for non mucinous epithelial ovarian cancer. It has a sensitivity of 50–60% for stage I disease, which increases to 91% for stage IV disease. The low sensitivity and specificity makes it inappropriate for screening of ovarian cancer. However, it is a good marker for prognosis and surveillance during and after the treatment.

CEA (Carcinoembryonic antigen) is elevated more often in mucinous (88%) than non-mucinous (19%) cancers.

Newer epithelial tumor markers are CA 72-4, Lipid Associated Sialic Acid in plasma (LASA-P), Lysophosphatidic Acid (LPA) and Tumor Associated Trypsin Inhibitor (TATI).

Germ cell tumor (GCT) associated markers (Table III, in Chapter Benign Ovarian Tumors) are more specific. Young women with suspected germ cell tumor should be investigated for all these markers to plan the surgical treatment and surveillance, accordingly.

Sex cord stromal cell tumors (SCST)—inhibin A is found raised in granulosa cell tumors.

Role of Imaging

Role of ultrasonography in the diagnosis of ovarian cancer has been discussed in the previous chapter. Abdominopelvic CT or MRI add little to the diagnosis. CT or PET scan help in deciding the management plan depending upon the extent of the disease. USG is required in post-treatment surveillance of ovarian cancer.

Ascitic Fluid Cytology and Fine-needle Aspiration Cytology (FNAC)

These tests are useful only for cytologic diagnosis of cases planned for neoadjuvant chemotherapy.

Treatment of Carcinoma Ovary

Once a woman is diagnosed to have ovarian cancer based on clinical features, imaging and tumor markers, she should be taken up for a staging laparotomy and appropriate surgery.

Staging laparotomy refers to assigning International Federation of Gynecology and Obstetrics (FIGO) stage (Table 1) to the disease by visual inspection, palpation and histological confirmation of spread of ovarian cancer.

Steps of Staging Laparotomy

- A midline vertical incision from pubic symphysis to about 3 finger breadths below the xiphisternum gives adequate access to upper abdominal viscera

Table 1: FIGO staging of ovarian cancer	
Stage I	Cancer limited to the ovaries
IA	Cancer is present in one ovary.
IB	Cancer is present in both ovaries.
IC	Cancer is present in one or both ovaries and one or more of the following is true: Cancer is found on the outside surface of one or both ovaries, or the outer covering of the tumor has ruptured, or cancer cells are found in the fluid or tissue linings of the abdomen.
Stage II	Cancer is present in one or both ovaries and has spread to other parts of the pelvic region.
IIA	Cancer has spread to the uterus and/or fallopian tubes.
IIB	Cancer has spread to other organs in the pelvic region such as the bladder, rectum, or sigmoid colon.
IIC	Cancer has spread to the uterus, fallopian tubes, bladder, sigmoid colon, or rectum. Additionally, cancer may be present in tissue and fluid samples of the linings of the abdominal cavity.
Stage III	Cancer is found in one or both ovaries and has spread to the abdomen.
IIIA	Cancer is found in one or both ovaries and has macroscopically spread to other parts of the abdominal peritoneum.
IIIB	Cancer has spread to the peritoneum in an amount less than 2 cm.
IIIC	Cancer has spread to the peritoneum more than 2 cm and/or has spread to the lymph nodes.
Stage IV	Cancer is found in one or both ovaries and has spread to parts of the body beyond the abdomen, or in the liver parenchyma.

➲ Any fluid present in peritoneal cavity is taken for cytology. In absence of any fluid, peritoneal cavity and pelvis is irrigated with 200 mL of normal saline and this fluid is sent for cytology

➲ Involvement of bilateral ovaries and tubes is assessed followed by evaluation of uterus, peritoneal cavity, sigmoid colon, intestines omentum, undersurface of liver diaphragm and stomach. Para-aortic and pelvic lymph nodes are palpated after entering the retroperitoneum behind the round ligament.

Cytoreductive surgery: After staging is done, complete removal of the disease is done by total abdominal hysterectomy, bilateral salpingo-oophorectomy, omentectomy and pelvic lymphadenectomy to achieve optimal cytoreduction. All metastatic deposits from peritoneum, intestines and bladder are removed. Appendectomy is performed in mucinous tumors.

Para-aortic lymph nodes are inspected and palpated.

Role of lymphadenectomy is debatable in ovarian cancer due to high surgical morbidity and lack of proof of survival benefit. Systematic lymphadenectomy is advised if residual tumor is less than 1 cm. Nodal debulking is recommended only when tumors are larger than intra abdominal residuals.

Currently, optimal cytoreduction is defined as residual disease less than or equal to 1 cm. Recent studies have suggested that this definition should be changed to no gross residual disease owing to improved survival observed. Aggressive cytoreductive surgery increases the operative morbidity (5%) in advanced stage disease. Thus, the extent of cytoreductitve surgery should be decided upon judiciously with the joint expertize of gyn onc surgeon, gastrointestinal surgeon and urologist.

Exceptions to Primary Staging Laparotomy

➲ Advanced disease cases with liver metastasis, pleural effusion, infiltration of bladder or bowel where complete cytoreduction does not seem possible

➲ Woman with comorbidities—increasing her anesthesia risk to high morbidity.

Clients for Staging Laparotomy and Conservative Surgery

➲ Young women desirous of child bearing with germ cell tumors—Stage 1
➲ Stage IA epithelial ovarian cancer
➲ Borderline ovarian tumor—Nonmetastatic.

All above cases are managed with staging laparotomy/laparoscopy, followed by unilateral salpingo-oophorectomy, avoiding any peritoneal spillage. Fluid cytology and random biopsies are required to rule out advanced stage disease.

ADJUVANT CHEMOTHERAPY IN EPITHELIAL OVARIAN CANCER (EOC)

Observational studies have demonstrated 5 year overall survival rates more than 90% for FIGO stage IA and IB tumors without adjuvant chemotherapy.

Two trials international collaborative ovarian neoplasm (ICON) 1 and adjuvant chemotherapy in ovarian neoplasm (ACTION) provided strong evidence for the benefit of platinum based adjuvant CT in patients with (poor prognosis) early stage disease. The gynecologic oncologic group (GOG) III trial then showed that combination of paclitaxel and carboplatin (Table 2) has overall superior response rate and it is considered as the standard of care. Dose of carboplatin is calculated by Calvert's formula = (GFR + 25) AUC 6

$$\text{Where GFR} = \frac{(140 - \text{age}) \times \text{body weight in kg} \times 0.85}{72 \times \text{serum creatinine (mg\%)}}$$

NEOADJUVANT CHEMOTHERAPY (NAC)

This is a viable option for inoperable advanced stage cases. Neoadjuvant chemotherapy refers to giving three courses of chemotherapy followed by interval debulking surgery. Various studies have shown that this approach makes the patient operable, and possibility of complete cytoreduction is dramatically increased. Yet the benefit in overall survival rate of cases taken for upfront surgery and those for NAC, followed by interval debulking is a debatable topic. Prospective randomized trials are ongoing to resolve this issue.

CHEMOTHERAPY IN GCT AND SCST

All patients with completely resected tumors should be offered adjuvant CT, except patients with stage IA, IB grade I immature teratoma and stage IA dysgerminoma. Most effective and commonly used chemotherapy is bleomycin, etoposide, cisplatin (BEP) regimen (Table 3) with 96% disease free survival of 2 years. Incompletely resected tumors may be given more courses, optimal number is not yet specified.

For granulosa cell tumors and Sertoli-Leydig cell tumors, chemotherapy with BEP or carboplatin and paclitaxel is recommended for stage IC and above.

Table 2: First line adjuvant chemotherapy for carcinoma ovary

Drugs	Dose	Route	Day	Interval	Cycles
Paclitaxel	175 mg/m²	IV	1	3 weeks	6–8
Carboplatin	AUC 5–6	IV	2		

Table 3: BEP regimen for germ cell tumors

BEP Regimen	(Repeated every 21 day)
Cisplatin	20 mg/m² days 1–5
Etoposide	100 mg/m² days 1–5
Bleomycin	30 units IV weekly from day 1

INTRAPERITONEAL CHEMOTHERAPY (IPCT)

This involves placement of an IP (intraperitoneal) drug delivery device during the primary surgery. The ports should be placed on the inferior thorax at the midclavicular line. The catheter is tunneled under the cutaneous tissue above the fascia to a point 6 cm lateral to the umbilicus and then pulled into the peritoneal cavity through a small hole. This is an area of active research for first line chemotherapy of EOC. There is no consensus as yet on the standard drug and dose to be delivered and whether all or some special cases should receive IPCT.

SURVEILLENCE OF CARCINOMA OVARY

All treated cases of carcinoma ovary are monitored by clinical, biochemical and radiological parameters, as per the following schedule:

- Clinical and biochemical surveillance is done monthly in 1st year, every 2 months in 2nd year, every 3 months in 3rd year, every 4 months in 4th year, every 6 months in 5th year and annually thereafter
- USG is advised once in three months for first 3 years, six monthly in 4th and 5th year and annually thereafter
- Chest X-ray is advised annually and CT scan only when indicated by any of the above.

RESPONSE TO THERAPY

The above monitoring is done to assess the response to therapy and plan further management accordingly. The following terminologies are used to identify cases with different response to therapy.

Refractory disease: Cases which show disease progression or show no disease reduction in the tumor mass during chemotherapy are said to have refractory disease. Refractory cases are then treated with an alternate chemotherapy.

Relapse disease: When the disease free interval after completion of chemotherapy is less than six months, it is a case of disease relapse. These cases can be treated with more courses of same (1st line) chemotherapy.

Recurrent disease: When the disease free interval after completion of chemotherapy is more than 6 months, it is a case of disease recurrence.

Cases with long duration of disease free survival (at least 12 months) respond well to secondary debulking if optimal debulking has been achieved, although there have been no prospective studies.

ALTERNATE CHEMOTHERAPY

These drugs are used in refractory and recurrent diseases. They include cytotoxic drugs like paclitaxel poliglumex, trabectedin, epothilones, canfosfamide, phenoxodiol and karenitecin. Targeted agents being tried are gefitinib, cetuximab, matuzumab, bevacizumab, sorafenib and aflibercept.

The anti-VEGF drug bevacizumab is considered most promising for future.

Gene therapy, immunotherapy and cytokines are other options under research.

Second look surgery: This term refers to laparotomy in patients with complete clinical remission with normal CA-125 and normal imaging to confirm the remission after chemotherapy. The surgery involves peritoneal cytology, random peritoneal biopsies and removal of any gross lesions. There is no clear recommendation for a second look surgery because presence of microscopic disease on second look surgery indicates disease progression and does not respond well to secondary debulking.

SCREENING FOR OVARIAN MALIGNANCY

General population screening for ovarian cancer is not yet recommended. In 1994, NIH recommended screening for those who had two or more family members affected with ovarian or breast cancer. Due to the elevated risk with BRCA1 and BRCA2 mutation, genetic testing is now recommended for these women.

Screening strategies have not been developed for ovarian cancer due to several challenges. Firstly, there is no defined in situ lesion and secondly confirmatory diagnosis requires a surgery (laparoscopy or laparotomy) for false positive cases. Two large prospective randomized trials conducted recently were the United Kingdom collaborative trial of ovarian cancer (UKCTOCS) and PLCOCS trials. Screening with annual transvaginal sonogram (TVS) and CA-125 (PLCOCS trial) did not reduce ovarian cancer mortality and there was high incidence of surgical complications (15%) in false-positive cases. The UKCTOCS trial showed encouraging preliminary results. The trial compared no screening with annual TVS and MMS (Multimodality screening by annual CA-125 followed by TVS). The specificity of MMS was significantly higher than other two groups. Another single arm study using ROCA (risk of ovarian cancer algorithm) shared a specificity of 99.7% and positive predictive value (PPV) of 37.5%.

These studies confirm that TVS has high specificity and PPV is used as a secondary tool but not as primary tool even in women with family history of ovarian cancer. In 2010 and 2011, US FDA has approved CA-125 and human epididymis (HE) 4 for early diagnosis of ovarian cancer in women with pelvic mass but not as screening test.

Currently, ACOG and Society of Gyne Oncologists recommend that there should be a high index of suspicion in women with symptoms like bloating, difficulty in eating, abdominal or pelvic pain, constipation or urinary symptoms. Women should be educated about these symptoms so that diagnostic work up can be done in these women. A symptom index screening tool has been prepared and its usefulness is being evaluated by Goff et al.

MANAGEMENT OF WOMEN AT HIGH RISK OF OVARIAN CANCER

Women with family history of ovarian or breast cancer should undergo genetic evaluation by BRCA1 and BRCA2 testing and counseling. NIH recommends that those tested positive, should have screening with CA-125 or TVS from the age of 35 years or 10 years earlier than the youngest age when a family member was diagnosed. Prophylactic bilateral salpingo-oopherectomy reduces the ovarian cancer risk by 92%. Younger women should be offered oral contraceptive pills. There is a decrease in risk of 10% after 1 year and 50% after 5 year use of oral contraceptive pills (OCPs). Tubal ligation decreases ovarian cancer risk in BRCA1 mutation carriers but not in BRCA2 mutation carriers. Trials are ongoing to find usefulness of retinoid for chemoprevention.

SUGGESTED READING

1. Ahmed N, Niaimi A, Ahmed M and Petersen CB. Epithelial ovarian Cancer in Obstetrics and Gynecology. Clinics of North America edited by CY Muller and WF Rayburn. Elsevier Publications. June 2012;39(2):269-84.
2. Berek JS, Longacre TA, Friedlander M. Ovarian, fallopian tube and peritoneal Cancer in Berek and Novak's Gynecology. Fifteenth edition, Lippin Williams and Wilkins Publication. 2012;p. 1350-425.
3. Fathalla MF. Incessant Ovulation. A factor in ovarian neoplasia? Lancet. 1971;2:163.
4. Fattaneh A, Tavassoli, Devilee A. Tumors of breast and female genital tract. WHO classification of tumors. Pathology and Genetics. IARC Lyon. 2003;113-97.
5. Goff BA. Ovarian cancer screening and early detection in Obstetrics and Gynecology clinics of North American edited by CY Muller and WF Rayburn. Elsevier Publication. June 2012;39(2):183-94.
6. Ovarian Cancer. NCCN practice guidelines in oncology. Vol1, 2007.
7. Sreedharan PS Intraperitoneal Chemotherapy for ovarian cancer in Comprehensive and Contemporary Management, Jaypee Publications, 1st edition. 2009;p. 223-7.
8. Wadhwa N. Etiopathogenesis of Ovarian tumors in Ovarian cancer Comprehensive and Contemporary Management, Jaypee Publications, 1st edition 2009;p. 3-10.

Chapter
52

Hydatidiform Mole

Neelam

Hydatidiform mole is the benign variety of gestational trophoblastic neoplasia (GTN) which also includes invasive mole and malignant entities such as choriocarcinoma and placental site trophoblastic tumor.

Its exact incidence is not known due to poor registry. In European women its incidence is 0.5–1/1000 pregnancies but it is more common in Asian women. Among Asians, the incidence is highest in the Chinese population (5.52/1000 deliveries, p<0.001).[1]

On the basis of morphology, histopathology and karyotype, it can be divided into partial hydatidiform mole (PHM) and complete hydatidiform mole (CHM). Partial hydatidiform mole consists of an embryo or foetus together with moles, whereas the complete variety has an absence of embryo or foetus. Its significance lies in the development of the complete mole into persistent gestational trophoblastic neoplasia which needs treatment with chemotherapy with no further confirmatory histopathological examination.[2]

PATHOLOGY

Hydatidiform mole is basically an abnormality of placental development. It is due to overexpression of paternally derived genes and is an example of imprinting abnormalities. They are associated with structural placental abnormalities and developmental defects in fetus. Thus, the hydatidiform mole can be differentiated from non-molar pregnancies by abnormal trophoblastic hyperplasia. CHM and PHM are differentiated on pathological and genetic features[3] which are described below.

Complete hydatidiform moles are almost always diploid, all chromosomal material is paternal in origin due to endo-reduplication, following mostly monospermic fertilization and rarely, dispermic fertilization of an anucleate oocyte. Rarely CHM of biparental variety also exists due to defect appearing as a result of imprinting abnormalities and over expression of paternal genome.[4]

Partial hydatidiform moles are always triploid, mostly due to dispermic fertilization of a normal oocyte. Maternal genome in PHM leads to less trophoblastic hyperplasia and more of the normal fetal development. Thus, in PHM there is an overexpression of the paternally transcribed genes.[4]

Histopathological examination is the gold standard for diagnosis in such cases. Heterogenic distribution of villus, trophoblastic hyperplasia, relative lack of villus hydrops, sheets of pleomorphic extravillus trophoblast, collapsed villus blood vessels and characteristic abnormal budding of villus architecture are the diagnostic features on histological examination in first trimester moles.[2] The rare classical presentation of a second trimester product of conception, showing marked villus hydrops with extensive hyperplasia of trophoblast at the periphery and cistern formation of villus at the centre is absent in first trimester.[2]

In cases of inconclusive histopathological diagnoses, auxillary diagnostic techniques may be utilized, including p57kip2 immunohistochemistry[5] (absence of staining in CHM, positive nuclear staining in others), assessment of ploidy using in-situ hybridization or flow cytometry[6] and microsatellite polymorphism analysis.[7] Extensive research to substantiate a genetic cause of hydatidiform mole (HM) has led to localization of a single gene NALP7 which is defective in HM. However, studies on gene defect and molecular basis of HM are still ongoing.[8]

CLINICAL FEATURES

The most common clinical feature is vaginal bleeding. This may be associated with excessive uterine enlargement, anemia, hyperemesis gravidarum, hyperthyroidism, toxemia of pregnancy, and theca lutein cyst.

In 97% of the cases, vaginal bleeding presents in early second trimester of pregnancy and is usually intermittent and prolonged. The excessive enlargement of uterus occurs due to separation of moles from the decidua leading to disruption of maternal blood vessels, which in turn, results in accumulation of a large volume of blood inside the uterine cavity. In about 50% of cases, patients may also present with anemia. In 23% of cases, hyperemesis gravidarum and early onset pre-eclampsia is observed. In 50% of cases, theca lutein cysts can be found on ultrasonography; these are usually bilateral, unilocular and thin walled and can also lead to ovarian torsion or rupture.

Tachycardia, tremor and warm skin (commonly associated with hyperthyroidism) may also be found in approximately 5% of patients. Hyperthyroidism can be diagnosed by detecting high levels of free thyroxin (FT4) and tri-iodothyronine (FT3). All the above symptoms and signs of hydatidiform mole are due to high levels of circulating serum human chorionic gonadotropin (HCG) and these disappear rapidly within 6–8 weeks once the uterus is evacuated.

DIAGNOSIS

Complete hydatidiform mole is always diagnosed by ultrasonography which demonstrates a typical appearance of "snow storm". This characteristic appearance is due to proliferation of chorionic villi with hydropic swelling producing characteristic vesicular pattern. This classic appearance is less commonly seen[9] as majority of simple, uncomplicated pregnancies and all patients presenting with bleeding in early pregnancy routinely undergo ultrasound examination which can diagnoses, either molar pregnancy or missed abortion, both of which are treated with evacuation of uterus.[4] The appearance in the first trimester is a typical complex, echogenic, intrauterine mass containing many small cystic spaces.[10] In one of the largest study in the UK, the average age for sonological diagnosis of hydatidiform mole was found to be 10 weeks.[11]

It can be differentiated from ectopic pregnancy by lack of pain, presentation in the second trimester and typical ultrasound features.

INVESTIGATIONS

Apart from routine laboratory investigations of complete blood count (CBC), blood grouping and typing, fasting and post-prandial (PP) blood sugar, HBsAg, and HIV status, special investigations like serum T3, T4, TSH, β-hCG estimation, X-ray of the chest, CT scan of brain, MRI of abdomen and pelvic doppler sonography may also be utilized when required.

MANAGEMENT

Suction evacuation is the mainstay of treatment which is aided later by infusion of 20 IU of oxytocin in 500 mL of lactated ringer. This should be followed by repeating the ultrasound examination to look for retained tissue a week later and if residual tissue is present, a second evacuation and curettage is recommended. At this stage, the uterus is firmer and much smaller so the risk of perforation is minimal. Rarely, Ashermann's syndrome may develop as a consequence of repeated curettage, but fertility in these patients can be restored by lysis of intrauterine adhesions.[12] In 27% of cases, acute respiratory distress syndrome (ARDS) has been reported after evacuation of uterus of more than 16 weeks, which is managed expectantly in the ICU. The predisposing factors are anemia, pre-eclampsia, fluid overload, hyperthyroidism and trophoblastic embolization, either alone or in combination.[13]

In cases where one of the twins is a mole and the other viable, the continuation of pregnancy may be an option, if so desired by the mother, after appropriate counseling. Counseling should include a detailed prognosis and estimation of the chances of achieving a viable pregnancy (about 40%) versus the associated risks including but not limited to pulmonary embolism and pre-eclampsia. Lastly, it has been noted that there is no added increase in the incidence of GTN after such twin pregnancy.[14]

FOLLOW-UP

Since the risk of undergoing malignant transformation with CHM is about 16% and with PHM 0.5%, it is imperative that all cases be followed up by serial HCG monitoring.[15] Moreover, it has been shown that the risk of development of a second and third complete molar pregnancy is 1:76 and 1:6.5 respectively.[16] Hence, the need for close clinical and laboratory monitoring for these patients cannot be over-emphasized.

After the second evacuation of uterus, patient should be clinically monitored on a weekly basis initially to rule out vaginal nodules (by pelvic examination) and to confirm regression in size of the uterus and theca lutein cysts and declining levels of serum β-hCG. Serum β-hCG level is measured fortnightly till it normalizes, after which urinary β-hCG examination may be done on a monthly basis. The risk of developing gestational trophoblastic neoplasia subsequently is greatest within the first 6 months of diagnosis so patients should be followed-up till at least 6 months after spontaneous β-hCG normalization.[17] Women should be strongly advised to avoid getting pregnant during this time interval. Initially, barrier contraceptive may be advised till the normalization of the serum β-hCG levels, after which hormonal oral contraceptive pills (OCPs) may be offered. This is because the use of OCPs before the normalization of β-hCG has been associated with an almost two fold increase in the incidence of postmolar tumor requiring chemotherapy.[18] However, it has been seen that using OCPs does not postpone the development of choriocarcinoma and that these woman run the same risks as their non-OCP counterpart of developing the disease, thus necessitating close follow-up.[10]

PARTIAL HYDATIDIFORM MOLE

Due to a paucity of data and histopathological reports, the true incidence of PHM is not known. In a study done in Malaysia, it was shown to be 30% of all the molar pregnancies.[19] Difficulty in diagnosis may also be attributed to the relative complex diagnostic criteria by an ultrasound. For a reliable diagnosis on ultrasound, it is essential to demonstrate cystic structures in the placenta and a ratio of transverse to anteroposterior diameter of gestation sac of >1.5.[20] Characteristic clinical features of complete mole may or may not be evident in these cases. PHM has not commonly been associated with choriocarcinoma,[21] however, malignant transformation have been reported infrequently.[22]

ROLE OF CHEMOTHERAPY

Chemotherapy is not routinely administered in all cases of molar pregnancy as about 80–90% of patients will not go on to develop persistent gestational neoplasia. It is usually reserved for the high-risk group which includes those with very slow decline in serum β-hCG levels, those with a subsequent rise in β-hCG levels after an initial decline and those showing an initial fall and then a plateau in serum β-hCG levels.

The patients falling in the above mentioned categories should receive methotrexate, prophylactic or low regimen chemotherapy[23] as this regimen has minimal toxicity and obviates the risk of resistance development by tumor cells due to the administration of the entire full course of chemotherapy until biochemical remission is achieved. Long-term follow-up has revealed that this therapy causes minimal interference with normal reproductive function and patients had normal offspring subsequently.[24]

The regimen compromises of administration of intravenous methotrexate 50 mg on day 1, 3, 5, 7, 9 coupled with 12 mg of oral folinic acid 24–30 hours after each dose of methotrexate. This course is repeated after 7–10 days until full biochemical remission has been demonstrated.[23] In one study patients receiving 'selective prophylactic chemotherapy' were shown to be free from disease at 10 year follow-up, thus proving the value of this regimen.[10]

ROLE OF HYSTERECTOMY

Prophylactic hysterectomy may be offered to patients with molar pregnancy if they have completed their family and are older than 40 years of age because of an unacceptably high rate of malignant transformation (3.5 times) in the subsequent years. This has been a common practice in many Asian countries.[10] This practice was also advocated by Tow et al[25] but metastasis to the brain following hysterectomy has been documented on long-term follow-up (as late as 9 years).[23] This again emphasizes the need for close monitoring and also questions the effectiveness of hysterectomy as radical treatment of the disease.

REFERENCES

1. Sivanesaratnam V. The President's lecture: Gestational trophoblastic disease-the Malaysian experience. Proceedings of the 3rd Malaysian Congress of Obstetrics and Gynecology, Kuala Lumpur, 1991.
2. Sibre J Neil. Gestational Trophoblastic Neoplasia. Ultrasonography in Obstetrics and Gynecology, 5th Edition. 2008;29:951-67.
3. Fisher RA. Genetics. In: Hancock BW, Newlands ES, Berkowitz RS, et al (eds): Gestational Trophoblastic Disease, 2nd edition. New York, International Society for the Study of Trophoblastic Diseases, 2003.
4. Fisher RA, Khatoon R, Paradinas FJ, et al. Repetitive complete Hydatidiform mole can be biparental in origin and either male or female. Hum Reprod. 2000;15:594.
5. Fisher RA, Hodges MD, Rees C, et al. The maternally transcribed gene p57 (KIP2) (CDNKIC) is abnormally expressed in both androgenic and biparental complete Hydatidiform moles. Hum Mol Genet. 2002;11:3267.
6. Berezowsky J, Zbieranowski I, Demers J, et al. DNA ploidy of Hydatidiform moles and nonmolar conceptus: a study using flow and tissue section image cytometry. Mod Pathol. 1995;8:775.
7. Fisher RA, Newlands ESL. Gestational Trophoblastic disease. Molecular and Genetic Studies. J Hum Reprod Med. 1998;43:87.
8. Jane Hook, Michael Seckl. Management of trophoblastic disease. Recent Advances in Obstetrics and Gynecology. 2009;10:135.
9. Paradinas FJ, Browne P, Fisher, RA, et al. A histopathological and flow cytometric study of 149 complete moles, 146 partial moles and 106 non molar hydropic abortions. Histopathology. 1996;28:101.
10. Sivanesaratnam V. The Essentials of Gynecology, 2nd edition 2011;40:470-8.

11. Fowler DJ, Liondsay I, Seckl MJ, et al. Routine pre evacuation ultrasound diagnosis of Hydatidiform mole: experience of >1000 cases from a regional referral centre. Ultrasound Obstet Gynecol. 2006;27:56.

12. Sivanesaratnam V. Ashermann's syndrome successfully treated by the insertion of a multiload copper 250 device. J Obstet Gynecol. 1986;7:22-3.

13. Twiggs LB, Morrow DP, Schlaerth JB. Acute pulmonary complication of hydatidiform mole. Am J Obstet Gynecol. 1979;135:189-94.

14. Saibre NJ, Foskett M, Paradinas FJ, et al. Outcome of twin pregnancies with complete hydatidiform mole and healthy co-twin. Lancet. 2002;359:2165-6.

15. Seckl MJ, Fisher RA, Saierno GA, et al. Choriocarcinoma and partial Hydatidiform moles. Lancet. 2000;356:36-9.

16. Bagshawe KD, Dent J, Webb J. Hydatidiform mole in the United Kingdom 1973-1983. Lancet. 1986;ii:673.

17. Saibre NJ, Foskett M, Paradinas FJ, et al. Outcome of twin pregnancies with complete hydatidiform mole and healthy co-twin. Lancet. 2002;359:2165-6.

18. Stone M, Dent J, Kardone A, et al. Relationship of oral contraception to development of trophoblastic tumour after evacuation of Hydatidiform mole. Br J Obstet Gynecol. 1976;83:913-6.

19. Cheah PL, Looi LM, Sivanesaratnam V. Hydatidiform molar pregnancy in Malaysian women, a histopathological study from the University Hospital, Kuala Lumpur: Malaysian Journal of pathology. 1993;15:59-63.

20. Fine C, Bundy AL, Berkowitz R, et al. Sonographic diagnosis of patient Hydatidiform mole. Obstet Gynecol. 1989;73:414-8.

21. Szulman AE. Trophoblastic disease: clinical pathology of Hydatidiform mole. Obstet Gyne clinics of North America. 1988;15:443-56.

22. Bagshawe KD. Trophoblastic Neoplasia – current results and therapeutic issues. In: Magreth 1 (Ed). New directions in Cancer Treatment. London: Springer. 1988;514.

23. Sivanesaratnam V. management of trophoblastic disease in developing countries. Best Practice and Research Clinical Obstetric and Gynecology. 2003;17:925-42.

24. Rustin GJ, Booth M, Dent J, et al. Pregnancy after cytotoxic chemotherapy for gestational trophoblastic tumors. Br Med J. 1984;288:183-206.

25. Tow WSH. The influence of the primary treatment of Hydatidiform mole and its subsequent course. J Obstet Gynecol Br Cwlth. 1966;77:544-52.

Management of Gestational Trophoblastic Neoplasia

Manju Gita Mishra, Mamta Singh

INTRODUCTION

Gestational trophoblastic neoplasia (GTN) are malignant lesions that arise from abnormal proliferation of placental trophoblast. The pathologic conditions that make up this entity include invasive partial and complete hydatidiform mole, choriocarcinoma, placental site trophoblastic tumor (PSTT), and epitheloid trophoblastic tumor (ETT). GTN most commonly follows a molar pregnancy but can follow a normal pregnancy, ectopic pregnancy, or abortion. The reported incidence of choriocarcinoma, the most aggressive form of GTN, in the United States is about 2 to 7 per 100,000 pregnancies. Fortunately, these malignancies are highly susceptible to chemotherapy and it is often possible to achieve cure while preserving the women's reproductive function.

RISK FACTORS

The risk of developing GTN after a complete hydatidiform mole (CHM) and a partial hydatidiform mole (PHM) is 15–20% and 1–4%, respectively. Following evacuation of a CHM, local uterine invasion occurs in approximately 15% and metastasis is observed in 4% of patients. Interestingly, patients with CHM who present with excessive uterine size and markedly elevated HCG levels (> 100,000 mIU/mL) develop GTN in 40–50% of cases and are considered high risk.

PATHOLOGY

Invasive moles: It is locally invasive, rarely metastatic lesions characterized by trophoblastic invasion of the myometrium and microscopically, there is hyperplasia of cytotrophoblast and syncytial elements and persistence of villus structures.

Choriocarcinoma: It is a malignant tumor of the trophoblastic epithelium, in which the uterine muscle and blood vessels are invaded with areas of hemorrhage and necrosis. Columns and sheets of trophoblastic tissue invade normal tissue and spread to distant sites, the most common of which are lungs, brain, liver, pelvis, vagina, spleen, intestines and kidney.

PSTT: It is a very rare tumor arising from the placental implantation site and resembles an exaggerated form of syncytial endometritis. Human placental lactogen is present in the tumor cells and hCG (human chorionic gonadotropin) is positive in only scattered cells. They are generally resistant to chemotherapy.

ETT: It is an extremely rare GTN. Pathologically, it has a monomorphic cellular pattern of epitheloid cells and may resemble squamous cell cancer of the cervix when arising in the cervical canal.

Trophoblastic tumors are perfused by fragile vessels and, as a result, metastases are often hemorrhagic, so biopsy is not recommended.

SIGNS AND SYMPTOMS

Patients with GTN usually present with continued vaginal bleeding in the post-delivery period. Patient may remain asymptomatic or present with dyspnea, chest pain, cough or hemoptysis with pulmonary metastasis. Patients with vaginal metastasis may present with irregular vaginal bleeding or purulent vaginal discharge. Cerebral involvement can cause increased intracranial pressure and intracerebral bleeding, which often leads to neurological symptoms like nausea, vomiting, headache, seizure, etc. Patients with liver metastasis may present with jaundice, intra-abdominal bleeding or epigastric pain.

DIAGNOSTIC EVALUATION

Patients newly diagnosed with GTN need a thorough evaluation to know the extent of disease that includes a history and physical examination, serum quantitative hCG level, a complete blood count, and hepatic and renal function tests. To know the extent of uterine involvement, pelvic ultrasound is often needed and this may identify women who are at risk for uterine perforation or who would benefit from a hysterectomy to reduce tumor burdens.

A chest X-ray should be obtained to evaluate lung metastasis. If this is negative, a chest computed tomography (CT) scan may be performed since it may detect micrometastases in 40% of patients with a negative chest X-ray. If a patient has a drug resistant disease, a 18-fluorodeoxyglucose positron emission tomography (FDG-PET) scan help determine if a persistent radiographic finding has viable, active tumor.

FIGO STAGING SYSTEM IN GTN (TABLES 1 AND 2)

The Federation International de Gynecologic et d' Obstetrique (FIGO) staging system incorporates a modified WHO (World Health Organization)

Table 1: FIGO anatomical staging	
Stage	
I	Disease confined to the uterus
II	GTN extends outside of the uterus, but is limited to the genital structures (adnexa, vagina, broad ligament)
III	GTN extends to the lungs, with or without known genital tract involvement
IV	All other metastatic sites

Table 2: Modified WHO prognostic scoring system as adapted by FIGO				
Scores	*0*	*1*	*2*	*4*
Age	<40	≥40	–	–
Antecedent pregnancy	Mole	Abortion	term	–
Interval months from index pregnancy	<4	4–6	7–12	>12
Pretreatment serum hCG (IU/L)	$<10^3$	$10^3–10^4$	$10^4–10^5$	$>10^5$
Largest tumor size (including uterus)	<3	3–4 cm	≥5 cm	–
Site of metastases	Lung	spleen, kidney	gastrointestinal	liver, brain
Number of metastases	–	1–4	5–8	>8
Previous failed chemotherapy	–	–	single drug	≥2 drugs

prognostic scoring system in management of GTN. A FIGO score of 6 or less indicates low-risk GTN where as a score of 7 or more identifies high-risk disease.

According to FIGO, GTN is diagnosed after a molar gestation if any of the following is observed.[1] (1) Four values or more of hCG plateau over at least three weeks (day, 1, 7, 14 and 21), (2) a rise in hCG of 10% or greater for three or more values over at least two weeks (day 1, 7 and 14), (3) the presence of histological choriocarcinoma, (4) persistence of hCG six months after molar evacuation.

TREATMENT OF LOW-RISK GTN

Patients with stage I and low-risk stage II and III GTN and FIGO prognostic score of ≤6 generally respond well to single-agent chemotherapy. There is no consensus on the best chemotherapy regimen for initial management of low-risk GTN, and firstline regimens vary by geography and institutional preference. Even if there are differences in initial remission rate among the regimens, salvage with alternate regimens is very effective, and the ultimate cure rates are generally 99% or more.

Commonly uses treatment regimens include the following: (1) the 8-day Charing Cross Regimen, MTX (50 mg IM on days 1, 3, 5 and 7) and folinic acid (7.5 mg orally on days 2, 4, 6 and 8). This may be the most common regimen worldwide but it has not been directly compared with other regimens. (2) Biweekly pulsed dactinomycin (1.25 mg/m^2 IV). (3) Weekly MTX 30 mg/m^2 IM.

Despite the effectiveness of MTX and ACT-D in treating low-risk GTN, some experience resistance to both agents. Recent data from Charing Cross Hospital indicates that patients with a low-risk FIGO score but with an hCG value exceeding 100,000 mIU/mL, frequently require combination chemotherapy.[2] These women are often treated with MAC (MTX, ACT_D and cyclophosphamide) or EMACO (Etoposide, MTX, ACT-D cyclophosphamide and vincristine). MAC is preferred as the initial combination chemotherapy regimen since Etoposide, which is a component of EMACO, is associated with an increased risk for secondary malignancies. In addition to medical therapy, surgical management may be useful in cases where GTN continues to be resistant to combination chemotherapy.

TREATMENT OF HIGH-RISK, STAGE II AND III GTN

Patient with stage II or III GTN and FIGO prognostic score ≥7 have a high-risk disease and are unlikely to be cured with single-agent therapy. Therefore, they should be treated with combination chemotherapy for high-risk, metastatic GTN, MAC in inadequate as primary treatment as it induces remission in only half the patient.

Although EMACO (Table 3) in the most common uses combination chemotherapy, other regimens have been used in the management of high-risk GTN. In a retrospective analysis of four chemotherapeutic regimens, Kim et al. compared the effectiveness of MFA (MTX, folinic acid, ACT-D), MAC, CHAMOCA (cyclophosphamide, hydroxycarbamide, doxorubicin, ACT-D, MTX, melphalan, and vincristine) and EMACO, They reported remission rates of 63%, 68%, 71% and 91%, respectively.[3] These results

Table 3: Specifics of the EMACO regimen

Day	Drug	Dose
1	Etoposide	100 mg/m^2 IV for 30 min
	Dactinomycin	0.5 mg IV push
	Methotrexate	300 mg/m^2 IV for 12 hours
2	Etoposide	100 mg/m^2 IV for 30 min
	Dactinomycin	0.5 mg IV push
	Folinic Acid	15 mg or PO every 12 hours × 4 doses, beginning 24 hours after the start of methotrexate
8	Cyclophosphamide	600 mg/m^2 IV infusion
	Vincristine	0.8–1.0 mg/m^2 IV push (maximum dose 2 mg)

support EMACO's effectiveness as primary therapy for patients with high-risk disease. Combination chemotherapy is often administered at two to three week intervals and timely administration is essential. Delay in treatment and decrease in dose should be avoided as it may result in tumor resistance and treatment failure. These patients should have serial hCG measurement. After the first undetectable hCG level, 2 to 4 additional chemotherapy courses are given to decrease the risk of relapse.

Patients with disease resistant to EMACO can be treated using EMAEP- a regimen that substitutes cyclophosphamide and vincristine on day 8, with cisplatin and etoposide.[4]

In some women, chemotherapy alone may not successfully treat GTN, and they may benefit from adjuvant surgical excision of the chemoresistant tumor. Clark et al. reported that 25 of 33 women (76%) with chemoresistant uterine tumor achieved complete remission with hysterectomy. An additional benefit to surgical treatment is that it may reduce tumor mass and may decrease the dose and length of administration of chemotherapy.

TREATMENT OF PSTT AND ETT

Hysterectomy is considered as firstline treatment strategy in women with stage I PSTT and ETT because of their inherent chemoresistance. Patients with metastatic PSTT may still achieve remission with intensive combination chemotherapy after surgical intervention, when they are diagnosed within 4 years of the antecedent pregnancy.

MANAGEMENT OF COMPLICATIONS FROM GTN

Women with GTN may present with complications related to their disease and may result in urgent surgical interventions. Hysterectomy may become essential to control profuse uterine hemorrhage or to remove an infected tumor focus. Vaginal metastases are highly vascular and friable and may bleed profusely. Bleeding is often controlled by packing the vagina. Other methods may become necessary such as wide local excision of the lesion or angiographic embolization of the hypogastric vessels. In rare instances, hepatic resection may be required to control intraperitoneal hemorrhage.

FOLLOW-UP PATIENTS WITH GTN

All patients with GTN should be followed with weekly serum quantitative hCG levels until normal for 3 consecutive weeks, then monthly for 12 months for women with stage I, II and III GTN and of 24 months for stage IV disease, during which the patient is advised not to conceive. This is necessary for accurate interpretation of the hCG levels and also for the well-being of the subsequent gestation.

RECURRENT GTN

Women with history of GTN have a potential risk of disease recurrence that is largely dependent on their initial stage. Mutch et al. reported recurrence rates of 2% in patients with nonmetastatic GTN, 4% in patient with low-risk metastatic GTN, and 13% in patients with high-risk, metastasis disease. Fortunately, recurrent GTN is often curable.

SUBSEQUENT PREGNANCIES

The risk of developing a subsequent molar pregnancy increases from a baseline of 1/1000 to 1/100. So, it is necessary to obtain serum hCG value and a pelvic ultrasound in the first trimester of all subsequent pregnancies to confirm normal gestational development. In additional, hCG levels should be measured 6 weeks after the completion of each future pregnancy to exclude the presence of occult trophoblastic disease.

CONCLUSION

Significant progress has been made over the past decades in the diagnosis and management of women with GTN. GTN is highly curable disease that can be effectively managed with single or multiagent chemotherapy. Careful follow up all women with GTN is important to ensure that recurrence is detected promptly, at a time when it is curable.

REFERENCES

1. Kohorn EI. Negotiating a staging and risk factor scoring system for gestational trophoblastic Neoplasia: a progress report. J Reprod Med Obstetrician Gynecologist. 2002;47(6):445-50.
2. Reusin GJS, Newlands ES, Lutz JM, et al. Combination but not single agent methotrexate chemotherapy for gestational trophoblastic tumors increase the incidence of second tumors," Journal of clinical oncology. 1996;14(10):2769-73.
3. Kim SJ, Bae SN, Kim JH, Kim CT, Han KT, Lee JM. Effects of multiagent chemotherapy and independent risk factors in the treatment of high-risk GTT – 25 years experiences of KRI-TRD, Int J Gynecol Obs. 1998;60:885-96.
4. Xiang Y, Sun Z, Wan X, Yang X. EMA/EP chemotherapy for chemorefractory gestational trophoblastic tumor, J Reprod Med Obstetrician and Gynecologist. 2004;49(6):443-6.

Index

Page numbers followed by '*f*' refer to figure and '*t*' refer to table

E

J

Q

R